PHYSICAL ASSESSMENT OF THE NEWBORN

A Comprehensive Approach to the Art of Physical Examination

2nd Edition

Ellen P. Tappero, RNC, MN, NNP
Mary Ellen Honeyfield, RNC, MS, NNP

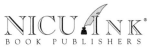

NICU INK
BOOK PUBLISHERS

1410 Neotomas Ave., Suite 107
Santa Rosa, CA 95405-7533

Editor-in-Chief: Charles Rait, RN, MSEd, PNC
Managing Editor: Suzanne G. Rait, RN
Editorial Coordinator: Tabitha Parker
Reviewer: Susan Tucker Blackburn, RN,C, PhD, FAAN
Editors: Beverley DeWitt, BA
Janine Stanich, RNC, BA
Lynn Stansbury, MD, MPH
Sylvia Stein Wright, BA
Proofreader: Jane Holly Love, MA
Indexer: Eleanor Lindheimer

Book design and composition by:
Marsha Godfrey Graphics

Cover art by: Sarah M. Waldron

LIBRARY OF CONGRESS CATALOGING-IN-PUBLICATION DATA
Physical assessment of the newborn: a comprehensive approach to the art of physical
examination/ (edited by) Ellen P. Tappero, Mary Ellen Honeyfield.—2nd ed.
     p.   cm.
    Includes bibliographical references and index.
    ISBN 1-887571-00-0 : 39.95
    1. Infants (Newborn)—Medical examinations.   2. Infants (Newborn)—Diseases—
Diagnosis. I. Tappero, Ellen P., 1952–. II. Honeyfield, Mary Ellen, 1944–.
    (DNLM: 1. Physical Examination—in infancy & childbood. 2. Infant, Newborn.
3. Physical Examination—methods. 4. Neonatal Nursing—methods. WS 420 P5775
1996)
RJ255.5.P435   1996
618.92 ' 01—dc20
DNLM/DLC
for Library of Congress   96-9065
                                                       CIP

ISBN: 1-887571-00-0

TABLE OF CONTENTS

CONTRIBUTING AUTHORS

Debbie Fraser Askin, RNC, MN
St. Boniface General Hospital
Winnipeg, Manitoba

Barbara E. Carey, RNC, MN, NNP, CPNP
UCLA School of Nursing
Los Angeles, California

Terri A. Cavaliere, RNC, MS, NNP
North Shore University Hospital
State University of New York
Stony Brook, New York

Garris Keels Conner, RN, DSN
The Children's Hospital
Birmingham, Alabama

Mary Ellen Honeyfield, RNC, MS, NNP
Innovative HealthCARE, Inc.
NNP Services of Colorado, Inc.
Denver, Colorado

Cynthia Boyer Johnson, RNC, MS, NNP
The Children's Hospital
Denver, Colorado

Elizabeth Kirby, RNC, MS, NNP
St. Peter's Medical Center
New Brunswick, New Jersey

Connie Rusk, RNC, MS, NNP
Columbia/HCA Corporation
Presbyterian/St. Luke's Medical Center
Denver, Colorado

Ellen P. Tappero, RNC, MN, NNP
Lutheran Medical Center
Wheat Ridge, Colorado

Carol Wiltgen Trotter, RNC, MPH, NNP
St. John's Mercy Medical Center
St. Louis, Missouri

Lyn Vargo, RNC, MSN, NNP
St. John's Mercy Medical Center
St. Louis, Missouri

Catherine Witt, RNC, MS, NNP
Presbyterian/St. Luke's Medical Center
Denver, Colorado

Foreword

The past few decades have brought many advances in neonatal care. Techno-
logical improvements and increased understanding of neonatal problems have
significantly reduced mortality and morbidity and improved outcome. Earlier discharge of both low- and high-risk infants has made care more family centered.
Despite these changes, however, one component remains the cornerstone of neonatal care. That component is physical assessment.

Systematic physical assessment has remained a critical component of neonatal
care because many problems in the neonate—such as early signs of sepsis, metabolic alterations, necrotizing enterocolitis, hyperbilirubinemia, or changes in skin
integrity—can be detected by an astute nurse or physician with good assessment
skills long before electronic monitors or other equipment record them. Accurate,
ongoing physical assessment is critical to the management of neonates across all
settings. Yet because assessment skills are such an integral aspect of practice, many
practitioners take them for granted. To maintain excellence, however, practitioners must continue to expand, update, and validate their skills.

Assessment is critical in evaluating the neonate's transition to extrauterine life,
in recognizing subtle indicators or changes that may be harbingers of serious problems, and in evaluating a plethora of clinical findings. The purposes of neonatal
assessment range from identifying the influences of the prenatal environment, to
obtaining baseline information after birth, to distinguishing between problems and
normal variations. Assessment can identify early signs of physiological problems
and subtle behavioral and neurological cues that indicate infant neurobehavioral
status. Assessment is also essential in care planning and parent teaching.

Physical Assessment of the Newborn is a valuable resource for all those involved in
neonatal care—and a long-needed addition to the neonatal literature. Editors Ellen
Tappero and Mary Ellen Honeyfield have brought together in one comprehensive
yet readable volume a wealth of detailed information on assessment of the newborn. The numerous tables, figures, and illustrations—a major strength—enhance

the book's usefulness as a clinical resource. The chapter authors clearly identify areas for assessment, provide the scientific basis for and rationale underlying various assessment techniques, and define and exemplify normal and abnormal findings and common variations. The book not only illustrates the skills needed to gather assessment data systematically and accurately but also provides a knowledge base for interpretation of these data.

This text is both an excellent teaching tool and a resource for anyone who does newborn examinations—including nurses, neonatal and pediatric nurse practitioners, nurse-midwives, physicians, and therapists. It should be a core text for any program preparing individuals for advanced roles in neonatal care, and it should be available as a resource in every setting providing care to neonates. Individual practitioners have varying degrees of familiarity and comfort with the many areas of newborn assessment. This text can serve as an in-depth, systematic introduction to the major components of and techniques for assessing all the major systems. For more experienced practitioners, it can reinforce, update, and improve knowledge and techniques. At all levels of practice, it serves as a convenient reference to common variations and less commonly seen abnormalities.

Understanding of the unique physical, physiologic, neurologic, and behavioral findings in the neonate helps practitioners recognize alterations and prevent or minimize their effects. Skillful newborn assessment reduces the risks associated with the transition to extrauterine life and the pathophysiologic problems of the neonatal period. The editors and authors are to be highly congratulated for this landmark publication—a significant contribution to neonatal care.

Susan Tucker Blackburn, RN,C, PhD, FAAN
Coauthor of Maternal, Fetal, and Neonatal Physiology:
    A Clinical Perspective.

Introduction

Physical assessment of the newborn infant is both a challenge and an opportunity. The practitioner is challenged to assimilate an immense body of knowledge and develop the technical and problem-solving skills necessary to apply that knowledge to clinical practice. Upon completion of this assessment, the practitioner has the opportunity to provide information about the infant that affects both the newborn and his family. Most often that information confirms the parents' dream of a perfect baby. Sometimes the practitioner must convey information about an unusual or abnormal finding and initiate the appropriate follow-up care for the infant. The practitioner's introduction to the principles of newborn physical assessment may forever influence his or her attitude toward this task. The goal of this book is to make the task of physical assessment an exciting challenge.

After performing and teaching newborn physical assessment for the past two decades and reviewing numerous chapters on the subject, we became acutely aware no text was available to staff nurses, nurse practitioners, nurse midwives, and medical students written with sufficient depth to guide the practitioner through the basics of a newborn physical examination and to show how the information is clinically applicable.

This text is a primer for the assessment of the term or near term infant. The authors believe that practitioners must be confident in their knowledge and demonstrate clinical competence with "well" newborns before they move on to the study of ill infants. We have been impressed over the years with how much pathology presents in the "routine" physical examination of newborns. This text should be used in combination with other resources to expand the practitioner's knowledge of pathogenesis and management of clinical pathology. We hope that this book arouses the interest of beginning students in newborn physical examination and allows experienced practitioners to further refine their assessment skills.

All texts are "works in progress." In writing this second edition, we have incorporated the comments we received from the students, faculty, reviewers, and practitioners who enjoyed reading the first edition. The new chapter, *Evaluating and Recording the Neonatal History,* reviews the importance of the maternal, family, and birth history as a first step in physical assessment of the newborn. Two chapters—*Genitourinary Assessment* and *Behavioral Assessment*—have received extensive revision.

The 13 chapters are organized in a head-to-toe approach. The authors undertook writing their chapters in individual ways, and no attempt has been made to enforce a uniform format. There is overlap of subject material between some chapters, but the somewhat different viewpoints presented and the cross-references noted in the chapters have persuaded us to permit these minor repetitions. The text concludes with a glossary of all important terms and a cross-referenced index.

The contributing authors have many years of accumulated experience. We have tried to combine the experiences of professionals devoted to the study of newborns with those who participate in day-to-day care of infants. This collective expertise provides the reader with a synopsis of essential information in language that is easy for students to understand. The many photographs and drawings illustrate important concepts and techniques to further enhance understanding.

This book was made possible because of the special help of many individuals. Thanks go to our teachers, who introduced us, as novices, in a positive way to the challenge of newborn physical assessment. We also wish to thank Charles Rait, whose comments and suggestions stimulated us to begin this work and whose interest sustained us throughout. Thanks to the authors who were committed to improve this second edition. We offer thanks for the many shared photographs to Dr. David Clark, Dr. Jacinto Hernandez, Dr. Barbara Quissell, Dr. Peter Honeyfield, and Dr. Eva Sujansky. The illustrations were done by Elizabeth Massari, a talented medical illustrator at UCLA, whose detailed anatomic drawings have made a substantial contribution to facilitating the study of newborn assessment.

Finally, this second edition comes to print because of the untiring efforts, skill, patience, and always cheerful encouragement of Suzanne Rait and Tabitha Parker. They, with Beverly DeWitt, Sylvia Stein Wright, and other members of the editorial staff, carefully read, edited and typed each chapter draft. They worked personally with each author and have the amazing ability to set the most impossible deadlines and have everyone meet them. Thanks!

Ellen P. Tappero
Mary Ellen Honeyfield

ACKNOWLEDGEMENTS

It is always hard to know where to start when writing a dedication to the people who were so supportive and who helped in so many ways to make this project possible. Certainly, I will always be grateful to my parents, John and Sarah Paysinger, who never thought anything was impossible for me to accomplish and who are proud of the achievements I have had. A special thanks to my husband, Charlie, for never complaining about missed meals or the lack of conversation when all I could think of were deadlines. This edition is also dedicated to the many mentors who were instrumental in my choice of neonatal nursing as my specialty area and Drs. John Curran, Andrew Wertz and Tom Ciszak who helped shape my career.

Ellen Tappero

This edition is dedicated to the Level I nurses at "St. Luke's." We have worked together in the "well baby" nursery for some 17 years. For those nurses still there from the early days, Ruth, Marge, Pat, Rosemary, Eunice, Bonnie and Patrice, I thank you for giving me the gift of observation. With yours and Teri Joyer's help I was able to overcome my intensive care mentality and learned the significance of the special role you have in the assessment and care of new babies and their families.

Mary Ellen Honeyfield-Rupert

1 Principles of Physical Assessment

Mary Ellen Honeyfield, RNC, MS, NNP

The importance of approaching the newborn physical examination with a sense of anticipation cannot be overemphasized. This first exam offers a unique opportunity for early recognition of any problems the infant may have. Seeing each infant as a mystery to be unraveled requires curiosity on the part of the examiner. The inability of the newborn to provide verbal information tests the acuity of the examiner's skills. When the examiner views this responsibility as a diagnostic challenge, newborn physical assessment provides both personal and professional satisfaction, even though the majority of infants examined are normal.

Initially, the inexperienced examiner finds physical assessment time-consuming. Lack of familiarity with the tools and limited practice with the techniques both slow assessment. In fact, the student often views the infant as a series of systems to be examined. Repetition and experience help the practitioner learn to see the newborn as a whole and to process multiple observations while examining individual systems. For example, if the infant begins to cry during palpation of the abdomen, the experienced examiner continues the abdominal exam but also notes the quality of the cry, the infant's color while crying, respiratory effort, facial movements, the tongue, intactness of the palate, and movement of the extremities.

Clinical expertise develops throughout a practitioner's career. With experience, each practitioner develops a unique approach to newborn physical examination. The sequence of how the exam is performed is not as important as that each practitioner develop a consistent and organized approach. Performing the examination in the same organized manner each time a newborn is examined maximizes the information gained from each exam, thus adding to the knowledge base, and insuring that portions of the assessment will not be forgotten. Consistency maximizes the information gained from every examination performed and adds new data to the knowledge base.

TECHNIQUES OF PHYSICAL ASSESSMENT

OBSERVATION

Observation is the most important physical assessment technique for the practitioner to master. It is also often the most difficult skill for the fledgling examiner to incorporate into

TABLE 1-1 ▲ Observations for Physical Assessment

To Assess	Observe
Distress	Facial expression, respiratory effort, activity, tone
Color	Tongue, mucous membranes (centrally pink vs cyanotic), nail beds, hands, feet (peripherally pink vs cyanotic), skin (jaundice, pallor, ruddiness, mottling), perfusion, meconium staining
Nutrition status	Subcutaneous fat, breast nodule
Hydration status	Skin turgor, anterior fontanel
Gestational age	Skin (smooth vs peeling), ear cartilage, areola and nipple formation, breast nodule, sole creases, descent of testes, rugae, labia
Neurologic status	Posture, tone, activity, response to stimuli, cry, state, state transition, reflexes
Respiratory/chest status	Respiratory rate and effort, retractions, nasal flaring, grunting, audible stridor or wheezing, chest shape, nipples (number and position), skin color
Cardiovascular status	Precordial activity, visible point of maximal intensity, skin perfusion and color
Abdomen	Size (full, distended, taut, shiny), shape (round, concave), distension (generalized or localized), visible peristaltic waves, visible bowel loops, muscular development/tone, umbilical cord, umbilical vessels, drainage from cord, periumbilical erythema (redness)
Head	Size, shape, anterior fontanel, hair distribution, condition of hair
Eyes	Shape, size, position, pupils, blink, extraocular movements, color of sclera, discharge, ability to fix and follow
Ears	Shape, position, external auditory canal, response to sound
Nose	Shape, nares, flaring, nasal bridge
Mouth	Shape, symmetry, movement, philtrum, tongue, palate, natal teeth, gums, jaw size
Neck	Shape, range of motion, webbing
Genitalia (male)	Scrotum, descent of testes, rugae, inguinal canals, foreskin, penile size, urine stream, meatus, perineum, anus
Genitalia (female)	Labia majora, labia minora, clitoris, vagina, perineum, inguinal canals, anus
Skin	Color, texture, firmness, vernix caseosa, masses, lanugo, lesions (pigmentary, vascular, trauma-related, infectious)
Extremities	Posture, range of motion (involuntary movement), digits, palmar creases, soles of feet, nails

the clinical approach. In 1860, Florence Nightingale wrote these thoughts about the art and skill of observation:

In the case of infants, everything must depend upon the accurate observation of the nurse or mother.... For it may safely be said, not that the habit of ready and correct observation will by itself make us useful…, but that without it we shall be useless with all our devotion.... If you cannot get the habit of observation one way or [the] other, you better give up…being a nurse, for it is not your calling, however kind and anxious you may be.[1]

Using the visual and auditory senses, the practitioner observes the infant and then assesses and makes decisions about what has been seen or heard. A specific observation may alert the examiner to assess a particular system more thoroughly. For example, the observation of an active precordium (visual cardiac pulsations) directs the examiner to careful auscultation of the heart. Auscultation may reveal a heart murmur. This finding suggests that the examiner palpate the precordium and peripheral pulses and obtain four extremity blood pressures, actions not normally part of the exam of an otherwise healthy-appearing newborn.

The practitioner can collect most of the information needed for a complete physical assessment solely through observation (Table 1-1).

AUSCULTATION

Auscultation is the technique of listening to sounds produced by the body (i.e., the lungs,

FIGURE 1-1 ▲ **Bimanual inspection of the kidneys.**

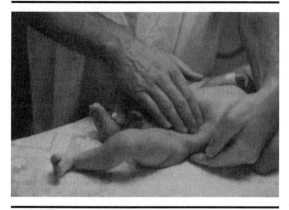

From: Coen RW, and Koffler H. 1987. *Primary Care of the Newborn.* Boston: Little, Brown, 30. Reprinted by permission.

FIGURE 1-2 ▲ **Transillumination of hydrocele.**

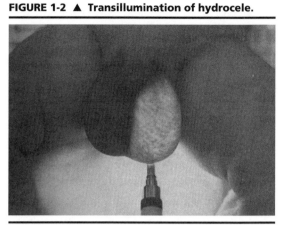

From: Coen RW, and Koffler H. 1987. *Primary Care of the Newborn.* Boston: Little, Brown, 33. Reprinted by permission.

heart, and gastrointestinal tract). *Direct auscultation* involves application of the examiner's ear to the body surface being assessed. Some sounds, such as stridor, wheezing, expiratory grunting, and Grade VI heart murmurs, may be heard simply by being near the infant. *Indirect (mediate) auscultation* utilizes a stethoscope to listen to these same sounds.

Accurate indirect auscultation of the newborn requires a stethoscope fitted with a pediatric-sized double-headed chest piece with an open bell and a closed diaphragm. The stethoscope should be placed firmly on bare skin rather than over the infant's clothes. A quiet infant and environment as well as a warm room and warm stethoscope facilitate auscultation.

PALPATION

Palpation is a technique in which the examiner uses the sense of touch to assess both superficial and deeper body characteristics. During palpation, the tips, palmar, and lateral surfaces of the fingers of both hands are used to assess external structures (i.e., skin, hair texture, neck), vibrations (i.e., peripheral pulses, precordial activity, and point of maximal impulse of the heart against the chest wall), and internal structures (i.e., liver, spleen, and kidneys). One hand

can be used, or a bimanual technique may enhance the palpation of deeper organs, such as the kidneys (Figure 1-1).

For accurate palpation, the infant should be quiet and relaxed at the beginning of the abdominal exam. Warm hands, a pacifier, progressing from superficial to deeper palpation, and elevating the infant's hips off the bed keep the abdominal muscles relaxed. The examiner should take care not to palpate too deeply for superficial abdominal organs such as the liver and spleen because the fingertips may be palpating stool-filled intestine or abdominal wall muscle mass rather than the organ itself.

In palpation of the extremities and genitalia, a grasping action of the fingers is used to evaluate such accessible features as skin texture, skin lesions, descent of testes into the scrotum, and muscle strength.

PERCUSSION

Percussion is tapping or striking a part of the body to put the underlying tissue into motion. This movement produces audible sounds and palpable vibrations, which are then assessed for the quality and duration of their tone and notes.

Indirect (mediate) percussion is performed (for a right-handed person) by hyperextending the middle finger of the left hand and placing only the distal interphalangeal joint firmly on the part of the body to be percussed. Contact by any other part of the hand will alter the sounds produced. The right wrist is then hyperextended and the middle right finger partially flexed and "cocked" upward in a position to strike the middle left finger. With a quick wrist motion downward, the tip of the right middle finger strikes the left middle finger's distal joint. Vibrations are transmitted through the bones of this joint to the underlying tissue being percussed.

Direct percussion is performed by directly striking the body surface to be assessed with the tip of the middle right finger.

The translation of sounds heard during percussion into descriptive words is difficult at best. It takes practice and multiple examinations of normal infants and those with pathology to develop skill in describing percussed sounds.

Although the technique of percussion is commonly taught to students, in practice, it is not a technique universally used on the newborn. When the examiner suspects pathologies like effusion or air leak, which might be assessed by percussion, the more common approach in the newborn is to confirm the suspected diagnosis by x-ray. A description of the comparative sounds produced during percussion has therefore been omitted.

TRANSILLUMINATION

Transillumination is the technique of applying a high-intensity light directly to a body part, such as the head, chest, or scrotum, and assessing the amount of pink light that can be seen as a corona (halo) around the cuffed flashlight or fiberoptic device.

Transillumination of the enlarged scrotum of an infant with a hydrocele reveals a fluid-filled mass that transmits light rather than a solid mass that does not transmit light, as in the case of an inguinal hernia (Figure 1-2).

As with the other physical assessment techniques described, practice enables the examiner to recognize the difference between normal and abnormal halos of light.

TIMING OF THE EXAM

Timing of newborn physical assessment often depends on circumstance and hospital guidelines. A quick overall exam should be done in the delivery room: It is disconcerting when the parents are the first to discover a problem. A more complete exam is done during the first few hours after birth. Daily and discharge exams are completed thereafter.

BASICS OF PHYSICAL ASSESSMENT

Certain themes recur throughout this text in the discussions of assessment of each system. The repetition is intentional and reflects the importance of these activities. These basic principles of physical assessment include the following:

▶ **Review the perinatal history for clues to potential pathology.** The newborn's history begins with conception and includes events that occurred throughout gestation, labor, and delivery. The newborn is also affected by the genetic histories of both parents and of their families. For example, a maternal history that includes diabetes mellitus directs the experienced practitioner to carefully assess the cardiovascular and neurologic systems and the extremities because infants of diabetic mothers show an increased incidence of abnormalities in these systems. The labor and delivery history may reveal that the mother received medication for pain relief just before delivery; that may account for the depression of the newborn's respiration. With this knowledge, the examiner need not pursue a more serious etiology for the depressed respirations, as long as the respiratory pattern improves over time or with the aid of a narcotic antagonist.

▶ **Assess the infant's color for clues to potential pathology.** The infant's color provides important information about several body systems. For example, the very red or ruddy infant may have polycythemia and may be more prone to complications, such as respiratory distress, that are associated with this phenomenon. The infant whose tongue and mucous membranes are pale or blue (central cyanosis) may be anemic or may have a heart lesion or respiratory disease. Proper lighting is essential for accurate assessment of color.

▶ **Auscultate only in a quiet environment.** It is difficult to assess the sounds produced by the body if there are noises, such as people talking or a radio playing, in the room. External interferences inhibit accurate evaluation of heart and breath sounds.

▶ **Keep the infant warm during examination.** After undressing the infant, prevention of heat loss is crucial to the infant's comfort and to the maintenance of a normal temperature and glucose homeostasis. The undressed infant is examined in a warm environment with an external heat source, such as an overhead radiant warmer. To keep from startling the newborn and to maintain a stable metabolic status, warm the stethoscope and, especially, your hands.

▶ **Have the necessary tools at hand.** A stethoscope, an ophthalmoscope, and a tape measure are used in all newborn examinations. Having them ready saves time.

▶ **Calm the infant before beginning the exam.** A quiet infant provides the best opportunity for data gathering. If a crying infant must be examined, patience—and possibly the aid of a second person to help calm the infant—is required.

▶ **Handle the infant gently.** The newly born infant is amazingly cooperative when the examiner is gentle. A soothing voice and a soft touch often allow the examiner to complete the entire physical assessment without disturbing the infant greatly or at all. Parents enjoy watching their infant interact with the examiner and appreciate the gentleness of touch. Certain portions of the examination cause the infant more distress than others. Examination of the hips is usually the most disturbing part of the exam; it is therefore performed last.

▶ **Complete the exam.** Re-dress the infant to maintain a normal temperature. Notify the primary caregiver that the exam is over and of any abnormalities that were found or observations that need to be made.

A SAMPLE APPROACH

One method of organizing the examination of the newborn is described here—as a guide for the inexperienced examiner. As mentioned earlier, with practice, each examiner develops a personal style. It is assumed that the infant is unclothed and supine under a radiant warmer.

OBSERVATION

It can be very difficult for a practitioner to just stand at the crib and observe an infant. The immediate inclination is to touch and talk to the infant. This natural response must be postponed until later in the examination, however, because observation alone produces important information about every organ system. These initial observations allow the practitioner to develop a visual differential diagnosis before employing other assessment techniques (auscultation, palpation). Table 1-1 catalogs the many observations the skilled examiner must process in this initial assessment of the infant's status.

If these multiple observations prove normal, the examiner is less likely to find a significant abnormality upon auscultation and palpation. Each observation of normality serves to reassure the examiner—just as an observation of abnormality should heighten the examiner's suspicion that further inspection is necessary.

Observation is not an isolated technique for use only at the outset of the exam. Although it is important to spend a moment or two observing the infant at the bedside before touching him, observation of the infant's responses takes place throughout the exam. Depending on the infant's state and responses, all the observations listed in Table 1-1 can be made during the hands-on examination. The examiner must learn to take advantage of every opportunity the infant's behavior offers for observation. If, for example, the infant awakens spontaneously during the exam, the examiner should take advantage of that opportunity to examine the eyes.

Hands-on inspection includes measurements and tactile inspection of the skin. Maneuvers to assess symmetry and reflexes are also done.

AUSCULTATION

After observing the infant closely, many examiners next auscultate the chest, heart, and abdomen. To separate the sounds of the heart from those of the lungs, it is important to concentrate. Listen first to one type of sound, then to the other. For example, listen first to the heart—its rate, rhythm, regularity, and any added sounds. Then listen to breath sounds, ignoring the cardiac sounds.

PALPATION

The exam continues with palpation. Palpating certain parts of the body disturbs the infant more than palpating others. An ordered approach keeps the infant calm through much of the process.

Because femoral pulses are difficult to assess in a crying infant, palpate them first. Then palpate the brachial pulses. Next palpate the abdomen, beginning with the more superficial liver and spleen. (Learning to palpate the liver and spleen with the tips of the fingers as well as with the lateral edges of the index fingers facili-

tates examination from either side of the bassinet.) Palpate for abdominal masses; then use deeper palpation for the kidneys. At this point, the infant may be disturbed and crying, but this will not impede the remainder of the exam.

THE INTEGRATED EXAM

The skilled examiner integrates examination tasks. For example, after palpating the head, neck, clavicles, arms, and hands, the examiner can perform the pull-to-sit maneuver to assess palmar grasp, arm strength, and tone. At that point, the infant is being held in an appropriate position to elicit the Moro reflex. Genitalia can be examined next, before progressing to the lower extremities. While the infant is positioned prone on the practitioner's hand to assess truncal tone and the truncal incurvation reflex, the back can also be examined. These shortcuts facilitate multiple inspections and save time. The hips should be examined last because this procedure causes the most stress to the infant.

It is usually not necessary to assess reflexes as a separate step. The examiner will most likely have observed root and suck by this point. Moro and palmar grasp can be incorporated into the upper extremity exam, as just explained.

Although an extremely cooperative infant may sleep through the entire exam, the assessment is not complete until the infant has been observed through the various behavioral states. Facial asymmetry, for example, cannot be seen until the infant cries.

Ideally, the parents should observe the first complete examination. Parents appreciate demonstration of their infant's normality and uniqueness as well as early identification of unusual or abnormal findings.

EQUIPMENT

OPHTHALMOSCOPE

In addition to developing hands-on confidence with the newborn and with performing the exam in the parents' presence, the student must become proficient with what may be unfamiliar equipment. Facility with the tools reduces stress to both infant and examiner. Again, practice is the key.

If the ophthalmoscope is not already intact, attach the head of the device to the handle by pushing the head toward the handle and turning the head clockwise. To turn the ophthalmoscope on, depress the on/off button, usually on the neck of the handle, at the same time turning the button clockwise. To gain familiarity with the various apertures, project the light onto the palm of the hand or a piece of paper. The smallest of the full spots is the only aperture necessary to assess the red reflex in newborns.[2,3] The lens selector compensates for visual acuity of the individual examiner. Adjust the lens selector dial to bring the structure being examined into focus.

Examination of the undilated eye of the newborn includes assessment of pupillary constriction and the red reflex. The most opportune time to examine a newborn's eyes is when the infant is in the quiet alert state. An infant who is in light sleep will often open the eyes if the room is darkened. To examine the infant's eyes, hold the ophthalmoscope in the right hand, with the viewing aperture as close as possible to the right eye, and use the right index finger to turn the lens selector dial to the appropriate lens for proper focus. While positioning the infant's head with the free hand, align the illuminating light along the infant's visual plane. The red reflex appears as a homogenous bright red-orange color. Any opacity along the central optical pathway will block all or part of the red reflex. Note that in dark-skinned infants, the reflex appears pale rather than red. Use the ophthalmoscope to observe pupillary constriction after assessing the red reflex.[2]

STETHOSCOPE

The acoustical stethoscope excludes environmental sounds, making it easier for the examiner to hear sounds coming from the infant; it does not magnify these sounds. The earpieces and connecting binaurals should be angled toward the wearer's nose to project sound onto the examiner's tympanic membrane. To minimize sound distortion, the tubing should be no longer than 12 inches. The chest piece of the stethoscope often has a double head: a flat, closed diaphragm and an open bell. The diaphragm is used to assess high-frequency sounds and the bell, low frequency. Use the diaphragm to assess breath sounds by applying it firmly to the infant's skin so that it moves with the chest wall. Both the diaphragm and the bell are used to assess heart sounds. Do not compress the bell against the chest so firmly that it fills with tissue and acts like a diaphragm (Chapters 6 and 7).[2]

OTOSCOPE

The infant's ears should be assessed for size, shape, and placement. Otoscopic examination is not normally done in the newborn period because the ear canals are often filled with vernix. Use of the otoscope is not discussed.

SUMMARY

Each newborn examination is as different as each infant. This text explains basic techniques for examining each body system—to guide examiners with limited experience in performing a thorough newborn physical assessment. Only through experience, however, do practitioners develop clinical expertise. As their experience and confidence grow, most examiners develop their own unique approach to physical examination, along with the flexibility to adapt their approach to different situations. As long as the necessary equipment is available and basic principles are kept in mind, an infant can be examined in any setting.

REFERENCES

1. Nightingale F. 1969. *Notes on Nursing.* New York: Dover, 112–113.
2. Malasanos L, et al. 1986. *Health Assessment,* 3rd ed. St. Louis: Mosby-Year Book, 18–22.
3. Vaughan D, et al. 1989. *General Ophthalmology.* Norwalk, Connecticut: Appleton & Lange, 30–36.

BIBLIOGRAPHY

- Bates B. 1991. *A Guide to Physical Examination and History Taking,* 5th ed. Philadelphia: JB Lippincott.
- Malasanos L, et al. 1986. *Health Assessment,* 3rd ed. St. Louis: Mosby-Year Book.
- Sapira JD. 1990. *The Art and Science of Bedside Diagnosis.* Baltimore: Williams & Wilkins.
- Scanlon JW, et al. 1979. *A System of Newborn Physical Examination.* Baltimore: University Park Press.
- Vaughan D, et al. 1989. *General Ophthalmology.* Norwalk, Connecticut: Appleton & Lange.
- Whaley LF, and Wong DE. 1987. *Nursing Care of Infants and Children,* 3rd ed. St. Louis: Mosby-Year Book.

NOTES

2 Evaluating and Recording the Neonatal History

Barbara E. Carey, RNC, MN, NNP, CPNP

A comprehensive physical examination of the newborn, performed no later than 12 to 18 hours after birth by the health care provider, physician, nurse practitioner, or physician assistant, is a standard of perinatal care.[1] The physical examination must be preceded by a thorough review of the history of the pregnancy; mother's past obstetrical history; intrapartum history; maternal medical, family medical, and social histories; and immediate neonatal adaptation history.[2] It is recommended that admitting nursery personnel evaluate the neonate's status and assess risks, through a review of the history documented in the antepartum and intrapartum records, no later than 2 hours after birth.[1] Assessment is the gathering of accurate, detailed data, and it includes four components: (1) reviewing the history, (2) reviewing the results of the physical examination, (3) reviewing available laboratory or other data, and (4) formulating an impression. The practitioner then develops a plan of care and monitors the newborn for actual or potential problems.

IMPORTANCE OF THE HISTORY

A comprehensive history is the prerequisite for adequate assessment. When the physical examination is performed without knowledge of the complete history, the information necessary for accurate formulation of an impression may be inadequate.

Knowledge of the history can also be useful in allaying parental anxiety when performing the physical examination. A mother whose ultrasound at 20 weeks revealed the possibility of her fetus having a fluid-filled gastrointestinal mass but whose subsequent ultrasounds appeared to be normal is likely to have an increased level of concern about the status of her neonate's gastrointestinal tract. Knowledge of this pertinent history allows the examiner to emphasize the normal GI findings, discuss the history of the positive ultrasound findings, and reassure the mother.

The history also alerts the examiner to potential problems and may indicate the need for more frequent repeat examinations. A cardiac murmur in a neonate with a history of maternal anticonvulsant use throughout pregnancy is of more concern than a murmur in a neonate with a negative history. Embryonic exposure to anticonvulsant therapy increases the risk for structural congenital cardiac malformations.[3]

The history is the context in which neonates with identified problems and disorders must be analyzed. Lack of a history or an incomplete history can lead to more extensive testing than would otherwise be necessary, or an incorrect impression or diagnosis. The following case exemplifies the need for obtaining an accurate history.

Baby Joe, a 36-week, 3 kg neonate, was admitted to the nursery at 1 AM following vaginal delivery to a 34-year-old, gravida 4, para 3 mother with a history of preeclampsia. His Apgars were 7 and 8 at one and five minutes. His admission was uneventful; his examination revealed slightly decreased tone and spontaneous activity. Re-evaluation at one and two hours of life revealed continued poor tone and decreased spontaneous activity, with no other abnormal findings on the physical examination. At two and a half hours, apnea was noted. After being notified, the on-call health care provider requested that a complete blood count and C-reactive protein be drawn. On the neonate's next examination, the findings were consistent with decreased tone and activity. Blood and spinal fluid were obtained for culture and sensitivity, and antibiotics were begun. The maternal chart with antepartum and intrapartum history was subsequently delivered to the nursery; it revealed that the mother had received magnesium sulfate. The neonate's magnesium level was obtained and found to be elevated. Review of the history would have given a more accurate context in which to view this infant's poor tone and activity and would have led to an earlier identification of hypermagnesemia, perhaps avoiding unnecessary testing.

THE SUPPLEMENTAL INTERVIEW

Sometimes the mother, or both parents, may need to be interviewed for information not found in the records. Before approaching the parents, review all available medical records and identify the specific information needed. Remember that the first contact with the mother or parents is one of the most important contacts. It's essential to introduce yourself and to inform the mother of the reason for your questions. Be sure she is comfortable and maintain a normal conversational distance. Asking what name has been chosen for the baby helps establish a friendly atmosphere.

It's important to make and maintain eye contact and to present questions without reading them. Allow time for the mother to respond to your questions without interrupting her or checking your watch or the clock. Avoid technical language as much as possible and also the tendency to overexplain or lecture. If you must take notes, make them brief. Copious note taking detracts from your listening and observing abilities and may be intimidating.[4] Be an active listener: Show that you understand the responses and request clarification if appropriate. Periodically or at the end of the interview, summarize what you have been told. Evaluate answers to questions for content—*what* was said—and also for affect or tone—*how* it was said. A parent who avoids answering a question or answers incompletely may be embarrassed or upset by the question.[5] When giving the parents information about the neonate's health status, have them repeat at the end of the interview what they believe the neonate's health status or problems to be so you can clarify any misunderstandings immediately if needed.

ELEMENTS OF A COMPLETE HISTORY

Gathering historical information is not enough. It must be organized and presented in a systematic format commonly used by other professionals. All pertinent information must be included. Elements of a complete history start with the identifying data, followed by the chief complaint, and then the interim history of the neonate or the history of the presenting problem or illness if one exists. This is followed by the antepartum history; past

TABLE 2-1 ▲ Categorization of High-Risk Pregnancy Factors

Socioeconomic Factors
1. Inadequate finances
2. Poor housing
3. Severe social problems
4. Unwed, especially adolescent
5. Minority status
6. Nutritional deprivation
7. Parental occupation

Demographic Factors
1. Maternal age under 16 or over 35 years
2. Overweight or underweight prior to pregnancy
3. Height less than 5 feet
4. Maternal education less than 11 years
5. Family history of severe inherited disorders

Medical Factors

A. Obstetric History
1. Infertility
2. Ectopic pregnancy or spontaneous abortion
3. Grand multiparity
4. Stillborn or neonatal death
5. Uterine/cervical abnormality
6. Multiple gestation
7. Premature labor/delivery
8. Prolonged labor
9. Cesarean section
10. Low birth weight infant
11. Macrosomic infant
12. Midforceps delivery
13. Baby with neurologic deficit, birth injury, or malformation
14. Hydatidiform mole or choriocarcinoma

B. Maternal Medical History/Status
1. Cardiac disease
2. Pulmonary disease

3. Metabolic disease—particularly, diabetes mellitus, thyroid disease
4. Chronic renal disease, repeated urinary tract infections, repeated bacteriuria
5. Gastrointestinal disease
6. Endocrine disorders (pituitary, adrenal)
7. Chronic hypertension
8. Hemoglobinopathies
9. Seizure disorder
10. Venereal and other infectious diseases
11. Weight loss greater than 5 pounds
12. Malignancy
13. Surgery during pregnancy
14. Major congenital anomalies of the reproductive tract
15. Mental retardation, major emotional disorders

C. Current OB Status
1. Late or no prenatal care
2. Rh sensitization
3. Fetus inappropriately large or small for gestational age
4. Premature labor
5. Pregnancy-induced hypertension
6. Multiple gestation
7. Polyhydramnios
8. Premature or prolonged rupture of the membranes
9. Antepartum bleeding
   a. Placenta previa
   b. Abruptio placenta
10. Abnormal presentation
11. Postmaturity
12. Abnormality in tests for fetal well-being
13. Anemia

D. Habits/Habituation
1. Smoking during pregnancy
2. Regular alcohol intake
3. Drug use/abuse

From: Aumann GM, and Baird MM. 1986. Screening for the high-risk pregnancy. In *High-Risk Pregnancy: A Team Approach*, Knuppel RA, and Drukker JE, eds. Philadelphia: WB Saunders, 12. Reprinted by permission.

obstetrical history; intrapartum history; and the maternal medical, family medical, and social histories. In some institutions, these data may be recorded on computerized forms; in other institutions, a written or dictated history is formulated. After the history is compiled, the physical exam data are recorded, followed by any laboratory or radiology studies obtained. An impression or assessment of the neonate is then formulated, and a plan for care is outlined.

IDENTIFYING DATA

The identifying data are the patient's name, birth date, and referral source. Both the referring obstetric care provider and the primary care pediatric provider should be listed so that they will receive a copy of the admission history and physical examination. If the patient is admitted to the neonatal intensive care unit, telephone numbers for the primary care providers should be included so that they can receive updates on

TABLE 2-2 ▲ Maternal Medications and Toxins: Possible Effects on the Fetus and/or Newborn

Medication/Toxin	Effect on Fetus/Newborn
Analgesics and Anti-inflammatories	
Aspirin	Hemorrhage, premature closure of ductus arteriosus, pulmonary artery hypertension
Codeine	Neonatal drug withdrawal reported
Indomethacin	Closure of fetal ductus arteriosus, pulmonary artery hypertension
Meperidine	Respiratory depression peaks 2–3 hours after maternal dose
Propoxyphene	Drug withdrawal reported, possible increased risk of anomalies
Anesthetics	
General anesthesia	Respiratory depression of infant at delivery if anesthesia is prolonged before delivery
Lidocaine	High fetal serum levels cause CNS depression; accidental direct injection into fetal head causes seizures
Antibiotics	
Aminoglycosides	Ototoxicity reported after first trimester use of kanamycin and streptomycin
Cephalosporins	Some drugs in this group displace bilirubin from albumin
Isoniazid	Risk for folate deficiency
Metronidazole	Potential teratogen
Tetracycline	Yellow-brown staining and caries of teeth
Sulfonamides	Some drugs in this group displace bilirubin from albumin
Streptomycin	Damage to the eighth cranial nerve, hearing loss
Anticonvulsants	
Phenobarbital	Withdrawal symptoms, hemorrhagic disease
Phenytoin	Hemorrhagic disease, fetal hydantoin syndrome
Trimethadione	Fetal trimethadione syndrome, cleft lip and palate, cardiac and genital anomalies
Valproic acid	Myelomeningocele, facial and cardiac anomalies
Anticoagulants	
Warfarin (Coumadin)	Warfarin embryopathy
Antineoplastics	
Aminopterin	Cleft palate; hydrocephalus, myelomeningocele, growth retardation
Cyclophosphamide	Growth retardation, cardiovascular and digital anomalies
Methotrexate	Absent digits
Antithyroid Drugs	
Iodide-containing drugs	May cause hypothyroidism
Methimazole	May cause hypothyroidism, cutis aplasia
Propylthiouracil	May cause hypothyroidism
Cardiovascular Drugs and Antihypertensives	
β-blockers (propranolol)	Neonatal bradycardia, hypoglycemia
Calcium channel blockers	If maternal hypotension occurs, could affect placental blood flow
Digoxin	Fetal toxicity with maternal overdose
Methyldopa	Mild, clinically insignificant decrease in neonatal blood pressure
Diuretics	
Furosemide	Increases fetal urinary sodium and potassium
Thiazides	Thrombocytopenia

TABLE 2-2 ▲ Maternal Medications and Toxins: Possible Effects on the Fetus and/or Newborn (continued)

Medication/Toxin	Effect on Fetus/Newborn
Hormonal Drugs	
Corticosteroids	Cleft palate reported in animals
Diethylstilbestrol (DES)	DES daughters: genital tract anomalies, increased rate of premature delivery
	DES sons: possible increase in genitourinary anomalies
Estrogens, progestins	Uncertain teratogenic potential, virilization of female fetuses reported with progestins
Sedatives, Tranquilizers, and Psychiatric Drugs	
Barbiturates (short-acting)	Theoretic risk for hemorrhage and drug withdrawal
Benzodiazepines	Hypotonia, impaired thermoregulation
Lithium	Cardiac anomalies (Ebstein's), diabetes insipidus, thyroid depression, cardiovascular dysfunction
Thalidomide	Limb reduction and other anomalies
Tricyclic antidepressants	Association with limb reduction defects (causation unproven)
Tocolytics	
Magnesium sulfate	Respiratory depression, hypermagnesemia
Ritodrine	Neonatal hypoglycemia
Terbutaline	Neonatal hypoglycemia
Vitamins and Related Drugs	
A	Excessive doses are teratogenic
D	Megadoses may cause hypercalcemia
Menadione (vitamin K_3)	Hyperbilirubinemia and kernicterus at high doses
Isotretinoin	Ear, cardiac, CNS, and thymic anomalies
Miscellaneous	
Antiemetics	Doxylamine succinate and/or dicyclomine hydrochloride with pyridoxine hydrochloride reported to be a teratogen, but this is unproven
Irradiation	Fetal death, microcephaly, growth retardation
Methyl mercury	Mental retardation, microcephaly
Oral hypoglycemics	Neonatal hypoglycemia
Social and Illicit Drugs	
Alcohol	Fetal alcohol syndrome or effects
Amphetamines	Withdrawal, prematurity, decreased birth weight and head circumference
Cocaine	Decreased birth weight; microcephaly; prematurity; abruptio placenta with possible asphyxia, shock, stillbirth, cerebral hemorrhage
Heroin	Increased incidence of low birth weight and small for gestational age, drug withdrawal, impaired postnatal growth, behavioral disturbances
Marijuana	Associated with decreased fetal growth and increased incidence of acute nonlymphoblastic leukemia in childhood
Methadone	Increased birth weight as compared to heroin, drug withdrawal (worse than with heroin alone)
Phencyclidine (PCP)	Irritability, jitteriness, hypertonia, poor feeding
Tobacco smoking	Decreases birth weight by 175–250 gm; increased prematurity rate; increased premature rupture of membranes, placental abruption, and placenta previa; increased fetal death

Adapted from: Klaus M, and Fanaroff A. 1993. Recognition, stabilization, and transport of the high-risk newborn. In *Care of the High-Risk Neonate*, 4th ed. Philadelphia: WB Saunders, 66–67. Reprinted by permission.

TABLE 2-3 ▲ Recommended Intervals for Routine and Specialized Antepartum Tests

Time (week)	Assessment
Initial (as early as possible)	Hemoglobin or hematocrit measurement Urinalysis, including microscope examination and infection screen Blood group and Rh type determinations Antibody screen Rubella antibody titer measurement Syphilis screen Cervical cytology Hepatitis B virus screen
8–18	Ultrasound Amniocentesis Chorionic villus sampling
16–18	Maternal serum α-fetoprotein
26–28	Diabetes screening Repeat hemoglobin or hematocrit measurement
28	Repeat antibody test for unsensitized Rh-negative patients Prophylactic administration of Rho(D) immune globulin
32–36	Ultrasound Testing for sexually transmitted disease Repeat hemoglobin or hematocrit measurement

From: American Academy of Pediatrics, American College of Obstetricians and Gynecologists. 1992. *Guidelines for Perinatal Care*. Washington, DC: American College of Obstetricians and Gynecologists, 53. Reprinted by permission.

the neonate's problems and progress. If the patient is transferred in from another facility for care, the name of the referring health care facility should also be included.

CHIEF COMPLAINT

The chief complaint is a brief statement regarding the initial known status of the neonate, including age, sex, birth and current weights, gestational age by dates and examination, and any problems the infant might have. In the normal newborn, the chief complaint might simply be stated as: "3 kg female, 41 weeks by dates, appropriate for gestational age, now 2 hours of age." Or it may include identified problems, as in the following sample:

1. 2.5 kg male, 42 weeks by dates, SGA, 3 hours of age
2. Hypoglycemia
3. Tachypnea: rule out pneumonia versus retained lung fluid
4. Suspected sepsis

INTERIM HISTORY

The interim history or history of present illness chronologically records the neonate's his-

tory from the time of delivery until the present time and, in the well newborn, should include data regarding temperature stabilization, feeding, voiding, stooling, and behavioral adaptation. In the neonate with identified problems, the sequence of the newborn's problem or problems is discussed, as are laboratory or x-ray findings, interventions, and responses to treatment. The age of the mother, type of delivery, neonate's birth weight and current weight (if greater than one day of age), and Apgar scores are sometimes also included to give a more comprehensive picture.

ANTEPARTUM HISTORY

The antepartum history includes more specific historical data on the pregnancy: maternal age, gravidity, and parity; last menstrual period (LMP); and estimated date of confinement (EDC) or delivery (EDD). The date and gestational age at which prenatal care began, who provided the care, and the number of visits are recorded. Medical complications and high-risk pregnancy factors (Table 2-1), treatments, and monitoring are recorded. The antepartum history should also include information about

TABLE 2-4 ▲ Indications for Antepartum Fetal Assessment

Chronic hypertension

Pregnancy-induced hypertension

Chronic renal disease

Insulin-dependent diabetes mellitus

Maternal cyanotic congenital heart disease

Rh or other isoimmunization

Homozygous hemoglobinopathies

Maternal abuse of tobacco, alcohol, or drugs

Previous unexplained stillbirth

Fetal growth retardation

Fetal postmaturity

Hydramnios, oligohydramnios

Decreased fetal movement

Multiple gestation

Premature rupture of membranes

Third-trimester bleeding

Sickle cell anemia

Maternal collagen vascular diseases

From: Huddleston JE, and Brown PC. 1992. Estimation of fetal well-being. Part 2: Antepartum fetal surveillance. In *Neonatal-Perinatal Medicine: Diseases of the Fetus and Infant*, 5th ed., Fanaroff AA, and Martin RJ, eds. St. Louis: Mosby-Year Book, 113. Reprinted by permission.

exposure of the fetus to radiation; over-the-counter, prescribed, or illicit drug use; and cigarette and alcohol use (Table 2-2).

When reviewing the history of the antepartum period, the examiner should note the results of all tests performed on the mother and/or fetus and understand their implications. Usual prenatal screenings may include the following tests: maternal blood type and Rh, antibody screen, serology testing, rubella immunity, purified protein derivative (PPD), hepatitis screening, α-fetoprotein, and ultrasound. Abnormal findings on routine screening tests will prompt follow-up or specialized screenings. A schedule for routine general laboratory examinations during pregnancy appears in Table 2-3. Indications for antepartum fetal assessment are listed in Table 2-4. Appendix A, Antepartum Tests and Intrapartum Monitoring, explains many of the routine and some specialized antepartum screenings and also indicates what the results mean.

OBSTETRIC HISTORY

The mother's obstetric history is reviewed for the number of pregnancies, abortions, stillbirths, living children, types of deliveries, dates of birth or abortion, birth weights, and gestational ages at birth. Any neonatal problems or subsequent major medical problems of prior children should be noted. The present age and health status of living children are recorded. If any child is deceased, the cause and date are included.

INTRAPARTUM HISTORY

The intrapartum history is evaluated for duration of labor, if the labor was spontaneous or induced, medications and anesthetics used during labor and delivery, length of the first and second stages of labor, type of delivery, and whether delivery was spontaneous or required forceps or vacuum assistance. The time and duration of rupture of membranes and the status of the amniotic fluid volume and presence or absence of meconium are ascertained. Laboratory and monitoring data obtained during labor are reviewed and noted, as are any complications that occurred during this period (such as fever, bleeding, or hypertension) and the treatment provided. The presentation of the neonate at delivery, the Apgar scores, any resuscitative interventions performed, and the response to resuscitation are documented.

MATERNAL MEDICAL HISTORY

The maternal medical history is reviewed for chronic health problems and for diseases or disorders treated in the past and/or during the pregnancy. Potential consequences of maternal medical problems for the fetus and/or newborn are listed in Table 2-5. Infections past, present, and during the pregnancy as well as surgical procedures and hospitalizations that occurred before or during the pregnancy are included.

TABLE 2-5 ▲ Potential Effects of Maternal Medical Conditions on the Fetus and/or Newborn

Maternal Condition	Potential Fetal/Neonatal Effects
Endocrine/Metabolic	
Diabetes mellitus	Hypoglycemia, hypocalcemia, macrosomia, polycythemia, hyperbilirubinemia, increased risk for birth defects, birth trauma, small left colon syndrome, cardiomyopathy, RDS, fetal demise
Hypoparathyroidism	Fetal hypocalcemia, neonatal hyperparathyroidism
Hyperparathyroidism	Neonatal hypocalcemia and hypoparathyroidism
Hyperthyroidism	Fetal and neonatal hyperthyroidism, IUGR, prematurity, congestive heart failure, tachycardia
Obesity	Macrosomia, birth trauma
Phenylketonuria (PKU) (untreated pregnancies)	Mental retardation, microcephaly, congenital heart defects
Cardiopulmonary	
Asthma	Increased rates of prematurity, toxemia, and perinatal loss
Congenital heart disease	Effects of cardiovascular drugs (see Table 2-2)
Hypertension, preeclampsia	Premature delivery caused by uncontrolled hypertension or eclampsia; uteroplacental insufficiency, abruptio placenta, fetal loss; IUGR; thrombocytopenia; neutropenia
Cystic fibrosis	Prematurity, IUGR, fetal loss
Hematologic	
Severe anemia (hemoglobin <6 mg/dl)	Impaired oxygen delivery, fetal loss
Iron deficiency anemia	Reduced iron stores, lower mental and developmental scores in follow-up
Idiopathic thrombocytopenia purpura	Thrombocytopenia, CNS hemorrhage
Fetal platelet antigen sensitization	Thrombocytopenia, CNS hemorrhage
Rh or ABO sensitization	Jaundice, anemia, hydrops fetalis
Sickle cell anemia	Increased prematurity, IUGR, fetal distress
Infections	
Chlamydia	Conjunctivitis, pneumonia
Chorioamnionitis	Increased risk for neonatal sepsis, premature labor and delivery
Cytomegalovirus	IUGR, microcephaly, cytomegalovirus inclusion disease, hearing loss
Gonorrhea	Ophthalmia neonatorum
Hepatitis A	Perinatal transmission
Hepatitis B	Perinatal transmission, chronic hepatitis
Herpes simplex	Encephalitis, disseminated herpes (risk of neonatal disease is much higher when maternal infection is primary rather than recurrent)
HIV	Risk of infectious transmission
Rubella	Rubella embryopathy, cataracts, cardiac defects
Syphilis	Congenital syphilis, IUGR
Toxoplasmosis	IUGR, microcephaly, hydrocephalus, chorioretinitis, myocarditis
Tuberculosis	Perinatal and postnatal transmission
Varicella	Congenital varicella syndrome, rash, pneumonia, myocarditis, encephalitis
Inflammatory/Immunologic	
Systemic lupus erythematosus	Fetal death, spontaneous abortion, heart block, neonatal lupus, thrombocytopenia, neutropenia, hemolytic anemia, endocardial fibrosis
Inflammatory bowel disease	Increase in prematurity, fetal loss, fetal and neonatal growth retardation

TABLE 2-5 ▲ Potential Effects of Maternal Medical Conditions on the Fetus and/or Newborn (continued)

Maternal Condition	Potential Fetal/Neonatal Effects
Neuromuscular	
Maternal seizure disorder requiring anticonvulsants	Teratogenic effects of medications (see Table 2-2)
Seizure during pregnancy	Fetal hypoxia
Myasthenia gravis	Transient neonatal myasthenia, preterm delivery
Myotonic dystrophy	Neonatal myotonic dystrophy
Renal/Urologic	
Urinary tract infection	Prematurity
Chronic renal failure	Prematurity, IUGR, fetal loss
Transplant recipients	Prematurity, IUGR, possible effects of maternal immunosuppressive therapy and mineral disorders

IUGR = Intrauterine growth retardation

RDS = Respiratory distress syndrome

Adapted from: Klaus M, and Fanaroff A. 1993. Recognition, stabilization, and transport of the high-risk newborn. In *Care of the High-Risk Neonate,* 4th ed. Philadelphia: WB Saunders, 64. (Compiled from: Creasy RK, and Resnik R. 1989. *Maternal-Fetal Medicine: Principles and Practice*, 2nd ed. Philadelphia: WB Saunders; Barron WM, and Lindheimer MD, eds. 1985. Symposium on medical disorders during pregnancy. *Clinics in Perinatology* 12(3): 479–713; and Cotton DB, ed. 1986. Critical care in obstetrics. *Clinics in Perinatology* 13(4): 695–868.) Reprinted by permission.

Counseling for psychological or social problems should also be noted. Medication use for nonpregnancy-related health or medical problems should be ascertained.

FAMILY MEDICAL HISTORY

The family medical history is reviewed for ages of the infant's mother, father, and siblings; sex of the other children; and any diagnosed chronic disorders, disabilities, or known hereditary diseases. A genetic history may be required if the neonate is dysmorphic, and further information should be sought regarding other family members affected with a similar disorder. Information about familial disease or disorders can be elicited by asking if anyone else in the immediate or extended family has the same or a related problem or if any relative has a genetic

FIGURE 2-1 ▲ Genetic pedigree chart.

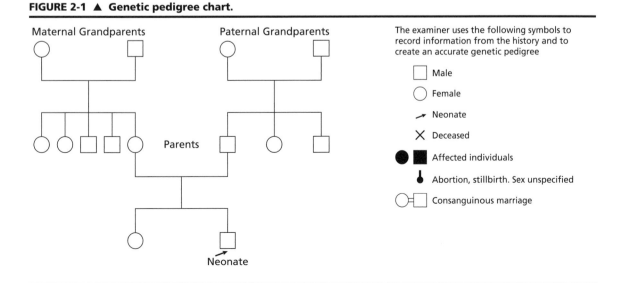

abnormality or an unusual disease or disorder. A finding such as a head circumference several standard deviations above normal with normal weight and length percentiles may raise the possibility of an intracranial abnormality. Review of the family history should include questions regarding any similar finding in the baby's parents when they were children. A grandparent can often provide or confirm this information. The most common cause of a large head in an otherwise normal newborn is benign familial megalencephaly, and one of the parents, usually the father, generally had the same finding in infancy.[6] Preparation of a genetic pedigree chart (Figure 2-1) often helps clarify the relationships of affected family members when the history is positive for similar findings in relatives. The question of consanguinity (mating of individuals related by blood) can be posed by asking the parents if they are related in any way besides by marriage and if there is anyone in the family who was related to both parents before their marriage.

SOCIAL HISTORY

The social history includes the mother's marital status, presence or support of the infant's father, and both parents' occupations and educations. The family's sources of support in the financial, housing, and care areas are noted. The family's religious affiliation and cultural heritage are included. The family unit should be defined, along with the number of people, family and nonfamily, living in the home. The health status of all household members should also be ascertained. Support agencies with which the family is now working and the family's current social service contacts are important. Members of the family or others who are planning to help with child care after discharge are included. If and when the mother plans to return to work and what arrangements for infant caretaking are planned should be elicited. Information regarding frequent or recent family moves, deaths in the family, and job changes also give an idea of the stressors affecting the family. This information will assist the practitioner in planning for necessary services following discharge or can point to the need for referral to social services.

REMAINING ELEMENTS

The physical examination is performed and recorded. Laboratory or radiology data that have been obtained should be noted. An assessment or impression of the infant's status is then made, including a statement of suspected or potential problems. Here is an example for an infant with problems:

1. 3.8 kg preterm female, 35 weeks gestation, large for gestational age, infant of a diabetic mother, 4 hours of age
2. Hypoglycemia
3. Cardiac murmur

An assessment statement for a well newborn with no complications might be similar to this one:

1. 3.5 kg term male, appropriate for gestational age, 4 hours of age
2. Teenage mother with little social support

A care plan addressing each of the identified problems should then be written.

SUMMARY

A thorough approach to history gathering coupled with analysis of antepartum and intrapartum data provides a comprehensive view of the neonate's present status and potential health problems. Taking the time to review the history lets the health care provider put problems in context and, in conjunction with the physical examination findings, to formulate a reasoned plan of care.

REFERENCES

1. American Academy of Pediatrics, American College of Obstetricians and Gynecologists. 1992. *Guidelines for Perinatal Care,* 3rd ed. Elk Grove Village, Illinois: American Academy of Pediatrics, 92–94.

2. Coen RW, and Koffler H. 1987. *Primary Care of the Newborn.* Boston: Little, Brown.

3. Creasy RK, and Resnik R. 1989. *Maternal-Fetal Medicine: Principles and Practice,* 2nd ed. Philadelphia: WB Saunders, 1076.

4. Barness LA. 1981. *Manual of Pediatric Physical Diagnosis.* St. Louis: Mosby-Year Book, 1–10.

5. Athreya BH, and Silverman BK. 1985. *Pediatric Physical Diagnosis.* Norwalk, Connecticut: Appleton & Lange, 17–28.

6. Goldbloom RB. 1992. *Pediatric Clinical Skills.* New York: Churchill Livingstone, 19.

BIBLIOGRAPHY

- Barron WM, and Lindheimer MD, eds. 1985. Symposium on medical disorders during pregnancy. *Clinics in Perinatology* 12(3): 479–713.

- Cotton DB, ed. 1986. Critical care in obstetrics. *Clinics in Perinatology* 13(4): 695–868.

- Jacobs MM, and Phibbs RH. 1989. Prevention, recognition and treatment of perinatal asphyxia. *Clinics in Perinatology* 16(3): 785.

- Harman CR. 1989. Fetal monitoring in the alloimmunized pregnancy. *Clinics in Perinatology* 16(3): 691–733.

- Robertson NR. 1986. *Textbook of Neonatology.* New York: Churchill Livingstone.

- Vulliamy DG, and Johnston PG. 1987. *The Newborn Child.* New York: Churchill Livingstone.

NOTES

NOTES

3 Gestational Age Assessment

Carol Wiltgen Trotter, RNC, MPH, NNP

Gestational age assessment is the process of estimating the postconceptional age of a neonate. An accurate determination of gestational age is important to the clinician for two reasons. First, knowledge of the neonate's age and the growth patterns appropriate to that age aid in identification of neonatal risks and in development of management plans. Second, an accurate determination of gestational age is essential when conducting neonatal research and applying the findings to clinical practice.[1]

There are three general methods of determining gestational age in the newborn: (1) calculation of dates based on the mother's last menstrual period, (2) evaluation of obstetrical parameters, and (3) physical examination of the neonate. Although evaluations based on menstrual dates and obstetrical methods are discussed briefly, this chapter focuses on determining gestational age through physical assessment.

The average pregnancy is usually described as lasting 280 days, or 40 weeks from the onset of the last menstrual period.[2] The accuracy with which the expected date of confinement (EDC) or delivery (EDD) can be determined based on the last menstrual period depends on the woman having regular menstrual cycles. If the

mother's menstrual cycles are irregular, in pregnancies occurring after cessation of oral contraceptive use, and in patients with medically induced ovulation, adjustments need to be made in dating the pregnancy.[3]

Reliance on obstetrical methods for assessing gestational age has become routine practice. These methods are summarized in Table 3-1, along with an indication of their accuracy and reliability.[3]

The physical assessment techniques used in the examination of the neonate for gestational age are inspection and palpation. When rapid assessment of gestational age is necessary, such as in the delivery room, a quick inspection of a few parameters will suffice. A detailed gestational age assessment, however, includes palpation and use of the ophthalmoscope.

HISTORICAL PERSPECTIVE

The gestational age assessment scoring system that provides the basis for many of the tools currently used was published in 1970 by Dubowitz, Dubowitz, and Goldberg.[4] The system is based on assessment of 10 neurologic and 11 external criteria (Tables 3-2 and 3-3). The external criteria were taken from charac-

TABLE 3-1 ▲ Prenatal Obstetrical Methods for Evaluating Gestational Age

Indicator	Appropriate Time During Gestation	Accuracy/Reliability
Last normal menstrual period	Entire pregnancy	± 14.6 days
Conception/ovulation date	Entire pregnancy	± 1 day
Pregnancy test		
Serum	Before 4 weeks	± 2–3 weeks
Urine	Before 6–7 weeks	± 2–3 weeks
Pelvic examination	Before 16 weeks	± 2.3 weeks
Detection of fetal heart tones by doppler stethoscope	Between 9 & 12 weeks	± 3 weeks
Ultrasound*		
Crown-rump length	Before 14 weeks	± 7–10 days
Biparietal diameter	Between 12 & 42 weeks	± 1–3 weeks
Femur length	Between 12 & 42 weeks	± 1–3.5 weeks
Uterus at umbilicus	20 weeks	± 15 days
Fundal height	Between 18 & 35 weeks	± 13–19 days
Fetal movement		
Primigravida	18–19 weeks	± 18 days
Multigravida	16–17 weeks	± 18 days
Detection of fetal heart tones by fetoscope	18–20 weeks	± 17 days

*Ultrasound becomes increasingly less accurate after 20 weeks of gestation and is most informative early in pregnancy.

Modified from: Attico NB, et al. 1990. Gestational age assessment. *American Family Physician* 41(2): 554. Reprinted by permission.

teristics defined by Farr and associates.[5] According to Dubowitz, Dubowitz, and Goldberg and Koenigsberger (as well as secondary sources), the development of neurologic criteria to assess gestational age originated in the work of the French schools in the 1950s under Andre Thomas and later Madame Sainte-Anne Dargassies.[4,6] During the 1960s, a number of other investigators helped better define the neurologic criteria. Dubowitz, Dubowitz, and Goldberg selected criteria from the data published by Koenigsberger, Amiel-Tison, and Robinson to develop the neurologic portion of their scoring system.[4,6–8]

Since publication of the system devised by Dubowitz, Dubowitz, and Goldberg, many variations of the tool have been used.[9,10] In 1978, Capurro and associates published a sim-plified method of gestational age assessment using seven of the original variables defined by Dubowitz, Dubowitz, and Goldberg. These investigators identified five physical and two neurologic criteria that most accurately determined gestational age.[11] In 1979, Ballard, Novak, and Driver published a tool using six neuromuscular criteria and six physical criteria.[12] In addition, other investigators have published reports of determination of gestational age by measuring hand and foot length as well as skin reflectance with an optical fiber spectrophotometer.[13,14]

More recently, both the Ballard and the Dubowitz tools have been criticized for overestimating the actual gestational age by two weeks.[15,16] Therefore, Ballard and colleagues expanded their tool to achieve greater accuracy and to include the extremely premature neonate.[17] This tool, according to its authors, overestimates gestational age by 0.3 to 0.6 weeks (2 to 4 days) at gestational ages less than 37 weeks. The "new" Ballard gestational age assessment tool will be used throughout this chapter.

PHYSICAL ASSESSMENT

There are two methods for determining gestational age by physical examination: (1) assessment of the anterior vascular capsule of the lens using the ophthalmoscope and (2) assessment of neuromuscular and physical criteria by inspection and palpation.

ANTERIOR VASCULAR CAPSULE OF THE LENS

The rationale and technique for examining the anterior vascular capsule of the lens to deter-

TABLE 3-2 ▲ External Criteria for Gestational Age Assessment

External Sign	0	1	2	3	4
			Score*		
Edema	Obvious edema of hands and feet; pitting over tibia	No obvious edema of hands and feet; pitting over tibia	No edema		
Skin texture	Very thin; gelatinous	Thin and smooth	Smooth; medium thickness; rash or superficial peeling	Slight thickening; superficial cracking and peeling, especially hands and feet	Thick and parchmentlike; superficial or deep cracking
Skin color	Dark red	Uniformly pink	Pale pink; variable over body	Pale; pink only over ears, lips, palms, soles	
Skin opacity (trunk)	Numerous veins and venules clearly seen, especially over abdomen	Veins and tributaries seen	A few large vessels clearly seen over abdomen	A few large vessels seen indistinctly over abdomen	No blood vessels seen
Lanugo (over back)	No lanugo	Abundant; long and thick over whole back	Hair thinning, especially over lower back	Small amount of lanugo and bald areas	At least half of back devoid of lanugo
Plantar creases	No skin creases	Faint red marks over anterior half of sole	Definite red marks over > anterior half; indentations over < anterior third	Indentation over > anterior third	Definite deep indentations over > anterior third
Nipple formation	Nipple barely visible; no areola	Nipple well defined; areola smooth and flat; diameter <0.75 cm	Areola stippled; edge not raised; diameter <0.75 cm	Areola stippled; edge raised; diameter >0.75 cm	
Breast size	No breast tissue palpable	Breast tissue on one or both sides; <0.5 cm diameter	Breast tissue both sides; one or both 0.5–1 cm	Breast tissue both sides >1 cm	
Ear form	Pinna flat and shapeless; little or no incurving of edge	Incurving of part of edge of pinna	Partial incurving whole of upper pinna	Well-defined incurving whole of upper pinna	
Ear firmness	Pinna soft, easily folded; no recoil	Pinna soft, easily folded; slow recoil	Cartilage to edge of pinna, but soft in places; ready recoil	Pinna firm, cartilage to edge; instant recoil	
Male genitals	Neither testis in scrotum	At least one testis high in scrotum	At least one testis down		
Female genitals with hips half abducted	Labia majora widely separated; labia minora protruding	Labia majora almost cover labia minora	Labia majora completely cover labia minora		

*If score differs on paired anatomic features (i.e., plantar creases, nipple formation, ear form), take the mean.

From: Dubowitz LMS, Dubowitz V, and Goldberg C. 1970. Clinical assessment of gestational age in the newborn infant. *Journal of Pediatrics* 77(1): 7. Reprinted by permission.

TABLE 3-3 ▲ Neurologic Criteria for Gestational Age Assessment

Neurologic sign	Score					
	0	**1**	**2**	**3**	**4**	**5**
Posture						
Square window	90°	60°	45°	30°	0°	
Ankle dorsiflexion	90°	75°	45°	20°	0°	
Arm Recoil	180°	90–180°	<90°			
Leg recoil	180°	90–180°	<90°			
Popliteal angle	180°	160°	130°	110°	90°	<90°
Heel to ear						
Scarf sign						
Head lag						
Ventral suspension						

From: Dubowitz LMS, Dubowitz V, and Goldberg C. 1970. Clinical assessment of gestational age in the newborn infant. *Journal of Pediatrics* 77(1): 4. Reprinted by permission.

mine gestational age was described in 1977 by Hittner, Hirsch, and Rudolph.[18] The hyaloid system and the tunica vasculosa lentis are transient embryologic vascular systems that invade the developing eye. The purpose of the vascular system is to nourish the eye during active growth. This system can be seen starting at approximately 27 weeks gestation and then atrophies progressively until it is gone after week 34. To visualize the vessels, the examiner uses a direct ophthalmoscope set between +6 and +12. These settings allow the examiner's eyes to focus on the lens rather than on the retina. To the novice practitioner, the image will initially appear blurry. As the ophthalmoscope is moved closer to the infant's eye (within 6 to 10 inches), the vascular system will come into view as the examiner focuses on the more anteriorly placed lens.

Figure 3-1 illustrates the grading system for gestational age assessment based on the pattern and presence of vessels noted. This examination must be performed within the first 24 to 48 hours of life because the vascular system atrophies rapidly after that period.[18]

NEUROMUSCULAR AND PHYSICAL CRITERIA

Ballard and colleagues have defined six neuromuscular and six physical criteria for evaluating gestational age in the newborn.[17] The criteria and the scoring tool are depicted in Figure 3-2. A discussion of each criterion follows, and photographs depicting assessment of the criteria accompany the text. Descriptions of the technique for assessment were taken from Dubowitz, Dubowitz, and Goldberg unless otherwise noted.[4]

Neuromuscular Criteria

Posture. The infant's posture is observed with the infant in a supine position. A score is assigned based on the degree of flexion of the arms, knees, and hips. The degree of hip adduc-

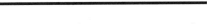

FIGURE 3-1 ▲ Gestational age assessment grading system: Anterior vascular capsule of the lens.

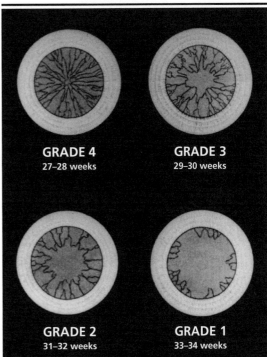

GRADE 4
27–28 weeks

GRADE 3
29–30 weeks

GRADE 2
31–32 weeks

GRADE 1
33–34 weeks

From: Hittner HM, Hirsch NJ, and Rudolph AJ. 1977. Assessment of gestational age by examination of the anterior vascular capsule of the lens. *Journal of Pediatrics* 91(3): 456. Reprinted by permission.

tion/abduction is also noted. The neonate demonstrates increasing flexion and hip adduction with advancing gestational age (Figures 3-3 through 3-5).

Square window. The infant's hand is flexed on the forearm between the thumb and index finger of the examiner. Enough pressure is applied to get as full a flexion as possible without rotating the wrist. The angle between the forearm and the palm is measured. The angle decreases with advancing gestational age (Figures 3-6 through 3-8).

Arm recoil. The neonate's arms are flexed for five seconds while he is in the supine position. The arms are then fully extended by pulling the hands and then released. The degree of arm flexion and the strength of the recoil are scored. A sluggish response with little or no

FIGURE 3-2 ▲ Gestational age assessment scoring system: Neurologic and physical criteria (New Ballard Score).

Maturational Assessment of Gestational Age (New Ballard Score)

Name_____ Date/time of birth _____ Sex_____

Hospital no._____ Date/time of exam_____ Birth weight _____

Race_____ Age when examined _____ Length _____

Apgar score: 1 minute_____5 minutes _____10 minutes _____ Head circ. _____

Neuromuscular Maturity

Examiner _____

Neuromuscular Maturity Sign	Score							Record Score Here
	−1	0	1	2	3	4	5	
Posture								
Square Window (Wrist)	>90°	90°	60°	45°	30°	0°		
Arm Recoil		180°	140°–180°	110°–140°	90°–110°	<90°		
Popliteal Angle	180°	160°	140°	120°	100°	90°	<90°	
Scarf Sign								
Heel to Ear								

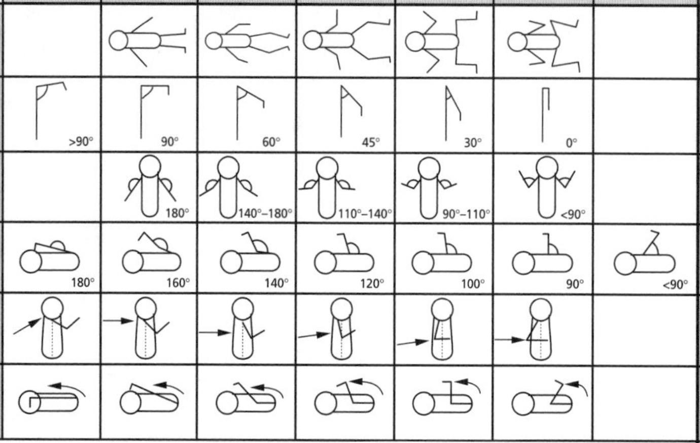

Total Neuromuscular Maturity Score

Score

Neuromuscular ____

Physical _____

Total _____

Maturity Rating

Score	Weeks
−10	20
−5	22
0	24
5	26
10	28
15	30
20	32
25	34
30	36
35	38
40	40
45	42
50	44

Gestational Age (weeks)

By dates _____

By ultrasound _____

By exam _____

Physical Maturity

Physical Maturity Sign	Score							Record Score Here
	−1	0	1	2	3	4	5	
Skin	sticky friable transparent	gelatinous red translucent	smooth pink visible veins	superficial peeling and/or rash, few veins	cracking pale areas rare veins	parchment deep cracking no vessels	leathery cracked wrinkled	
Lanugo	none	sparse	abundant	thinning	bald areas	mostly bald		
Plantar Surface	heel-toe 40–50 mm:-1 <40 mm:-2	>50 mm no crease	faint red marks	anterior transverse crease only	creases anterior 2/3	creases over entire sole		
Breast	imperceptible	barely perceptible	flat areola no bud	stippled areola 1–2 mm bud	raised areola 3–4 mm bud	full areola 5–10 mm bud		
Eye/Ear	lids fused loosely: -1 tightly: -2	lids open pinna flat stays folded	sl. curved pinna; soft; slow recoil	well-curved pinna; soft but ready recoil	formed and firm; instant recoil	thick cartilage ear stiff		
Genitals (Male)	scrotum flat, smooth	scrotum empty faint rugae	testes in upper canal rare rugae	testes descending few rugae	testes down good rugae	testes pendulous deep rugae		
Genitals (Female)	clitoris prominent & labia flat	prominent clitoris & small labia minora	prominent clitoris & enlarging minora	majora & minora equally prominent	majora large minora small	majora cover clitoris and minora		

Total Physical Maturity Score

From: Ballard JL, et al. 1991. New Ballard score, expanded to include extremely premature infants. *Journal of Pediatrics* 119(3): 418. Reprinted by permission.

FIGURE 3-3 ▲ **Posture score = 4.**

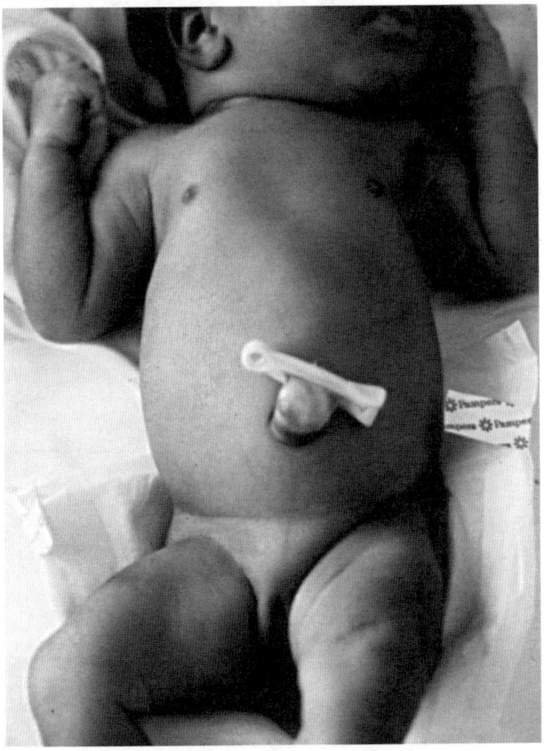

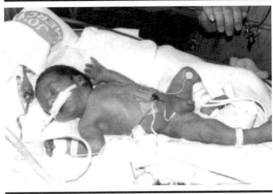

FIGURE 3-5 ▲ **Thirty-week male infant. Posture score = 2.**

Courtesy of St. John's Mercy Medical Center, St. Louis, Missouri.

flexion receives a low score. A brisk, fully flexed response receives a high score (Figures 3-9 through 3-11).

Popliteal angle. The neonate should be in a supine position with the pelvis on the mat-

FIGURE 3-4 ▲ **Preterm LGA female infant. Posture score = 3.**

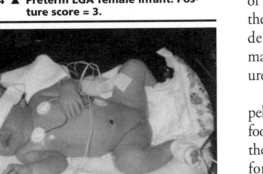

tress. With the thumb and index finger of one hand, the examiner holds the infant's knee adjacent to the chest/abdomen. At the same time, the examiner extends the leg gently with the other index finger. The popliteal angle (the angle between the lower leg and thigh, posterior to the knee) is measured. This angle decreases with advancing gestational age (Figures 3-12 through 3-14).

Scarf sign. With the neonate supine and the head in the midline position, the examiner grasps the infant's hand and pulls the arm across the chest and around the neck. The arm should be gently pulled posteriorly as far as possible around the opposite shoulder. The examiner scores this item based on the relationship of the elbow to the midline of the body when the arm is pulled across the chest. The neonate demonstrates increasing resistance to this maneuver with advancing gestational age (Figures 3-15 through 3-17).

Heel to ear. With the baby supine and the pelvis flat on the table, the examiner grasps one foot with the thumb and index finger and draws the foot as near to the head as possible without forcing it.[7] The examiner notes the distance between the foot and the head as well as the degree of knee extension. The neonate demonstrates increasing resistance to this maneuver

FIGURE 3-6 ▲ Square window in term neonate. Score = 4 (0 degrees).

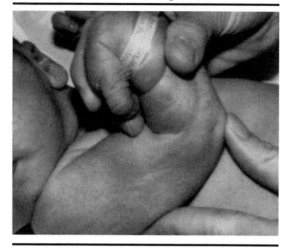

FIGURE 3-9 ▲ Eliciting arm recoil in a term infant. Arms are flexed for five seconds and then extended.

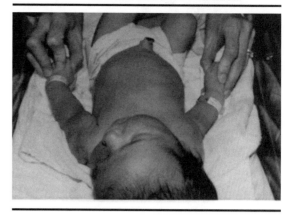

FIGURE 3-7 ▲ Square window in preterm infant. Score = 1 (60 degrees).

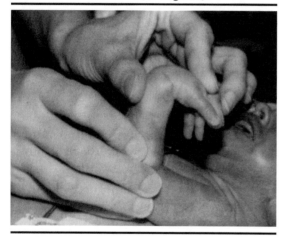

FIGURE 3-10 ▲ Arm recoil in term infant. After arms are extended (Figure 3-9), they are released, and the degree of arm flexion is scored. Score = 4 (<90 degrees).

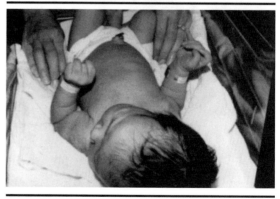

FIGURE 3-8 ▲ Square window in preterm infant. Score = 0 (90 degrees).

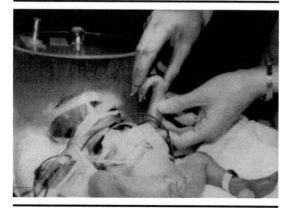

FIGURE 3-11 ▲ Arm recoil maneuver elicited Moro response in this preterm infant. Score = 2.

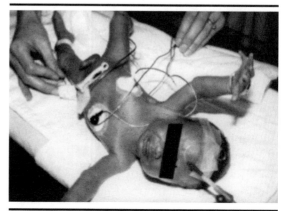

FIGURE 3-12 ▲ Popliteal angle in term infant. Score = 5 (<90 degrees).

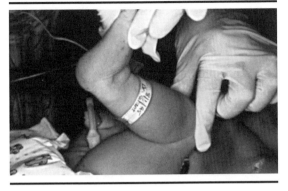

FIGURE 3-13 ▲ Popliteal angle in preterm infant. Score = 3 (100 degrees).

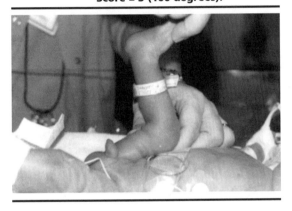

FIGURE 3-14 ▲ Popliteal angle in preterm infant. Score = 2 (120 degrees).

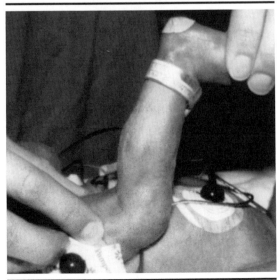

FIGURE 3-15 ▲ Scarf sign in term infant. Elbow does not reach the midline of the body. Score = 3.

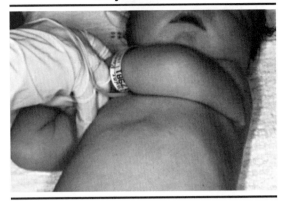

FIGURE 3-16 ▲ Scarf sign in term infant. Elbow drawn to midline of body. Score = 2.

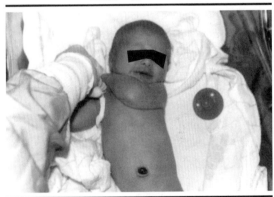

Courtesy of St. John's Mercy Medical Center, St. Louis, Missouri.

FIGURE 3-17 ▲ Scarf sign in preterm infant with elbow past midline. Score = 1.

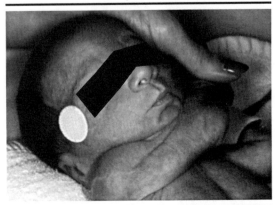

FIGURE 3-18 ▲ Heel to ear maneuver in a 37-week infant. Score = 3.

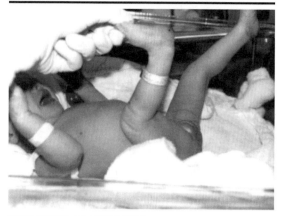

Courtesy of St. John's Mercy Medical Center, St. Louis, Missouri.

with advancing gestational age (Figures 3-18 through 3-20).

Physical Criteria

Skin. The examiner assesses skin texture, color, and opacity. As the neonate matures, more subcutaneous tissue develops. Veins become less visible, and the skin becomes more opaque (Figures 3-3, 3-4, 3-21, and 3-22).

Lanugo. Lanugo is the fine downy hair present on the body of the neonate. Lanugo development peaks at 28 to 30 weeks gestation and then declines as the infant matures.[19] It is most abundant over the back (particularly between the scapulae), although it will be noted over the

FIGURE 3-19 ▲ Heel to ear maneuver in preterm infant. Score = 3.

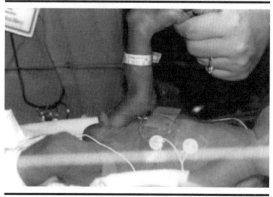

FIGURE 3-20 ▲ Heel to ear maneuver in preterm infant. Score = 2.

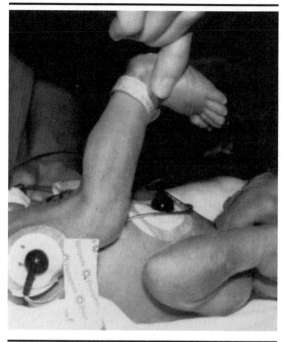

face, legs, and arms as well (Figures 3-23 and 3-24).

Plantar surface. In the extremely premature neonate, the examiner assesses the plantar surface of the foot for length and, as the neonate matures, for creases. Foot length is measured from the tip of the great toe to the back of the heel.[17] Creases should appear between 28 and 30 weeks gestation and should cover the entire plantar surface at or near term (Figures 3-25 through 3-27).

Breast. The breast is assessed for nipple size and development and for amount of breast tissue. Breast tissue increases and nipple development progresses with advancing gestational age (Figures 3-28 through 3-30).

Eye/ear. The ear is assessed on the basis of formation and amount of cartilage present in the pinna and for the recoil of the pinna when folded and released. At the earliest gestations, the eyes are evaluated based on fusion of the eyelids (Figures 3-31 and 3-32).

FIGURE 3-21 ▲ Skin of term infant. Score = 4.

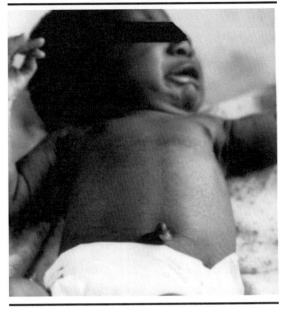

Genitalia. The male genitalia are assessed for the presence of the testes, the degree of descent of the testes into the scrotum, and the development of rugae on the scrotum. Rugae—creas-

FIGURE 3-22 ▲ Friable, transparent skin of extremely preterm infant. Score = –1.

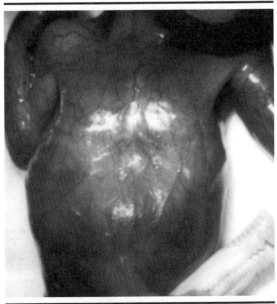

Photo courtesy of David A. Clark, MD, Louisiana State University Medical Center and Wyeth-Ayerst Laboratories, Philadelphia, Pennsylvania.

FIGURE 3-23 ▲ Lanugo over back of preterm infant. Score = 2.

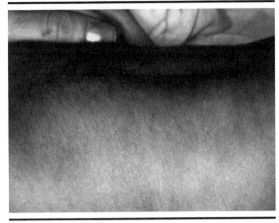

es that appear over the scrotum—become more prominent with advancing gestation (Figures 3-33 and 3-34). The female genitalia are assessed based on the prominence of the clitoris as well as the development of the labia minora and majora. With advancing gestational age, the labia majora and minora become more developed so that at term they completely cover the clitoris (Figures 3-35 and 3-36).

SCORING THE PHYSICAL EXAMINATION

After the infant has been examined and a score assigned to each criterion, a total score is

FIGURE 3-24 ▲ Lanugo noted over arm, shoulder, and chin of this preterm infant. Score = 1.

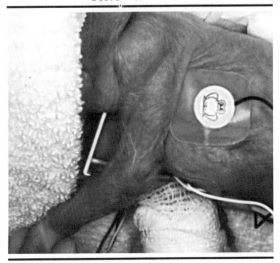

FIGURE 3-25 ▲ Sole creases covering the foot of this term neonate. Score = 4.

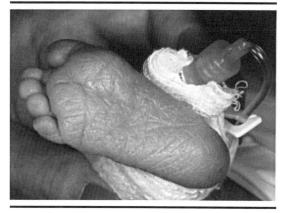

FIGURE 3-27 ▲ There are faint red marks over soles of the feet of this preterm infant. Score = 1.

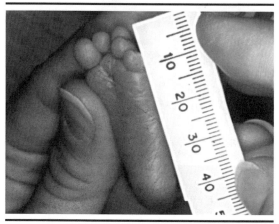

determined for the neuromuscular category and for the physical category. These two scores are added to obtain the final maturity rating score. As shown in Figure 3-2, the final maturity rating score (in the shaded area) is matched with

FIGURE 3-26 ▲ Sole creases covering the anterior two-thirds of this foot. Score = 3.

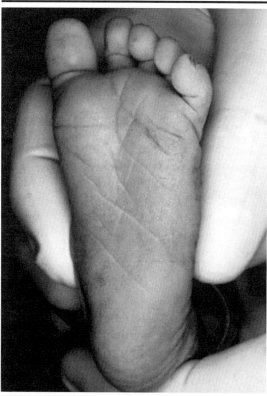

the corresponding gestational age in weeks (in the unshaded column to the right). If the maturity rating score is 15, for example, the infant is assigned a gestational age of 30 weeks. The new Ballard score authors do not give guidelines for what gestational age to assign when the maturity score falls between the numbers listed. At our institution, a gestational age that most closely approximates the maturity rating is chosen. For example, if the maturity rating score is 23, a gestational age of 33 weeks is assigned.

FIGURE 3-28 ▲ Evaluation of breast tissue in postterm infant. Score = 4.

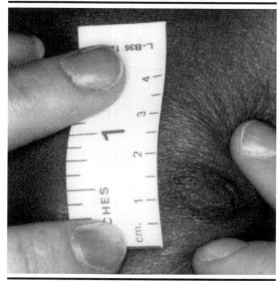

FIGURE 3-29 ▲ **Breast tissue in a term neonate. The breast bud is 3–4 mm, and the areola is raised. Score = 3.**

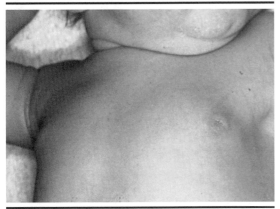

FIGURE 3-31 ▲ **Fully formed ear of term infant. Score = 4.**

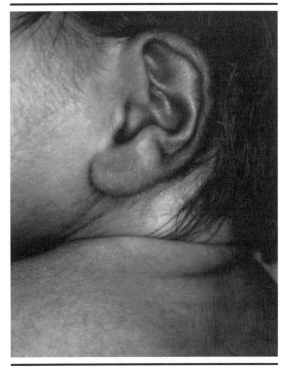

From: Mead Johnson. 1978. *Variations and Minor Departures in Infants.* Evansville, Indiana: Mead Johnson and Company, 32. Reprinted by permission.

Infants born before 37 completed weeks of gestation (less than 38 weeks) are considered preterm. Infants born between the beginning of week 38 and the completion of week 41 of gestation are considered term. Infants born after 42 weeks gestation are considered postterm.[20] These categories are depicted in Figure 3-37.

TIMING OF THE PHYSICAL EXAMINATION

There are no consistent, specific guidelines for optimal timing of the gestational age examination. Ballard and associates state that in

FIGURE 3-30 ▲ **Breast tissue in a preterm neonate. There is no breast bud, and the areola is flat. Score = 1.**

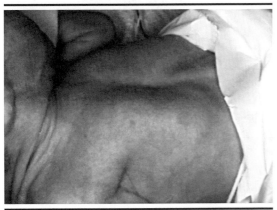

FIGURE 3-32 ▲ **Ear of preterm infant with a partially curved pinna. Score = 1.**

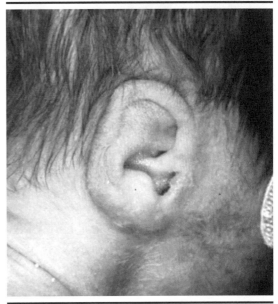

FIGURE 3-33 ▲ **Male genitalia in postterm infant. Score = 4.**

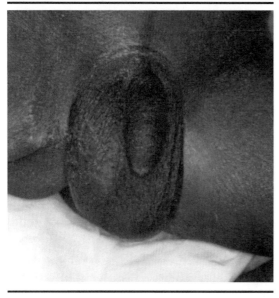

FIGURE 3-34 ▲ **Male genitalia in preterm neonate. Score = 1.**

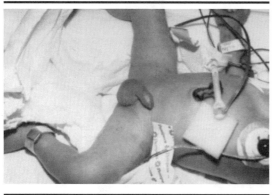

FIGURE 3-35 ▲ **Female genitalia in term infant. Score = 3.**

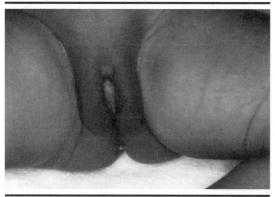

FIGURE 3-36 ▲ **Female genitalia in preterm infant. Score = 0.**

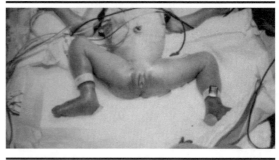

extremely premature neonates, prompt examination at a postnatal age of less than 12 hours is essential to ensure validity of the examination.[17] Ballard, Novak, and Driver previously recommended examining all infants between 30 and 42 hours of age.[12] This is to allow for stabilization and adjustment to extrauterine life. Koenigsberger states that the neurologic examination is of little value during the first 48 hours of life because tone and reflexes change rapidly with extrauterine adjustment.[6] Amiel-Tison suggests repeating the examination performed on the first day of age at two-to-three days of age because tone changes in the days following birth. Amiel-Tison also states that the optimal time for neuromuscular evaluation is one hour before feeding (when the infant is neither too sleepy nor too agitated) because both sleepiness and agitation affect tone.[7] When conducting their study, Dubowitz, Dubowitz, and Goldberg performed all assessments within five days of delivery. They found that when they performed multiple assessments on 70 neonates, the assessments were as reliable during the first 24 hours as during the subsequent four days of life.[4]

Much of the concern regarding gestational age assessment and timing of the exam relates to neuromuscular adjustment following birth. This is further complicated by conditions altering neuromuscular function, such as asphyxia or medications administered during the pre- and postnatal periods. In general, it is advisable

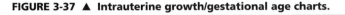

FIGURE 3-37 ▲ Intrauterine growth/gestational age charts.

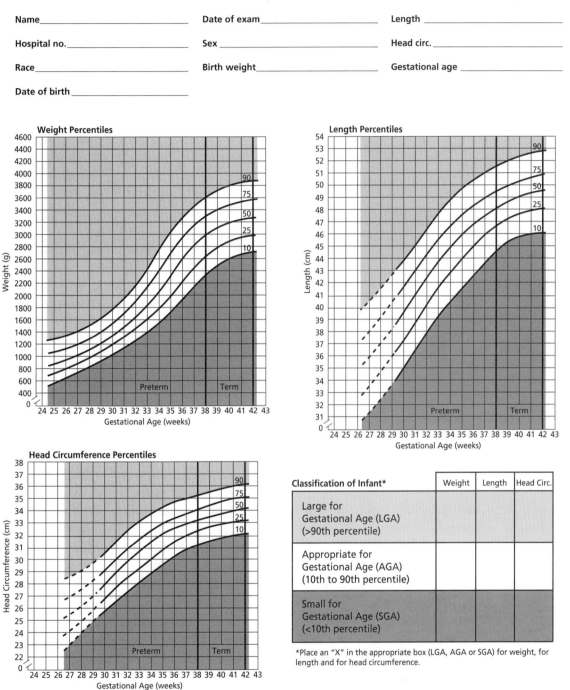

Classification of Newborns (both sexes) by Intrauterine Growth and Gestational Age

Name_____   Date of exam_____   Length _____

Hospital no._____   Sex _____   Head circ._____

Race_____   Birth weight_____   Gestational age _____

Date of birth _____

Classification of Infant*	Weight	Length	Head Circ.
Large for Gestational Age (LGA) (>90th percentile)			
Appropriate for Gestational Age (AGA) (10th to 90th percentile)			
Small for Gestational Age (SGA) (<10th percentile)			

*Place an "X" in the appropriate box (LGA, AGA or SGA) for weight, for length and for head circumference.

From: Ross Laboratories publication: 10–91; (0.05) A-58560, constructed from Battaglia FC, and Lubchenco LO. 1967. A practical classification of newborn infants by weight and gestational age. *Journal of Pediatrics* 71:159–163, and Lubchenco LO, Hansman C, and Boyd E. 1966. Intrauterine growth in length and head circumference as estimated from live births at gestational ages from 26 to 42 weeks. *Pediatrics* 37: 403–408. Reprinted by permission of Ross Laboratories, American Academy of Pediatrics, and Mosby-Year Book.

FIGURE 3-38 ▲ **Neonatal risk factors by birth weight and gestational age.**

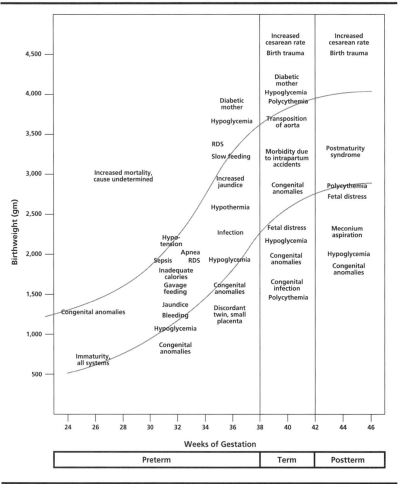

From: Lubchenco LO. 1976. *The High Risk Infant*. Philadelphia: WB Saunders. Reprinted by permission.

found that external characteristics scored collectively gave a better age index than the neurologic criteria. However, the total score using both parameters was the most accurate.

EVALUATION OF GROWTH INDICES

When the gestational age of the neonate has been determined, the examiner plots the gestational age by the neonate's weight, length, and occipital-frontal head circumference (OFC) on growth charts like those in Figure 3-37. For example, when using the weight chart, a neonate is defined as being appropriate for gestational age (AGA) if his weight falls between the tenth and ninetieth percentiles (the unshaded area of the weight graph in Figure 3-37). A small for gestational age (SGA) neonate is one whose weight falls below the tenth percentile for gestational age (heavily shaded area). A large for gestational age (LGA) neonate is one whose weight falls above the ninetieth percentile for his gestational age (lightly shaded area).[21] On the basis of the relationship between weight and gestational age, each neonate will fall into one of nine categories: preterm SGA, AGA, or LGA; term SGA, AGA, or LGA; or postterm SGA, AGA, or LGA. These classifications are important because neonatal risk factors are identified based on intrauterine growth patterns and the gestational age of the neonate.

that the initial examination be performed within the first 48 hours of life to ensure accuracy. Follow-up examinations may be necessary if the findings from the first examination disagree with gestational age assessments based on menstrual dates or obstetrical methods. If the neuromuscular condition of the neonate is unreliable at birth, the examiner may assess the physical criteria, multiply the score by a factor of two, and then assign a gestational age based on this total score. Although the validity of this approach has not been addressed, it is based on the fact that Dubowitz, Dubowitz, and Goldberg, when analyzing their data,

A low birth weight infant is defined as one with a birth weight of less than 2,500 gm. A very low birth weight infant is one weighing less than 1,500 gm.[22] An intrauterine growth retarded neonate (IUGR) is one who has not grown at the expected *in utero* rate for weight, length, or OFC. The term IUGR is often used synonymously with SGA. Practically speaking, IUGR infants are often SGA, but this is not always the case. Some neonates may be growth retarded yet not fall below the tenth percentile.[21]

Using the Ballard tool, a scorer may label an infant as AGA, LGA, or SGA for one, two, or all three of the growth parameters (Figure 3-37). An infant who is less than the tenth percentile—one who has not grown at the expected rate—for all three parameters (height, weight, and OFC) is referred to as *symmetrically growth retarded*. Factors that may produce this diminished overall growth rate typically exert their effects early in gestation. Examples include congenital viral infections, single-gene defects, and chromosomal disorders. These conditions have a significant impact on cell replication and overall growth potential.[23] An infant who falls below the tenth percentile or who has not grown at the expected rate for one parameter only is referred to as *asymmetrically growth retarded*. Asymmetrically growth retarded infants are typically those with normal OFC and length measurements but who have a relatively low weight. These infants appear thin and wasted, with a head that is disproportionately large when compared with body size. This pattern of growth retardation is associated with impaired uteroplacental function or nutritional deficiencies occurring during the third trimester. Conditions predisposing the neonate to asymmetrical growth retardation include maternal preeclampsia, poor caloric intake during pregnancy, and chronic fetal distress.[23]

LGA infants are frequently born to diabetic mothers with poor glucose control. Maternal hyperglycemia results in fetal hyperglycemia and hyperinsulinemia. The high insulin levels result in hypoglycemia postnatally and act as a fetal growth hormone causing macrosomia.[24] Risks associated with preterm, term, and postterm SGA, AGA, and LGA infants are summarized in Figure 3-38. A detailed discussion of each is beyond the scope of this chapter.

SUMMARY

Assessment of the neonate's gestational age is an essential component of the neonatal physical examination. Knowledge of gestational age and appropriate growth patterns assists the practitioner in identifying potential risks to the neonate. With experience and a cooperative neonate, the examiner should be able to perform the gestational age examination in five minutes. Infants born with altered neuromuscular states may require reassessment at a later date.

REFERENCES

1. DiPietro JA, and Allen MC. 1991. Estimation of gestational age: Implications for developmental research. *Child Development* 62(5): 1184–1199.

2. Taylor CM, and Pernoll M. 1991. Normal pregnancy and prenatal care. In *Current Obstetric and Gynecologic Diagnoses and Treatment*, Pernoll ML, ed. Norwalk, Connecticut: Appleton & Lange, 186.

3. Attico NB, et al. 1990. Gestational age assessment. *American Family Physician* 41(2): 553–560.

4. Dubowitz LMS, Dubowitz V, and Goldberg C. 1970. Clinical assessment of gestational age in the newborn infant. *Journal of Pediatrics* 77(1): 1–10.

5. Farr V, et al. 1966. The definition of some external characteristics used in the assessment of gestational age in the newborn infant. *Developmental Medicine and Child Neurology* 8(5): 507–511.

6. Koenigsberger MR. 1966. Judgment of fetal age. Part I: Neurologic evaluation. *Pediatric Clinics of North America* 13(3): 823–832.

7. Amiel-Tison C. 1968. Neurological evaluation of the maturity of newborn infants. *Archives of Disease in Childhood* 43(227): 89–93.

8. Robinson RJ. 1966. Assessment of gestational age by neurological examination. *Archives of Disease in Childhood* 41: 437–447.

9. Bhagwat VA, Dahat HB, and Bapat NG. 1990. Determination of gestational age of newborns: A comparative study. *Indian Pediatrics* 27(3): 272–275.

10. Eregie CO. 1991. Assessment of gestational age: Modification of a simplified method. *Developmental Medicine and Child Neurology* 33(7): 596–600.

11. Capurro H, et al. 1978. A simplified method for diagnosis of gestational age in the newborn infant. *Journal of Pediatrics* 93(1): 120–122.

12. Ballard JL, Novak KK, and Driver M. 1979. A simplified score for assessment of fetal maturation of newly born infants. *Journal of Pediatrics* 95(5): 769–774.

13. Kumar GP, and Kumar UK. 1993. Estimation of gestational age from hand and foot length. *Medicine, Science and the Law* 34(1): 48–50.

14. Lynn C, et al. 1993. Gestational age correlates with skin reflectance in newborn infants of 24–42 weeks gestation. *Biology of the Neonate* 64(2-3): 69–75.

15. Sanders M, et al. 1991. Gestational age assessment in preterm neonates weighing less than 1,500 grams. *Pediatrics* 88(3): 542–546.

16. Alexander GR, et al. 1992. Validity of postnatal assessments of gestational age: A comparison of the method of Ballard JL, et al. and early ultrasonography. *American Journal of Obstetrics and Gynecology* 166(3): 891–895.

17. Ballard JL, et al. 1991. New Ballard score, expanded to include extremely premature infants. *Journal of Pediatrics* 119(3): 417–423.

18. Hittner HM, Hirsch NJ, and Rudolph AJ. 1977. Assessment of gestational age by examination of the anterior vascular capsule of the lens. *Journal of Pediatrics* 91(3): 455–458.

19. Robertson A. 1979. Commentary: Gestational age. *Journal of Pediatrics* 95(5): 732–734.

20. Blackburn S. 1990. The first six hours after birth. Module 4D in *Assessment of Risk in the Newborn: Neonatal Growth and Maturity,* series 1, 2nd ed. White Plains, New York: March of Dimes.

21. Sparks JW, and Cetin I. 1992. Intrauterine growth and nutrition. In *Fetal and Neonatal Physiology,* vol. 1, Polin RA, and Fox WW, eds. Philadelphia: WB Saunders, 179.

22. Behrman RE, and Shiono PH. 1992. Neonatal risk factors. In *Neonatal-Perinatal Medicine: Diseases of the Fetus and Infant,* 5th ed., vol. 1, Fanaroff AA, and Martin RJ, eds. St. Louis: Mosby-Year Book, 4.

23. Kliegman R. 1992. Intrauterine growth retardation: Determinants of aberrant fetal growth. In *Neonatal-Perinatal Medicine: Diseases of the Fetus and Infant,* 5th ed., vol. 1, Fanaroff AA, and Martin RJ, eds. St. Louis: Mosby-Year Book, 167–168.

24. Coustan DR. 1992. Diabetes in pregnancy. In *Neonatal-Perinatal Medicine: Diseases of the Fetus and Infant,* 5th ed., vol. 1, Fanaroff AA, and Martin RJ, eds. St. Louis: Mosby-Year Book, 199.

NOTES

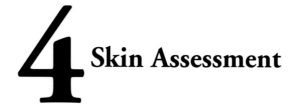

Skin Assessment

Catherine Witt, RNC, MS, NNP

Assessment of the skin is a very important element of the newborn physical exam. Valuable information regarding the neonate's health and well-being can be obtained by observing the color, integrity, and characteristics of the skin. Close examination can aid the practitioner in determining gestational age, nutritional status, functioning of organ systems, and the presence of cutaneous or systemic disease.

Newborn rashes, birthmarks, and lesions can be a source of questions and anxiety for parents. Those caring for newborns must be well versed in normal and abnormal variations, for both educational and diagnostic purposes.

A complete examination of the skin involves both inspection and palpation. Most skin variations can be noted by inspection alone, but palpation is essential to avoid missing less obvious problems. Palpation is also important for determining the thickness, turgor, and consistency of the skin.

ANATOMY AND PHYSIOLOGY

The skin serves a number of basic functions in the neonate. These include physical and immunologic protection, heat regulation, sense perception, and self-cleaning. An understand-

ing of the skin's structure is essential to careful examination and to recognition of irregularities in appearance or function.

FIGURE 4-1 ▲ Cross-section of human skin and the anatomic relationships among the various structures.

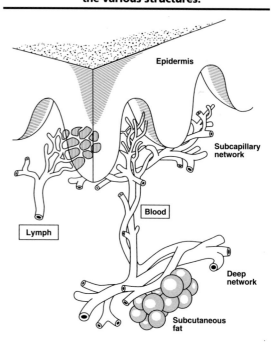

From: Nasemann T, Sauerbrey W, and Burgdorf W. 1983. *Fundamentals of Dermatology.* New York: Springer-Verlag, 11. Reprinted by permission.

The skin consists of three layers: the epidermis, the dermis, and the subcutaneous layer (Figure 4-1). The epidermis, or outermost layer, is subdivided into five layers. On top is the stratum corneum, consisting of dead cells that are constantly being brushed off and replaced. The lower layers of the epidermis contain keratin-forming cells and melanocytes.

The dermis lies directly under the epidermis. It consists of fibrous and elastic tissues, sweat glands, sebaceous glands, and hair shafts as well as blood vessels and nerves.

The third layer of the skin consists of subcutaneous fat. This fat layer serves as insulation, protection for internal organs, and calorie storage.

The skin of the newborn is similar to that of the adult in its basic structure. As with any other organ, however, the less mature the infant, the less mature the function of the skin.

The more immature the skin, the thinner and more permeable it is. Fibrils, which connect the dermis and the epidermis, are more fragile in term and preterm skin than in adult skin, and the stratum corneum is thinner.[1] Sweat glands, although present at birth, do not reach full adult functioning until the second or third year of life.

Fetal skin is covered *in utero* with vernix caseosa, a greasy white or yellow material composed of sebaceous gland secretions and exfoliated skin cells. Vernix is present during the third trimester, gradually decreasing as the infant approaches 40 weeks gestation.

In utero the fetus is covered with a fine, soft, downy type of hair called lanugo. Lanugo first appears at approximately 20 weeks gestation and covers most of the body, including the face. Most of it will disappear by 40 weeks gestation.

BEGINNING THE EXAMINATION

Several factors influence the appearance of the newborn's skin and affect the examiner's ability to note normal and abnormal variations. A consistent, systematic approach to examining the skin increases the likelihood of gathering all the information.

A family and maternal history and an account of the labor and delivery are useful to the examiner because they may highlight items that should be inspected with extra care. For example, a forceps or vacuum extraction may lead to disruption of skin integrity. A family history of neurofibromatosis would alert the examiner to search for café au lait spots.

Before beginning the exam, it is important to consider the infant's environment. The amount and type of light and the temperature of the room both affect the appearance of the skin. Adequate lighting, preferably bright natural light, is important. Ideally, the infant should be examined under a radiant heat source so that the infant can be completely undressed. This allows the examiner to observe vascular changes.

To begin the exam, undress the infant, and inspect the general color, consistency (smooth, peeling), thickness, and opacity of the skin. Note distribution of hair and any obvious markings or anomalies. Then begin a closer inspection of the infant. It is important to follow the same pattern every time to avoid missing subtle deviations. Many examiners find it easiest to begin at the head and progress downward toward the feet. While looking closely at the skin, note the size, color, and placement of any discolorations, markings, or variations. The infant should be turned over for a complete examination of the back. Inspect all skin crevices, including the axillae and the groin.

Palpation is an equally important aspect of the exam. It permits examination of the underlying dermis, thickness of the skin and subcutaneous fat, presence of edema, and any irregularities in texture or consistency. Palpation is also necessary to determine the size or configuration of certain lesions or variations that may be observed during the exam. Blanching of lesions should be assessed by pressing the pad of the thumb against the lesion for a few seconds and observing for color changes.

Hydration and nutrition can also be assessed by examination of the skin. Poor skin turgor or loose, hanging skin indicates dehydration or poor nutritional status. Excessive fluid, or edema, can be noted by pressing the pad of the thumb into the skin and looking for pitting. Edema may be especially notable in dependent areas or on the scalp if the delivery was difficult. Most newborns will have some edema around the face and eyes due to excess fluid volume after delivery.

To determine the amount of subcutaneous fat, pinch a skin fold between thumb and forefinger. Loose skin folds will be present in the term baby who has a decreased amount of fat—for example, the infant who has intrauterine growth retardation or the postterm infant who has lost some weight in the week or two before delivery.

USING CORRECT TERMINOLOGY

When reporting skin irregularities, correct terminology facilitates accurate description of observations. The following terms are commonly used to define skin irregularities.

Bulla: A vesicle greater than 1 cm in diameter

Crust: A lesion consisting of dried serous exudate, blood, or pus

Cyst: A raised, palpable lesion with a fluid or semisolid filled sac

Ecchymosis: A large area of subepidermal hemorrhage, initially bluish black in color, then changing to greenish brown or yellow, that does not blanch with pressure

Lesion: An area of altered tissue

Macule: A discolored, flat spot less than 1 cm in diameter that is not palpable

Nodule: An elevated, palpable lesion with indistinct borders, some of the lesion is palpable below the skin outside the elevated area

Papule: An elevated, palpable lesion, solid and circumscribed, less than 1 cm in diameter

Patch: A macule greater than 1 cm in diameter

Petechia: A small, purplish hemorrhagic spot on the skin, pinpoint in size

Plaque: An elevated, palpable lesion with circumscribed borders greater than 1 cm or a fusion or coalescence of several papules

Purpura: A small hemorrhagic spot larger than a petechia, 1–3 mm in size

Pustule: An elevation of the skin filled with cloudy or purulent fluid

Scale: An exfoliation of dead or dying bits of skin; can also result from excess keratin

Vesicle: An elevation of the skin filled with serous fluid and less than 1 cm in diameter (blister)

Wheal: A collection of fluid in the dermis that appears as a reddened, solid elevation of the skin

RECOGNIZING COMMON VARIATIONS IN NEWBORN SKIN

A number of changes occur in the newborn skin during the first few days and weeks after birth. Most are benign, transient lesions that do not require therapeutic intervention. It is important to be familiar with these normal changes and to be able to distinguish them from signs of serious disease.

COLOR VARIATIONS

Acrocyanosis

Acrocyanosis refers to bluish discoloration of the palms of the hands and the soles of the feet. Most infants present with acrocyanosis at birth. It may persist for up to 48 hours after delivery and is exacerbated by low environmental temperatures. It is benign in the otherwise normal infant. Circumoral (around the

FIGURE 4-2 ▲ Harlequin color change.

Sharply demarcated red color seen in the dependent half of the body. It is of no pathological significance.

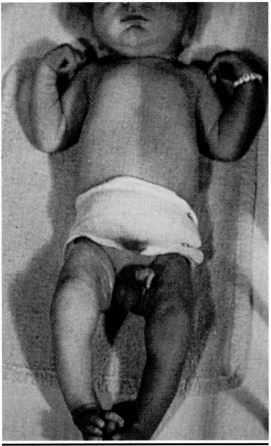

From: Solomon LM, and Esterly NB. 1973. *Neonatal Dermatology*. Philadelphia: WB Saunders. Reprinted by permission.

mouth) cyanosis may also be present during the first 12 to 24 hours after birth. Acrocyanosis that persists beyond the first few days after birth or circumoral cyanosis lasting longer than 24 hours should be investigated.

Plethora

Plethora describes the ruddy or red appearance present in some newborns. It may be indicative of a high level of red cells to blood volume. Infants who are ruddy, or plethoric, at birth should have their hemoglobin and hematocrit checked by heelstick or central venipuncture if the peripheral hematocrit is greater than

65 percent. Newborns with central hematocrits greater than 65 percent are considered polycythemic and should be watched closely for symptoms such as hypoglycemia, cyanosis, respiratory distress, and jaundice.[2]

Jaundice

Jaundice is the term used to describe a yellow coloring of the skin and the sclera. The color is caused by the deposition of bile pigment due to hyperbilirubinemia, or excess bilirubin in the blood. The presence of jaundice in a newborn should be noted, with particular attention paid to the age of the infant and the degree of jaundice present. As a general rule, jaundice first appears in the head or face, then progresses head to toe as the bilirubin level rises. Because it is difficult, if not impossible, to estimate serum bilirubin levels on the basis of clinical appearance, laboratory measurements must be made to determine the extent of hyperbilirubinemia.

Cutis Marmorata

The bluish mottling or marbling of the skin seen in response to chilling, stress, or overstimulation is called cutis marmorata. It is caused by the dilatation of capillaries and venules and usually disappears when the infant is warmed. Persistent cutis marmorata may be seen in infants with trisomy 21, trisomy 18, and Cornelia de Lange syndrome.[3]

Harlequin Color Change

Seen only in the newborn period, harlequin color change appears to be more common in the low birth weight infant.[4] When the infant is lying on one side, a sharply demarcated red color is seen in the dependent half of the body, with the superior half appearing pale (Figure 4-2). If the infant is rotated to the other side, the color reverses.

The color change may last anywhere from 1 to 30 minutes and disappears slowly if the infant is returned to the back or abdomen. This

FIGURE 4-3 ▲ Erythema toxicum.

Benign rash seen in approximately 70 percent of term newborns.

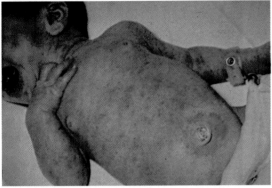

Courtesy of Barbara Quissell, MD, Presbyterian/St. Luke's Medical Center, Denver, Colorado.

FIGURE 4-4 ▲ Milia.

Yellow or pearly white papules caused by accumulation of secretions of sebaceous glands.

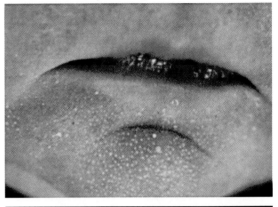

From: Mead Johnson. 1978. *Variations and Minor Departures in Infants.* Evansville, Indiana: Mead Johnson and Company, 5. Reprinted by permission.

phenomenon occurs in both healthy and sick infants and is of no pathological significance.[4-6] It has been attributed to a "temporary imbalance of [the] autonomic regulatory mechanism of the cutaneous vessels."[5]

COMMON NEWBORN SKIN LESIONS

Erythema Toxicum

This benign rash is found in up to 70 percent of term newborns.[4,6] Erythema toxicum consists of small white or yellow papules or vesicles with an erythematous base. The rash may be found on any part of the body, but it is most commonly seen on the face, trunk, or extremities (Figure 4-3). This rash often disappears and then reappears moments or hours later on a different part of the body. It may last anywhere from a few hours to several days. The peak incidence is from 24 to 48 hours of life, but it can occur up to three months of age. The cause is unknown; however, it may be exacerbated by handling or chafing of linen.

Diagnosis is generally made by visual recognition of the eruption. A definitive diagnosis may be made by the presence of numerous eosinophils in a smear of an aspirated papule.

Milia

Milia are multiple yellow or pearly white papules about 1 mm in size (Figure 4-4). They are usually found on the brow, cheeks, and nose of up to 40 percent of newborns.[4] When found in the mouth, they are called Epstein's pearls. Milia are epidermal cysts caused by accumulation of sebaceous gland secretions. They resolve spontaneously during the first few weeks of life.

Sebaceous Gland Hyperplasia

Sebaceous gland hyperplasia is characterized by numerous tiny (less than 0.5 mm) white or yellow papules found on the nose, cheeks, and upper lips. These enlarged sebaceous glands are caused by maternal androgenic stimulation. They will spontaneously decrease in size after birth and require no treatment.

Miliaria

Miliaria is caused by obstruction of the sweat ducts as a result of an excessively warm, humid environment. It is seen primarily over the forehead, on the scalp, in creases, or in the groin area. Depending on its severity, miliaria is classified as one of four types. *Miliaria crystallina* consists of clear, thin vesicles, 1–2 mm in diameter, that develop in the epidermal portion of

FIGURE 4-5 ▲ Hyperpigmented macule.

Skin lesion caused by infiltration of melanocytes in the dermis.

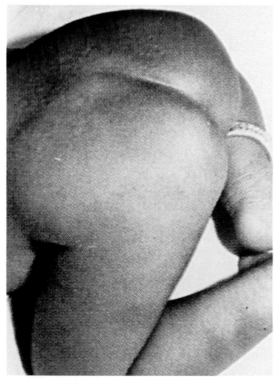

Courtesy of Barbara Quissell, MD, Presbyterian/St. Luke's Medical Center, Denver, Colorado.

FIGURE 4-6 ▲ Multiple papules present in neonatal pustular melanosis.

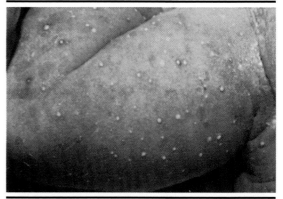

From: Weston W, and Lane A. 1991. *Color Textbook of Pediatric Dermatology*. St. Louis: Mosby-Year Book. 226. Reprinted by permission.

Sebaceous Nevus

The sebaceous nevus is a small yellow or yellowish orange papule or plaque. It is most often found on the scalp or face, but it may be seen on other parts of the body. It consists of immature hair follicles and sebaceous glands. It is devoid of hair when found on the scalp because of the rudimentary hair follicles found in the lesion. The sebaceous nevus may remain unchanged until puberty, when it enlarges and becomes raised. Occasionally, it transforms into a basal cell epithelioma; therefore, surgical removal is recommended.[4,5]

COMMON PIGMENTED LESIONS

Hyperpigmented Macule (Mongolian Spot)

The most common pigmented lesion in the newborn, the hyperpigmented macule is seen in up to 90 percent of African American, Asian, and Hispanic infants and up to 10 percent of Caucasian infants.[4] These large macules or patches are seen most commonly over the buttocks, flanks, or shoulders (Figure 4-5). They are gray or blue-green in color. Because hyperpigmented macules may be mistaken for bruising due to their color and location, it is important to document the size and location

the sweat glands. Prolonged obstruction of the ducts of the sweat glands, leading to release of sweat into adjacent tissue, is termed *miliaria rubra* and is accompanied by a prickly sensation (prickly heat). *Miliaria rubra* appears as small erythematous papules.

Continued occlusion causes progression to *miliaria pustulosa,* caused by leukocyte infiltration of the papule. If the condition is not resolved, it can lead to a secondary infection of the deeper dermal portions of the sweat glands. This condition, termed *miliaria profunda,* is extremely rare.

Treatment of miliaria consists of eliminating precipitating factors, such as excessive heat and humidity. Keeping the infant clean and dry causes the lesions to resolve within a few hours.

FIGURE 4-7 ▲ Pigmented nevus.

This brown or black macule is most commonly seen on the lower back or buttocks, but it may occur anywhere on the body.

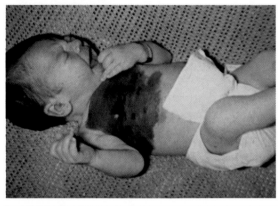

Courtesy of Peter Honeyfield, MD, Presbyterian/St. Luke's Medical Center, Denver, Colorado.

FIGURE 4-8 ▲ Café au lait spots.

Light tan or brown macules. If large or more than six in number, they may indicate cutaneous neurofibromatosis.

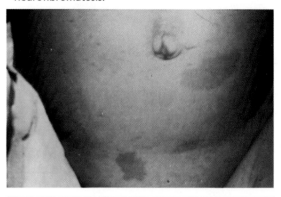

Courtesy of Eva Sujansky, MD, associate professor of pediatrics, University of Colorado Health Sciences Center.

of the lesion to avoid later suspicion of non-accidental trauma.

Hyperpigmented macules are caused by melanocytes that infiltrate the dermis. The macules tend to fade gradually over the first three years of life, but some may persist into adulthood.

Transient Neonatal Pustular Melanosis

Transient neonatal pustular melanosis begins with superficial, vesiculopustular lesions (Figure 4-6), often causing some alarm when present at birth. These vesicles rupture within 12 to 48 hours after birth, leaving small pigmented macules. The macules are often surrounded by very fine white scales. These small hyperpigmented macules may remain for up to three months after birth.

Transient neonatal pustular melanosis is benign, requiring no treatment. Aspiration of the vesicles reveals numerous neutrophils and almost no eosinophils. This skin lesion is found in up to 5 percent of African American infants and about 0.2 percent of Caucasian infants.[7,8]

Pigmented Nevus

A dark brown or black macule, the pigmented nevus is most commonly seen on the lower back or buttocks, but it may occur anywhere on the body (Figure 4-7). These lesions are generally benign, but malignant changes may occur in up to 10 percent. They should therefore be observed closely for changes in size or shape. Surgical excision may be required.[4,9]

Café au Lait Patches

Café au lait patches are tan or light brown macules or patches with well-defined borders (Figure 4-8). When less than 3 cm in length and less than six in number, they are of no pathologic significance. Up to 19 percent of normal children have one café au lait spot. Larger spots or more than six may indicate cutaneous neurofibromatosis.[4,10–12]

Neurofibromatosis (von Recklinghausen disease) is a condition in which tumors of various sizes form on peripheral nerves. Cranial nerves may also be affected. It is an autosomal-dominant disorder, with a positive family history present in 50 percent of all cases. Ninety percent of patients with neurofibromatosis have café au lait patches.[10,11] Neurofibromas, small skin-colored nodules, may be present at birth or may not appear until adolescence in children with neurofibromatosis.

FIGURE 4-9 ▲ Forcep marks.

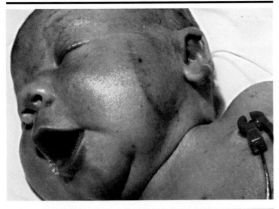

Courtesy of Peter Honeyfield, MD, Presbyterian/St. Luke's Medical Center, Denver, Colorado.

FIGURE 4-10 ▲ Subcutaneous fat necrosis.

Subcutaneous nodule caused by trauma, asphyxia, or cold.

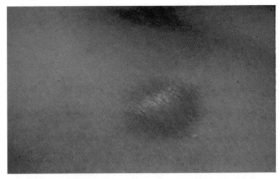

Courtesy of Barbara Quissell, MD, Presbyterian/St. Luke's Medical Center, Denver, Colorado.

Tuberous Sclerosis

Tuberous sclerosis is a hereditary disease characterized by seizures, developmental delays and behavioral problems. It presents with hypopigmented, white macules that may be thumb or leaf shaped. They are sometimes referred to as ash leaf macules. They may number up to 100 and are found anywhere on the newborn's skin, most often on the trunk and buttocks. Infants who present with unexplained seizures should be examined closely for these lesions because most patients with tuberous sclerosis will have these macules at birth or soon afterward. Because of their light color, they may not be readily apparent in fair-skinned infants. A Wood (ultraviolet) light may be helpful in illuminating white or hypopigmented lesions.

SKIN LESIONS SECONDARY TO TRAUMA

Forcep Marks

Forcep marks may be seen on the cheeks, scalp, and face of infants born following the use of forceps (Figure 4-9). The marks are generally red or bruised areas where the forceps were applied. The skin may also be abraded. The infant should be examined for other complications of birth trauma, such as facial palsy, fractured clavicles, or skull fractures.

Subcutaneous Fat Necrosis

Subcutaneous fat necrosis is a subcutaneous nodule that is hard, nonpitting, and sharply circumscribed (Figure 4-10). It may have a red or purplish color. It is thought to be caused by trauma, cold, or asphyxia. The nodule appears during the first weeks of life, grows larger over several days, and then resolves on its own over several weeks. There may be more than one lesion present. Occasionally, hypercalcemia may occur in infants with more than one nodule. Serum calcium levels should be monitored and intervention may be necessary.[13]

Subcutaneous fat necrosis usually requires no treatment, with the exception of correcting any underlying cause, such as hypoglycemia or asphyxia.

Sucking Blisters

Vesicles or bullae may appear on the lips, fingers, or hands of newborns as a result of vigorous sucking, either *in utero* or after birth. These sucking blisters (Figure 4-11) may be intact or ruptured and require no treatment.

Scalp Lesions

Scalp abrasions or lacerations due to trauma during delivery or the insertion of a scalp electrode may be noted. Application of a suction cup for vacuum extraction or scalp pH

FIGURE 4-11 ▲ Sucking blister.

Small vesicle resulting from vigorous sucking, either *in utero* or after birth.

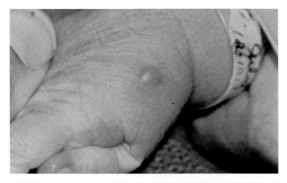

Courtesy of Peter Honeyfield, MD, Presbyterian/St. Luke's Medical Center, Denver, Colorado.

FIGURE 4-12 ▲ Nevus simplex.

Most common of vascular birthmarks, seen in up to 50 percent of newborns.

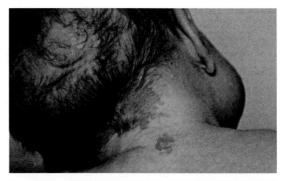

Courtesy of Barbara Quissell, MD, Presbyterian/St. Luke's Medical Center, Denver, Colorado.

sampling may also result in abrasions. Treatment generally consists of keeping the area clean and dry and observing for secondary infections. Facial bruising may also be significant following delivery.

VASCULAR SKIN LESIONS

Nevus Simplex

The nevus simplex, or stork bite, is the most common of the vascular birthmarks. It is seen in up to 50 percent of newborns.[6] The nevus simplex is an irregularly bordered pink macule composed of dilated, distended capillaries (Figure 4-12). The lesion is most often found on the nape of the neck, the upper eyelids, the bridge of the nose, or the upper lip. Nevi simplex blanch with pressure and frequently become more prominent with crying. They generally fade by the second year after birth, although those on the nape of the neck may persist.

Port Wine Nevus (Nevus Flammeus)

The port wine nevus is a flat pink or reddish purple lesion consisting of dilated, congested capillaries directly beneath the epidermis. (In African American infants, it is a jet black color.) It has sharply delineated edges and does not blanch with pressure (Figure 4-13). The port

wine nevus does not grow in size or spontaneously resolve. It may be small or may cover almost half of the body. It is usually unilateral but may occasionally cross the midline. Unfortunately, the lesion most often occurs on the face, but it may appear on other parts of the body.

Initially, the best treatment is to cover the lesion with a water-repellent cosmetic cream. Laser therapy has been somewhat successful in eliminating or reducing port wine nevi. The pulsed-dye laser is reported to work well in small children, producing less scarring than the argon laser.[14–16]

Most port wine nevi are isolated, but those that follow a pattern similar to the branches of

FIGURE 4-13 ▲ Port wine nevus.

Permanent lesion caused by dilated, congested capillaries directly beneath the dermis.

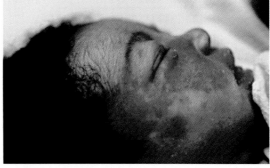

Courtesy of David A. Clark, MD, Louisiana State University.

FIGURE 4-14 ▲ Strawberry hemangioma.

Red, lobulated tumor caused by dilated capillaries and endothelial proliferation.

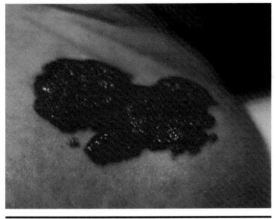

Courtesy of David A. Clark, MD, Louisiana State University.

FIGURE 4-15 ▲ Cavernous hemangioma.

Similar to strawberry hemangioma with larger vessels involving the dermis and subcutaneous tissues.

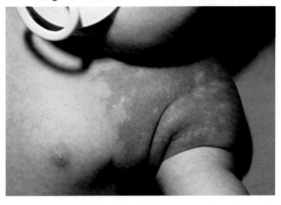

Courtesy of Barbara Quissell, MD, Presbyterian/St. Luke's Medical Center, Denver, Colorado.

the trigeminal nerve (the forehead and upper eyelid) may be associated with Sturge-Weber syndrome. This disorder causes a proliferation of endothelial cells, particularly in the small blood vessels. Intracerebral calcifications and atrophic changes may be present.

Children with Sturge-Weber syndrome may present with seizures, mental retardation, hemiparesis, and glaucoma. The cause of this syndrome is unknown. It does not appear to be hereditary.

Strawberry Hemangioma

A strawberry hemangioma is a bright red, raised, lobulated tumor that occurs on the head, neck, trunk, or extremities. It is soft and compressible, with sharply demarcated margins (Figure 4-14). The tumor may also occur in the throat, causing airway obstruction. Strawberry hemangiomas occur in up to 10 percent of newborns.[16,17]

The lesion is caused by dilated capillaries, with associated endothelial proliferation in the dermal and subdermal layers. Twenty to 30 percent are present at birth; the remainder are usually apparent by six months of age.[16,17] It is not

uncommon for an infant to have more than one of these lesions.

The strawberry hemangioma gradually increases in size for approximately six months and then gradually begins to regress spontaneously. Complete regression may take several years.

Complications of strawberry hemangiomas include bleeding, ulceration, infection, or compression of vital organs or orifices. Treatment consists of allowing natural spontaneous regression. If the lesion is interfering with vital functions (such as the airway or vision), systemic corticosteroids may be helpful.[16,17]

Cavernous Hemangioma

The cavernous hemangioma is similar to the strawberry hemangioma but consists of larger, more mature vascular elements lined with endothelial cells and involving the dermis and subcutaneous tissues. The overlying skin is bluish red in color. On palpation, the cavernous hemangioma is soft and compressible, with poorly defined borders (Figure 4-15).

The cavernous hemangioma usually increases in size during the first 6 to 12 months, then involutes spontaneously. Treatment is unnecessary unless the lesion is interfering with vital

FIGURE 4-16 ▲ Klippel-Trenaunay-Weber syndrome.

Vascular nevus with hypertrophy of the bone and soft structures of the extremity.

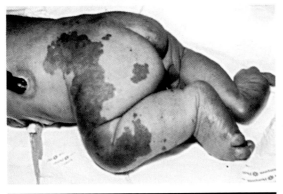

Courtesy of Peter Honeyfield, MD, Presbyterian/St. Luke's Medical Center, Denver, Colorado.

FIGURE 4-17 ▲ Blisters on trunk seen with neonatal herpes.

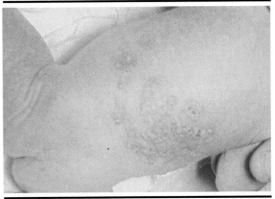

From: Weston W, and Lane A. 1991. *Color Textbook of Pediatric Dermatology.* St. Louis: Mosby-Year Book. 84. Reprinted by permission.

functions. In those cases, treatment with systemic corticosteroids has been shown to cause some shrinkage.[4,17]

Two syndromes may be associated with cavernous hemangiomas. The first, Kasabach-Merritt syndrome, is a cavernous hemangioma associated with sequestration of platelets and thrombocytopenia. Treatment consists of platelet transfusions as necessary and administration of corticosteroids.[16,17]

The second, Klippel-Trenaunay-Weber syndrome, consists of a vascular nevus with hypertrophy of the bone and soft structures of an extremity (Figure 4-16). The hypertrophy is probably due to excess blood flow and malformed vessels in the extremity.[16] This is a rare congenital anomaly, seen more frequently in males.[4,16] Prognosis depends on the severity of the limb involvement.

INFECTIOUS LESIONS

Thrush

A common infection in the newborn, thrush is an oral fungal infection caused by the organism *Candida albicans.* It appears as patches of white material scattered over the tongue and mucous membranes. The material is adher-

ent and cannot be scraped off with a tongue blade. Thrush is treated with an oral form of nystatin.[18]

Candida Diaper Dermatitis

Diaper dermatitis is common in newborns and generally needs no treatment other than frequent diaper changes and keeping the area clean and dry. However, it can occasionally be caused by, or associated with, *Candida albicans.* This rash is a moist, erythematous eruption with small white or yellow pustules. Small areas of skin erosion may also be seen. It is found primarily over the buttocks and perianal region, occasionally spreading to the thighs. Treatment consists of keeping the area clean and dry and applying a nystatin cream several times a day. If the rash is persistent or severe, an oral nystatin solution may be recommended.[18]

Herpes

Neonatal herpes is one of the most serious viral infections in the newborn, with a mortality rate of up to 60 percent.[19] The rash appears as vesicles or pustules on an erythematous base (Figure 4-17). Clusters of lesions are common. The lesions ulcerate and crust over rapidly. Fifty to 70 percent of infants with neonatal herpes eventually develop this characteristic rash, but not always before they exhibit other signs and

FIGURE 4-18 ▲ Scalded skin syndrome secondary to staphylococcal infection.

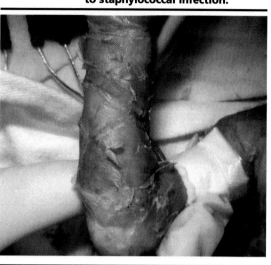

Courtesy of Dr. David A. Clark, Louisiana State University Medical Center and Wyeth-Ayerst Laboratories. Philadelphia, Pennsylvania. Reprinted by permission.

FIGURE 4-19 ▲ Aplasia cutis congenita.

Congenital anomaly resulting in absence of some or all layers of the skin.

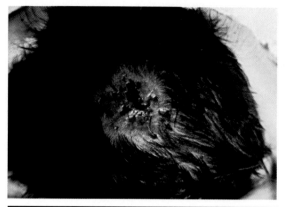

Courtesy of Peter Honeyfield, MD, Presbyterian/St. Luke's Medical Center, Denver, Colorado.

symptoms. Absence of vesicles does not rule out the presence of the disease.[6,19,20]

Treatment includes use of an antiviral agent such as acyclovir, both topically and intravenously. Other signs and symptoms, such as seizures, should be treated as they occur. Precautions for blood and body secretions must be observed.[6,19]

Staphylococcal Scalded Skin Syndrome

Staphylococcal scalded skin syndrome begins with a generalized, tender erythema, followed by bullous eruption and peeling of the epidermis, often in large sheets (Figure 4-18). The eruption is due to *Staphylococcus aureus* infection, which produces a toxin damaging to epidermal cell walls. Treatment includes systemic antistaphylococcal antibiotics and isolation to prevent spread of the infection. There may be extensive insensible water loss, so fluids and electrolytes should be closely monitored.

Other Congenital Viral Infections

Viral infections such as rubella or cytomegalovirus may present with dermatological findings. Most frequently, these consist of jaundice and petechiae or purpura (small red or purple hemorrhagic spots) seen on the head, trunk, and extremities. Often described as "blueberry muffin" spots, these lesions are caused by thrombocytopenia and dermal erythropoiesis. One associated finding is hepatosplenomegaly. Treatment depends upon the type of disease present.

MISCELLANEOUS SKIN LESIONS

Cutis Aplasia

Aplasia cutis congenita (cutis aplasia) is a congenital abnormality characterized by the absence of some or all layers of the skin (Figure 4-19). It most often appears as an ulceration or scarred area on the scalp (on the parietal bones or near the sagittal suture), but it can occur on other parts of the body.

Cutis aplasia may be an isolated defect, or it may be associated with other anomalies, such as midline defects and chromosomal disorders (trisomy 13).[3,20,21] The cause is unclear, but it may be due to vascular disruptions, midline developmental disruptions, trauma, or uterine or amnionic abnormalities (amniotic disruption sequence). Treatment consists of keeping the area clean and dry. Use of antibacterial dressings may be helpful.[21] Large defects may require surgery.

INSPECTING THE NAILS

The examination of the skin is not complete without close attention to the nails on the hands and feet. The nail consists of hard keratin. Damage to the nail matrix can be caused by trauma, inflammation, or genetic problems. This damage can appear as pits, ridges, aplasia, or hypertrophy.[6] Most defects in the neonatal period are congenital rather than traumatic in origin.

ABSENCE OR ATROPHY OF NAILS

Absence or atrophy of nails is seen in a number of congenital syndromes. More well known ones include trisomy 13, trisomy 18, and Turner syndrome.[3] Inherited ectodermal dysplasias and skeletal anomalies may also be seen with absent or dystrophic nails.[21]

HYPERTROPHY OF NAILS

Hypertrophic nails are rarely seen in the newborn period. They may occur in diseases such as congenital hemihypertrophy or familial onychogryposis.

ABNORMALLY SHAPED NAILS

Spoon- or racquet-shaped nails may occur as a result of a congenital or hereditary anomaly. They may be associated with anomalies of the hair or skin. Spoon-shaped nails may also be a temporary finding in an otherwise healthy infant.[21]

SUMMARY

Careful assessment of the skin gives the examiner insight into the overall health of the newborn as well as underlying pathology. Although numerous other anomalies may occur in newborn skin, this overview of the most common variations should aid the examiner in performing a complete and thorough newborn skin examination.

REFERENCES

1. Weston W, and Lane A. 1991. *Color Textbook of Pediatric Dermatology.* St. Louis: Mosby-Year Book, 1–8, 41–53, 74–97, 223–254.
2. Blanchette V, et al. 1994. Hematology. In *Neonatology: Pathophysiology and Management of the Newborn,* 4th ed., Avery GB, Fletcher MA, and MacDonald MG, eds. Philadelphia: JB Lippincott, 952–999.
3. Jones KL. 1988. *Smith's Recognizable Patterns of Human Malformation,* 4th ed. Philadelphia: WB Saunders, 11, 16, 20, 80.
4. Margileth A. 1994. Dermatologic conditions. In *Neonatology: Pathophysiology and Management of the Newborn,* 4th ed., Avery GB, Fletcher MA, and MacDonald MG, eds. Philadelphia: JB Lippincott, 1229–1268.
5. Solomon LM, and Esterly NB. 1973. *Neonatal Dermatology.* Philadelphia: WB Saunders, 43–48, 60–80.
6. Weston WL. 1985. *Practical Pediatric Dermatology,* 2nd ed. Boston: Little, Brown, 319–364.
7. Ramamurthy RS, et al. 1976. Transient neonatal pustular melanosis. *Journal of Pediatrics* 88(5): 831–835.
8. Mallory SB. 1991. Neonatal skin disorders. *Pediatric Clinics of North America* 38(4): 745–761.
9. Hodgeman JE, Freedman RI, and Levan NE. 1971. Neonatal dermatology. *Pediatric Clinics of North America* 18(3): 713–734.
10. Hurwitz S. 1985. *The Skin and Systemic Disease in Children.* Chicago: Year Book Medical Publishers, 220–249.
11. Fienman NL, and Yakovac WC. 1970. Neurofibromatosis in childhood. *Journal of Pediatrics* 76(3): 339–346.
12. Mihara M, et al. 1992. Cutaneous nerves in café au lait spots with white halos in infants with neurofibromatosis. *Archives of Dermatology* 128(7): 957–961.
13. Cunningham K, and Paes BA. 1991. Subcutaneous fat necrosis of the newborn with hypercalcemia: A review. *Neonatal Network* 10(3): 7–14.
14. Apfelberg DB, Maser MR, and Lash H. 1984. Review of usage of argon and carbon dioxide lasers for pediatric hemangiomas. *Annals of Plastic Surgery* 12(4): 353–360.
15. Ashinoff R, and Geronemus RG. 1991. Capillary hemangiomas and treatment with the flash lamp-pumped pulsed dye laser. *Archives of Dermatology* 127(2): 202.
16. Morelli JG, Huff JC, and Weston WL. 1993. Treatment of congenital telangiectatic vascular malformations with the pulsed-dye lasar (585 nm). *Pediatrics* 92(4): 603–606.
17. Silverman RA. 1991. Hemangiomas and vascular malformations. *Pediatric Clinics of North America* 38(4): 811–834.
18. Ruis-Maldonado R. 1989. Neonatal skin diseases. In *Textbook of Pediatric Dermatology,* Ruis-Maldonado R, Parish LC, and Beare JM, eds. Philadelphia: Grune & Stratton, 66, 219–223.
19. Whitley RJ, et al. 1991. Predictors of morbidity and mortality in neonates with herpes simplex virus infections. The National Institute of Allergy and Infectious Diseases Collaborative Antiviral Study Group. *New England Journal of Medicine* 324(7): 450–454.
20. Blunt K, et al. 1992. Aplasia cutis congenita: A clinical review and associated defects. *Neonatal Network* 11(7): 17–27.
21. Pappert AS, Scher RK, and Cohen JL. 1991. Nail disorders in children. *Pediatric Clinics of North America* 38(4): 921–940.

NOTES

5 Head, Eyes, Ears, Nose, Mouth, and Neck Assessment

Cynthia Boyer Johnson, RNC, MS, NNP

Examination of the infant's head and neck requires visual inspection, palpation, use of an ophthalmoscope, brief auscultation, and in rare cases, transillumination. After initial close observation, the exam should proceed from the top of the head downward to the neck. Attention should be given to the infant's state: Examination of the eyes is easier when the infant is in the quiet alert state and examination of the oropharynx, when the infant is crying.

General initial observations should include the infant's state; color of the skin and mucous membranes; size and symmetry of the head and face; and obvious deformations, malformations, or evidence of birth trauma. Minor anomalies of the head and neck are common, occurring second in frequency to minor anomalies of the hands.[1] There is an increased incidence of an associated major malformation if three or more minor anomalies are noted on the complete physical exam.[1]

CRANIUM

HEAD SIZE

Measurement of the occipital-frontal circumference (OFC) is the first step in assessing head size. A nonstretchable tape measure should be used to obtain three measurements of the OFC; the largest measurement should be recorded. The normal OFC for a term infant is 31 to 38 cm.[2–4] A falsely small or large OFC may result from cranial molding, scalp edema, or hemorrhage under the periosteum (fibrous membrane covering the bones of the skull). The measurement should be within normal range several days after birth. The OFC should be plotted on a standard growth chart (Figure 3-37) and the percentile in which the measurement falls noted. The percentile of the OFC, along with those for weight and length for gestational age, are necessary to diagnose micro- or macrocephaly.[5]

Microcephaly (OFC below the tenth percentile for gestational age) is due to poor brain growth. The sutures often become prematurely fused due to lack of expansive force of brain growth that enlarges the cranial vault. Microcephaly can be an isolated finding, or it may be associated with a genetic syndrome or congenital infection.[3,5–7]

Macrocephaly is diagnosed when the OFC is above the ninetieth percentile with normal weight and length for gestational age. Macro-

FIGURE 5-1 ▲ Transillumination.

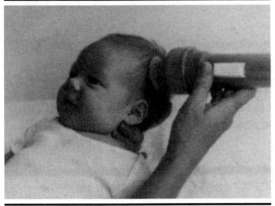

From: Jarvis C. 1992. *Physical Examination and Health Assessment.* Philadelphia: WB Saunders, 297. Reprinted by permission.

FIGURE 5-2 ▲ Molded head.

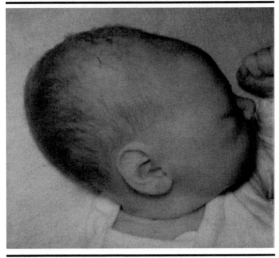

Courtesy of David A. Clark, MD, Louisiana State University.

cephaly may be familial, due to hydrocephalus, or associated with dwarfism or osteogenesis imperfecta.[5,8]

Transillumination of the skull is not part of the routine newborn physical exam, but it may be helpful when the infant's head has an unusual shape or size or the neurological exam is abnormal. A transilluminator or a flashlight with a rubber cuff may be placed flat against the infant's head in a dark room (Figure 5-1). A ring of light more than 2 cm larger than the light source implies increased fluid or decreased brain tissue in the cranium. A false positive transillumination may occur with a large caput because the scalp edema will transmit a halo of light. More definitive studies are necessary for diagnosis.[3,5]

HEAD SHAPE

The shape of the infant's head usually relates to molding of the skull during delivery (Figure 5-2). An infant delivered by cesarean section will usually have a well-rounded head. The breech position may cause the head to be molded posteriorly into an egg shape, with a prominent occiput. Prolonged diagonal pressure may cause the head to appear "out of round" when viewed from above. Parents can be reassured

that molding usually resolves within a few weeks after birth.[3,5,7,9]

SKULL

Inspection and careful palpation of the infant's skull are necessary to identify bones, sutures, and fontanels (Figure 5-3). Sutures separate bones, and fontanels occur where two sutures meet. The metopic suture extends midline down the forehead between the two frontal bones and intersects with the coronal suture, which separates the frontal and parietal bones. The anterior fontanel (AF) is formed at the intersection of the metopic, coronal, and sagittal sutures. The size of the AF varies from barely palpable to 4 to 5 cm across. Fontanels are measured diagonally from bone to bone rather than from suture to suture (Figure 5-4). The AF is normally described as flat and soft. A tense or bulging fontanel may be a sign of increased intracranial pressure or may occur when the infant is crying (Figure 5-5). If the examiner is uncertain whether the fontanel is flat or bulging, it should be palpated with the infant in an upright, sitting position. A sunken fontanel is a sign of severe dehydration and is rarely seen in the newborn nursery. A very large

FIGURE 5-3 ▲ Sutures, fontanels, and bones of the neonatal skull.

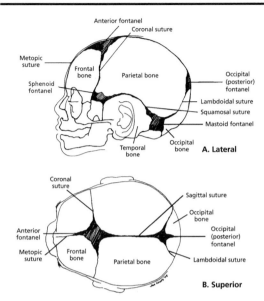

A. Lateral

B. Superior

From: Scanlon JW, et al. 1979. *A System of Newborn Physical Examination.* Baltimore: University Park Press, 47. Reprinted by permission of the author.

AF can be associated with hypothyroidism.[10] The AF normally closes by 18 to 24 months of age.[2,3,5]

The only auscultation necessary during examination of the head and neck is of the skull. Auscultation of a bruit (murmur-like sound) over the fontanels or the lateral skull may be a normal finding in an otherwise normal infant. In an infant with suspected cardiac failure, however, it may signify an intracranial arteriovenous malformation, which may be the cause of congestive heart failure.[5,11–13]

The sagittal suture extends midline between the two parietal bones to the posterior fontanel (PF). This fontanel is formed where the sagittal suture meets the lambdoidal suture, which extends posterolaterally to separate the occipital from the parietal bones. The PF is small and closes by approximately two to three months of age.[3,5] A third "fontanel" may occur along the sagittal suture between the anterior and posterior fontanels. This is really a defect of the

FIGURE 5-4 ▲ Measurement of the anterior fontanel: bone to bone.

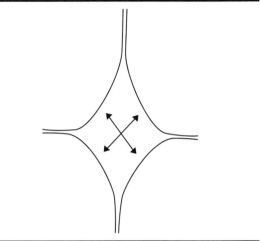

parietal bone and not a true fontanel. It can be a normal variant or may be associated with Down syndrome or congenital hypothyroidism.

The squamosal suture extends above the ear to separate the temporal bone from the parietal. This suture and the sphenoid and mastoid fontanels are usually apparent only when there is increased intracranial pressure, as with hydrocephalus, but may be palpable in the premature infant with rapid brain growth.[5]

FIGURE 5-5 ▲ Bulging anterior fontanel.

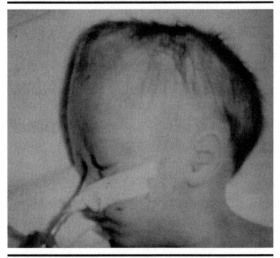

Courtesy of David A. Clark, MD, Louisiana State University Medical Center and Wyeth-Ayerst Laboratories, Philadelphia, Pennsylvania.

FIGURE 5-6 ▲ Cross-section of sutures: (a) Over-riding (b) Craniosynostosis.

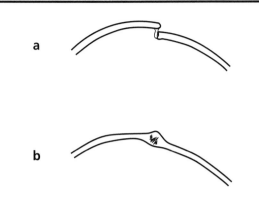
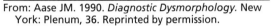

From: Aase JM. 1990. *Diagnostic Dysmorphology.* New York: Plenum, 36. Reprinted by permission.

Mobility of sutures is assessed by placing the thumbs on the bones on either side of the suture and gently pressing down alternately with one thumb and then the other. Normal sutures may be described as approximated and mobile. Sutures may be split (separated) up to 1 cm. More widely split sutures may indicate increased intracranial pressure and require further investigation. With molding, the edge of the bone on one side of the suture will feel as if it is on top of the edge of the opposing bone; these sutures are described as overriding. It is common for the lambdoidal sutures to be overriding, with the parietal bone on top of the occipital. It is important to differentiate an overriding suture from one that feels ridged and immobile. The latter finding implies premature fusion of the suture, or craniosynostosis (Figure 5-6).[5,6]

Premature closure of a suture stops bone growth perpendicular to the suture but allows continued parallel growth and compensatory expansion at the functional sutures, leading to abnormal head shape.[3,5–7,14,15] Abnormal head shape due to craniosynostosis may be noted at birth, or the premature fusion may not be suspected until later in infancy (Figure 5-7). Fused coronal sutures limit forward growth of the

FIGURE 5-7 ▲ Normal skull and shapes that result from craniosynostosis.

From: Disabato J, and Wulf J. 1989. Nursing strategies: Altered neurologic function. In *Family-Centered Nursing Care of Children*, Foster RL, Hunsberger MM, and Tackett JJ, eds. Philadelphia: WB Saunders, 1731. Reprinted by permission.

skull and lead to a broad skull (brachycephaly). Early closure of the sagittal suture limits lateral growth and results in a long, narrow head (scaphocephaly). Plagiocephaly is an asymmetric skull resulting from closure of the sutures on one side. The premature infant's head may develop the shape termed dolichocephaly, which is flattened side to side without craniosynostosis. Viewing the head from above aids in shape assessment. Craniosynostosis may be primary (isolated), associated with a genetic syndrome such as Apert or Crouzon, or the result of a metabolic disorder such as hyperthyroidism.[6,7,14,15] The incidence of isolated craniosynostosis in the U. S. is reported to be 0.4 to 1 per 1,000 live births.[6,15]

FIGURE 5-8 ▲ Cephalhematoma.

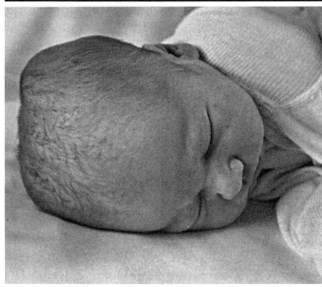

From: Mead Johnson. 1978. *Variations and Minor Departures in Infants.* Evansville, Indiana: Mead Johnson and Company, 10. Reprinted by permission.

Palpation of the skull may reveal areas of soft bone, or craniotabes. Pressing on the bone elicits a snapping sensation similar to pressing on a Ping-Pong ball. Craniotabes may be associated with pressure of the fetal head on the uterine fundus with breech position, associated with hydrocephalus, or an incidental finding.[3,5]

SCALP AND HAIR

While palpating the skull, the examiner also inspects the scalp to observe hair growth patterns and to look for birth trauma and other abnormalities. The most common form of trauma to the head is caput succedaneum (caput). This is edema of the presenting part of the scalp caused by pressure that restricts the return of venous and lymph flow during delivery. It can be accentuated by vacuum-assisted delivery. The edema pits on pressure, usually crosses suture lines, and has edges that are poorly defined. Caput is noted immediately after birth and resolves within a few days, which can help differentiate it from a cephalhematoma.[3,5,9]

A cephalhematoma results from collection of blood between the periosteum and the skull.

It may not be evident at birth because of associated caput. A cephalhematoma has clearly demarcated edges confined by suture lines (Figure 5-8). With time, it may liquefy and become fluctuant on palpation; it may take weeks or months to resolve completely. The most common locations for a cephalhematoma are the parietal and occipital bones. Associated depressed skull fractures are very rare.[2,3,5,9]

Other trauma to the scalp may include puncture from a scalp electrode; lacerations from fetal blood sampling or uterine incision; and bruises, abrasions, or subcutaneous fat necrosis from instrument delivery.[2,3,16] The trauma should be described by its appearance, size, and location near sutures or bones. Open scalp defects, known as cutis aplasia (Figure 5-9), are associated with trisomy 13, but they may also be seen as a normal variant.[10] Other skin lesions are described in Chapter 4.

Examination of the scalp should also include assessment of the hair for quantity, texture, distribution, and hair whorls. Low hairline, increased quantity of hair, and brittleness may be associated with congenital anomalies. The slope of each hair follicle appears to be associ-

FIGURE 5-9 ▲ Cutis aplasia.

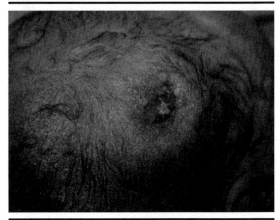

From: Blunt K, et al. 1992. Aplasia cutis congenita: A clinical review and associated defects. *Neonatal Network* 11(7): 18. Reprinted by permission.

FIGURE 5-10 ▲ Facial asymmetry.

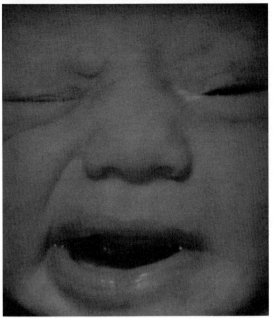

Courtesy of David A. Clark, MD, Louisiana State University Medical Center and Wyeth-Ayerst Laboratories. Philadelphia, Pennsylvania.

ated with the stretch of the skin during brain growth. The most rapid brain growth occurs at 16 to 19 weeks gestation and results in the formation of a hair whorl in the posterior parietal region. One or two hair whorls can be normal. An abnormally placed whorl, absence of hair whorl, or abnormal hair growth may be associated with abnormal brain growth and mental retardation.[10]

Malformation of the skull associated with incomplete neural tube closure results in an encephalocele. Central nervous tissue can protrude from a defect anywhere on the skull, most commonly in the occipital area.[3]

FACE

Examination of the face should begin with observing the relationships between all the facial components: eyes, ears, nose, and mouth. The forehead of a newborn takes up the upper half of the face, reflecting the large cranial volume needed for rapid brain growth. In childhood, the growth of the mid and lower face exceeds that of the upper face, eventually resulting in the face and skull shape of the adult.[7,14]

The shape and symmetry of the face, as well as evidence of any birth trauma, should be noted. Face or brow presentation or the presence of a nuchal cord may cause facial bruising or petechiae. Unusual flattening of facial features may occur as a result of prolonged intrauterine compression from oligohydramnios. Forceps application may cause bruises, abrasions, or subcutaneous fat necrosis.[3] The location and extent of any trauma should be carefully described. Other skin lesions that may be seen on the face are described in Chapter 4.

Many malformation syndromes have very distinctive facial features. These minor anomalies may serve as aids in the diagnosis of a particular syndrome.[1,10] The examiner should also

FIGURE 5-11 ▲ Normal external newborn ear (pinna).

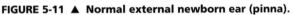
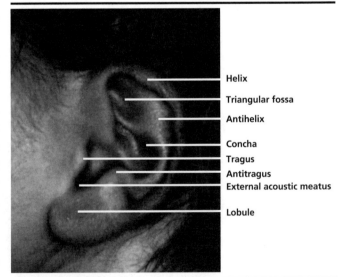

From: Mead Johnson. 1978. *Variations and Minor Departures in Infants.* Evansville, Indiana: Mead Johnson and Company, 32. Reprinted by permission.

FIGURE 5-12 ▲ Variations and minor malformations.

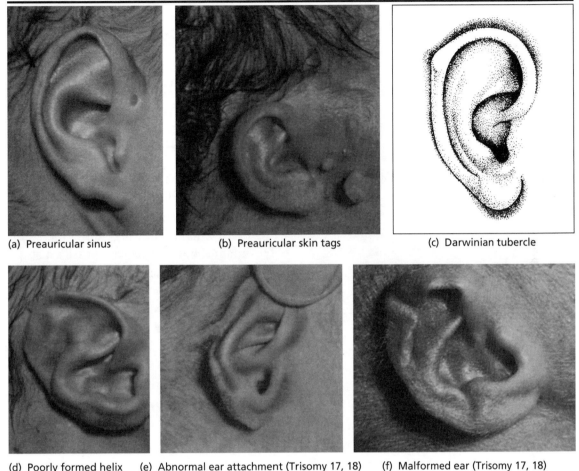

(a) Preauricular sinus   (b) Preauricular skin tags   (c) Darwinian tubercle

(d) Poorly formed helix   (e) Abnormal ear attachment (Trisomy 17, 18)   (f) Malformed ear (Trisomy 17, 18)

From: Mead Johnson. 1978. *Variations and Minor Departures in Infants.* Evansville, Indiana: Mead Johnson and Company, 34, 36. Reprinted by permission.

remember that unusual facial characteristics may be familial.

Facial movements during crying must be assessed for symmetry. Drooping of muscles on one side of the face could imply facial palsy, possibly as a result of nerve damage from forceps application (Figure 5-10). (Chapter 11 provides guidelines for a complete assessment.)

EARS

Abnormal formation or placement of the ears can be associated with chromosomal anomalies and syndromes; however, a wide variety of minor structural variations falls within the normal range. Ear anomalies are usually nonspecific and are supportive rather than diagnostic.[3,5,9,10] To describe abnormalities, the examiner should be familiar with the normal anatomy and nomenclature of the ear (Figure 5-11). In a term infant, the pinna should be well formed, with cartilage that recoils easily after folding (Chapter 3). Temporary asymmetry of the ears from unequal intrauterine pressure on the sides of the head is common.[10]

Minor malformations, such as pits and skin tags, may be familial or associated with other anomalies (Figure 5-12).[3,5,9,10,17] These minor malformations are usually located anterior to

FIGURE 5-13 ▲ The normal ear position.

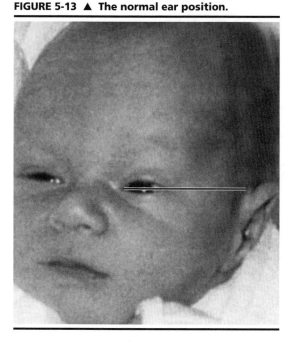

the tragus and are thought to be embryologic remnants of the first branchial cleft or arch. A preauricular sinus may be blind, or it may communicate with the internal ear or brain. Chronic infection could necessitate surgical removal of the entire sinus tract. Darwinian tubercle is a normal variant, appearing as a small nodule on the upper helix. A very poorly formed external ear should alert the examiner to possible chromosomal anomaly or syndrome.[9,10]

The position of the external ear on the head can be assessed by extending a line from the inner to the outer canthus of the eye toward the ear (Figure 5-13). If the insertion of the ear falls below this line, it is low set. It is important to assess both ears because one may be posteriorly rotated and give the appearance of being low set.[2,9,10]

The newborn infant's external auditory canal is short and may contain vernix, making otoscopic examination difficult. This is not part of the routine newborn exam; it can be done later at the first well-baby visit. The ear should

FIGURE 5-14 ▲ Anatomy of the eye.

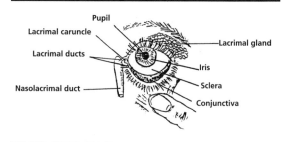

be inspected visually to assess presence and patency of the auditory canal.[2,3,5]

The examiner should attempt some assessment of the infant's hearing during the exam. The infant should startle, cry, or stiffen at the sound of a loud noise or alert to the sound of a voice. This can be a difficult assessment; the infant may be responding to air movement rather than noise and can quickly habituate to a repeated stimulus.[3,5] Any infant with a small or abnormally developed ear should be assessed for hearing loss in that ear. Hearing assessment of all infants by audiology is becoming routine in some nurseries.

EYES

Eyes are usually a major area of focus when parents are viewing their newborn infant. Parents will need reassurance about common eye trauma, such as bruises or edema of the eyelids and hemorrhages seen around the iris that can occur after a normal vaginal delivery. Conjunctival or subconjunctival hemorrhage results from rupture of a capillary of the mucous membrane that lines the eyelids and is reflected onto the eyeball (conjunctiva) (Figure 5-14). It is seen as a bright red area on the white part of the eye (sclera) near the iris and usually resolves within a week to ten days. Inflammation of the conjunctiva can be caused by prophylaxis of the eyes with silver nitrate drops.[2,3,8,9,18]

Malformation of the eyelids is uncommon but coloboma (a defect in closure of a portion

FIGURE 5-15 ▲ Eye measurements.

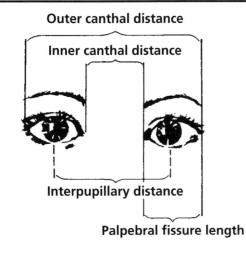

Outer canthal distance

Inner canthal distance

Interpupillary distance

Palpebral fissure length

From: Aase JM. 1990. *Diagnostic Dysmorphology.* New York: Plenum, 63. Reprinted by permission.

of the lid or eye) may be seen. Ptosis, a paralytic drooping of an eyelid when the lids are fully open, may also be seen. Nevus simplex is a common vascular birthmark seen on the eyelids and glabella (area above the nose and between the eyebrows) (Chapter 4).[9,19]

Tear formation does not usually begin until two to three months of age. The nasolacrimal duct is not fully patent until five to seven months, and purulent or mucoid eye drainage is common. Unless accompanied by redness or swelling, this drainage can generally be treated by lacrimal massage and gentle cleansing with water and a cotton ball.[2,3,5]

Abnormal placement of the eyes or small palpebral fissures (eye openings) may alert the examiner to the presence of a syndrome or chromosomal anomaly. The distance between the outer canthi can be divided into equal thirds, with one normal palpebral fissure length fitting into the inner canthal distance (Figure 5-15). Hypertelorism exists if the eyes are more widely spaced; hypotelorism is present if the eyes are more closely spaced. Small palpebral fissures can give the appearance of hypertelorism.[3,5,10,20]

If the outer canthus of the eye is higher than the inner canthus, the eye is said to have a mongolian slant; if the outer canthus is lower than the inner canthus, it is said to have an antimongolian slant. The epicanthal fold is a vertical fold of skin on either side of the nose that covers the lacrimal caruncle. Epicanthal folds with a mongolian slant are common in Asian infants but may suggest Down syndrome in other ethnic groups.[3,10]

The eyebrows normally extend above the eye in a curve approximately the length of the palpebral fissure. Eyebrows that meet at the glabella and abnormally long or tangled eyelashes are associated with some syndromes, such as Cornelia de Lange.[1,10]

Examination of the eyes is much easier if they are opened spontaneously by the infant. This may be accomplished at the beginning of the exam by giving an auditory stimulus, changing the infant's position from supine to upright, gently swinging the infant in an arc on the examiner's arm, or dimming the lights. If the eyes are forcefully pried open, the eyelids will often evert, making visualization impossible. The eye exam can also be more difficult if attempted after eye prophylaxis has been given.

A full ophthalmoscopic exam is not practical, so the examiner must be alert to obtain the information needed in a limited time.[2,3,19] The ophthalmoscope should first be adjusted for focus and then for supply of a round white beam of light. The examiner directs the light into the infant's pupils from a distance of about 6 inches to assess equality of size, pupillary reflex (constriction with bright light), and red retinal reflex. The notation "PERL" can be used if pupils are noted to be equal and reactive to light. When a bright light is directed at the newborn's lens, a clear red color is reflected from the retina back to the examiner. Opacity of the lens or cornea interrupts the reflection; lack of the red reflex could imply congenital

FIGURE 5-16 ▲ Congenital cataracts.

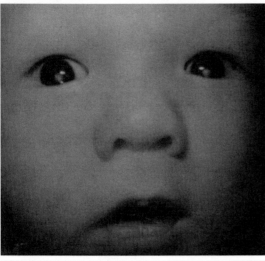

Courtesy of David A. Clark, MD, Louisiana State University Medical Center and Wyeth-Ayerst Laboratories. Philadelphia, Pennsylvania.

FIGURE 5-17 ▲ Strabismus.

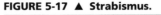

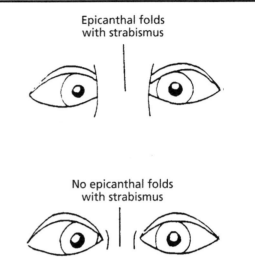

From: Alexander MM, and Brown MS. 1979. *Pediatric History Taking and Physical Diagnosis for Nurses*, 2nd ed. St. Louis: Mosby-Year Book, 97. Reprinted by permission of the authors.

cataract, retinoblastoma, or glaucoma (Figure 5-16).[3,5,19,21] In dark-skinned infants, the red reflex tends to be slightly pale. The lens vessels of the premature infant can be examined to help determine gestational age (Chapter 3). A keyhole-shaped pupil, also known as coloboma of the iris, may be associated with other anomalies.[2,3,5,19]

The iris of a newborn infant is generally dark gray, blue, or brown at birth and will acquire final pigment color at about six months of age. Brushfield spots are white specks scattered linearly around the entire circumference of the iris. They are associated with Down syndrome, but may be seen as a normal variant.[10] The sclera of a term infant is generally white to bluish white. A blue sclera is associated with osteogenesis imperfecta. The sclera may become jaundiced with hyperbilirubinemia. In a normal gaze, no sclera should be visible above the iris. The "sunset sign" is often seen in infants with hydrocephalus, where there is lid retraction and a downward gaze.[2,3,5,9,19]

Observation of eyeball movements during neurologic assessment is discussed in detail in

Chapter 11. Nystagmus is a rapid, searching movement of the eyeballs that usually disappears by three to four months of age. When it persists, it may be associated with an abnormal neurologic exam. Strabismus is due to muscular incoordination and gives the appearance of crossed eyes (Figure 5-17). Pseudostrabismus from a flat nasal bridge or epicanthal folds usually resolves by one year of age. Exophthalmos (abnormal protrusion of the eyeball) is associated with hyperthyroidism and congenital glaucoma.[3,9,19,21]

NOSE

Its size and shape may be familial, but the infant's nose is generally smaller and flatter than an adult's. The nose should be symmetric and placed vertically in the midline. Nasal flaring is abnormal and is a sign of respiratory distress. Sneezing is common and normal unless excessive or continuous. Nasal stuffiness can be normal in the newborn period; however, chronic breathing difficulty or chronic nasal discharge is abnormal.[2–5]

FIGURE 5-18 ▲ Nasal deformity.

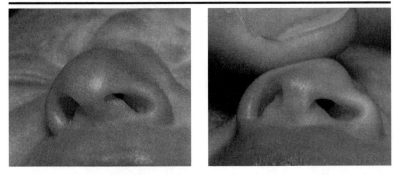

This infant incurred dislocation of the triangular cartilage of the nasal septum during delivery. Inspection of the nose reveals deviation of the septum to the right and asymmetry of the nares (left). When the septum is manually moved toward the midline, the asymmetry persists, confirming the dislocation (right).

From: Balsan MJ, and Holzman IR. 1992. Neonatology. In *Atlas of Pediatric Physical Diagnosis*, 2nd ed., Zitelli BJ, and Davis HW, eds. London, UK: Mosby-Wolfe Europe Limited, 2.11. Reprinted by permission.

A very low nasal bridge with a broad base may be associated with Down syndrome.[3,10] Deviation of the nasal septum to one side may be a deformation from position *in utero*, or it may be caused by a dislocated septum. If the septum won't easily straighten and the nares remain asymmetric when the tip of the nose is pushed to midline, the septum is dislocated and will require treatment (Figure 5-18).[5-6]

The examiner can elevate the tip of the nose slightly to view the nasal septum, the floor of the nose, and the turbinates.[18] Patency can be assessed by watching the infant breathe in a quiet state. Because infants are obligate nose breathers, bilateral choanal atresia (obstruction of the posterior nasal passages) will cause them to be cyanotic at rest and pink when crying and breathing through the mouth. If obstruction is suspected, a soft 5 French catheter can be gently passed through both nostrils to assess patency. If an infant has noisy, nasal respirations, a piece of cold metal can be held under the nose to observe for mist formation under both nares. If the turbinates are swollen from previous suctioning, passing a catheter to assess patency may only make the edema worse.[3,5]

MOUTH

The lips and mucous membranes of a healthy term infant should be pink. Mild circumoral cyanosis is normal.

Abnormal shape and size of the oral opening, lips, philtrum (midline groove between the nose and upper lip), and mandible may be associated with a syndrome. A small oral opening, known as microstomia, may be seen in some trisomies. Macrostomia is seen with storage diseases such as the mucopolysaccharidoses. A thin upper lip with a smooth philtrum and short palpebral fissures may be seen in fetal alcohol syndrome. Cleft lip may be unilateral or bilateral and may be small or extend to the floor of the nose. Micrognathia, or small lower jaw, is seen in Robin sequence and other syndromes (Figure 5-19).[3,5,10,15]

The infant's cry should be assessed during the exam for quality, strength, pitch, and hoarseness or stridor. The examiner should look for symmetry of facial movements during the cry and should test root and suck reflexes (Chapter 11).

Examining the inside of the mouth is easiest when the infant is crying. Use of a tongue depressor may stimulate a strong protrusion reflex, making visualization difficult. The mouth may be opened by gently pressing down on the chin. Abnormalities of the oropharynx are unusual, but a quick look is necessary to ensure absence of a structural abnormality or tumor. If possible, the uvula should be visualized at the back of the soft palate. A bifid uvula may be associated with other congenital anomalies.[3,10]

The tongue should fit well into the floor of the mouth. A large tongue (macroglossia) is associated with Beckwith-Wiedemann syndrome, hypothyroidism, and mucopolysaccharidosis.

FIGURE 5-19 ▲ **Robin sequence (micrognathia).**

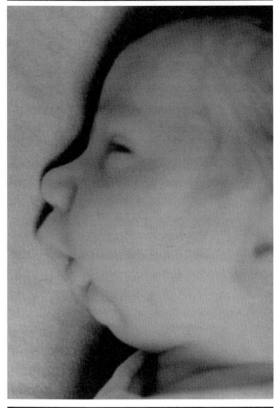

Courtesy of David A. Clark, MD, Louisiana State University.

FIGURE 5-20 ▲ **Cystic hygroma, with extension to the axilla.**

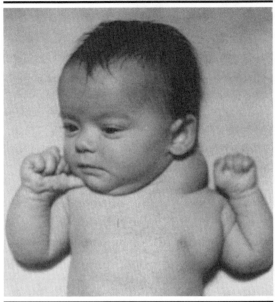

From: Koop CE. 1976. *Visible and Palpable Lesions in Children.* New York: Grune & Stratton, 35. Reprinted by permission of the author.

The frenulum attaches the underside of the tongue to the floor of the mouth, usually midway between the ventral surface of the tongue and the tip. A very thick or prominent frenulum, or "tongue tie," is rare. White patches on the tongue and mucous membranes may be from residual milk. If not easily removed with a tongue blade or cotton swab, they are lesions of candidiasis (oral thrush). A translucent or bluish swelling under the tongue is a mucocele or ranula. These mucous or salivary gland retention cysts usually resolve spontaneously.[3,9]

The gums should be pink and smooth. Natal teeth or eruption cysts with teeth appearing after birth (neonatal teeth) are usually seen in the lower incisor region. These are usually immature caps of enamel and dentine with poor root formation and may be very mobile. They may cause ulceration of the infant's tongue and pain with feeding, and there is a presumed risk of aspiration. For these reasons, removal is generally recommended, after consultation with the family. If the tooth is firmly implanted, the dentist may choose to leave it in place and do follow-up examinations to assess for any of the previously mentioned complications.[3,9,22,23]

A gloved finger should be inserted into the infant's mouth with the fingerpad up to ensure continuity of the hard and soft palates and to assess suck and gag reflexes. Small whitish yellow clusters of Epstein's pearls may be seen at the junction of the hard and soft palates and on the gums. These are masses of epithelial cells and usually disappear by a few weeks of age.[3,5,9]

Excessive oral secretions requiring frequent suctioning are abnormal in the newborn infant. The etiology could be esophageal atresia or poor swallow from a neurologic abnormality. Patency of the esophagus is easily assessed by passage of an orogastric tube in the delivery

FIGURE 5-21 ▲ **Webbed neck—Turner syndrome.**

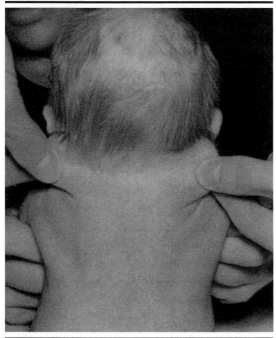

From: Milner RDG, and Herber SM. 1984. *Color Atlas of the Newborn,* Oradell, New Jersey: Medical Economics, 102. Reprinted by permission of Blackwell Scientific Publications.

room (or in the nursery) after the infant has stabilized.[3]

NECK

The infant's neck is normally short, but severe shortness may be associated with a syndrome. To observe shape and symmetry of the neck, the shoulders can be elevated, allowing the head to fall back slightly. Asymmetry is most likely due to *in utero* positioning.

The neck must be visualized and palpated anteriorly, laterally, and posteriorly. The thyroid gland is difficult to palpate unless it is enlarged. Goiter, caused by intrauterine deprivation of thyroid hormone, is very unusual.[3]

Cystic hygroma is the most commonly seen neck mass (Figure 5-20). It is caused by development of sequestered lymph channels, which dilate into large cysts. Cystic hygroma is soft and fluctuant, transilluminates well, and is usually seen laterally or over the clavicle. Its size

can range from only a few centimeters to massive, and it may cause severe feeding difficulties or airway compromise. Very small lesions may regress spontaneously, but surgical resection is usually required.[5,17]

A mass high in the neck may be a thyroglossal duct cyst or a branchial cleft cyst. A branchial sinus may also be seen anywhere along the sternocleidomastoid muscle. It may communicate with deeper structures, and infection may necessitate surgical removal of the entire sinus tract.[17]

During palpation of the neck, redundant skin or webbed neck may be noted. This is associated with Turner (Figure 5-21), Noonan, and Down syndromes.[2,5,10]

The clavicles should be palpated to assess for fracture. Movement of the bone ends may be felt soon after birth, or fracture may not be evident for weeks, until callus has formed and can be palpated as a mass over the clavicle.

Assessment of neck reflexes, range of motion, and tone, is described in Chapters 10 and 11.

SUMMARY

Minor anomalies of the head and neck are common and may provide evidence for a particular syndrome. Examination of the eyes and mouth requires cooperation of the infant, and the examiner needs to be alert for opportune times.

REFERENCES

1. Cohen MM. 1990. Syndromology: An updated conceptual overview. Part IX: Facial dysmorphology. *International Journal of Oral and Maxillofacial Surgery* 19(2): 81–88.
2. Robertson NR, ed. 1986. *Textbook of Neonatology.* New York: Churchill Livingstone, 134–136.
3. Seidel HM, et al. 1991. *Mosby's Guide to Physical Examination,* 2nd ed. St. Louis: Mosby-Year Book.
4. Perry S. 1991. Normal newborn. In *Essentials of Maternity Nursing,* 3rd ed., Bobak IM, and Jensen MD, eds. St. Louis: Mosby-Year Book, 441–481.
5. Scanlon JW, et al. 1979. *A System of Newborn Physical Examination.* Baltimore: University Park Press, 45–60.
6. Disabato J, and Wulf J. 1989. Nursing strategies: Altered neurologic function. In *Family-Centered Nursing Care*

of Children, Foster RL, Hunsberger MM, and Tackett JJ, eds. Philadelphia: WB Saunders, 1675–1732.

7. Griscom NT. 1978. Craniosynostosis. In *Skull, Spine, and Contents. Part II: Progress in Pediatric Radiology,* vol. 6, Kaufman JH, ed. Basel: Karger, 3–38.

8. Cole TR, and Hughes HE. 1991. Autosomal dominant macrocephaly: Benign familial macrocephaly or a new syndrome? *American Journal of Medical Genetics* 41(1): 115–124.

9. Mead Johnson. 1978. *Variations and Minor Departures in Infants.* Evansville, Indiana: Mead Johnson and Company.

10. Jones KL. 1988. *Smith's Recognizable Patterns of Human Malformation,* 4th ed. Philadelphia: WB Saunders.

11. Barber G, and Chin AJ. 1990. Volume loads except TAPVD. In *Fetal and Neonatal Cardiology,* Long WA, ed. Philadelphia: WB Saunders, 452–454.

12. Musewe NN, et al. 1992. Arteriovenous fistulae: A consideration of extracardiac causes of congestive heart failure. In *Neonatal Heart Disease,* Freedom RM, Benson LN, and Smallhorn JF, eds. New York: Springer-Verlag, 759–761.

13. Pellegrino PA, et al. 1987. Congestive heart failure secondary to cerebral arterio-venous fistula. *Child's Nervous System* 3(3): 141–144.

14. Marsh JL, and Vannier MW. 1985. *Comprehensive Care for Craniofacial Deformities.* St. Louis: Mosby-Year Book, 88–100, 122–172.

15. Snively SL. 1987. Craniofacial anomalies. Part II: Congenital syndromes and surgical treatment. *Selected Readings in Plastic Surgery* 4(25): 1–25.

16. Balsan MJ, and Holzman IR. 1992. Neonatology. In *Atlas of Pediatric Physical Diagnosis,* 2nd ed., Zitelli BJ, and Davis HW, eds. Philadelphia: JB Lippincott, 2.9–2.13.

17. Friedberg J. 1989. Pharyngeal cleft sinuses and cysts, and other benign neck lesions. *Pediatric Clinics of North America* 36(6): 1451–1469.

18. Swartz MH. 1989. *Physical Diagnosis.* Philadelphia: WB Saunders, 572–576.

19. O'Doherty N. 1985. *Atlas of the Newborn,* 2nd ed. Lancaster, England: MTP Press, 45–53.

20. Aase JM. 1990. *Diagnostic Dysmorphology.* New York: Plenum, 34–118.

21. Franks W, and Taylor D. 1989. Congenital glaucoma— a preventable cause of blindness. *Archives of Disease in Childhood* 64(5): 649–650.

22. King NM, and Lee AM. 1989. Prematurely erupted teeth in newborn infants. *Journal of Pediatrics* 114(5): 807–809.

23. Nik-Hussein NN. 1990. Natal and neonatal teeth. *Journal of Pedodontics* 14(2): 110–111.

NOTES

6 Chest and Lungs Assessment

Debbie Fraser Askin, RNC, MN

Physical assessment of the lungs should begin with a thorough review of the infant's history. Physical findings will vary greatly with the infant's gestational age and the time elapsed since delivery. Other important factors from the infant's prenatal, intrapartum, and postnatal history are outlined in Table 6-1.

Physical exam of the chest generally begins with observation so the infant is not disturbed before assessing breath sounds. Auscultation and palpation follow. Depending on the infant's physical condition, it may be necessary to allow him to rest between parts of the exam. Provisions should also be made to ensure that the infant does not become cold during the examination; cold stress will precipitate or further aggravate respiratory distress.

LANDMARKS AND STRUCTURE

The chest cavity is bounded by the sternum, 12 thoracic vertebrae, and 12 pairs of ribs (7 true vertebrocostal pairs and 5 false, or vertebrochondral dyads). The ribs in the neonate are much more cartilaginous than in the adult, accounting in part for increased chest wall compliance and for the retractions seen in respiratory distress. The lower boundary of the thorax

TABLE 6-1 ▲ Historical Factors the Examiner Should Note

Prenatal/Intrapartum History
Gestational age
Maternal drug ingestion
Fetal distress
Maternal health (i.e., diabetes, fever)
Prolonged rupture of membranes
Meconium-stained fluid
Delivery mode
Apgar scores

Postnatal History
Corrected age
Duration of mechanical ventilation
History of respiratory distress syndrome or broncho-pulmonary dysplasia
History of pneumonia
Difficulty feeding
Apnea

is formed by the diaphragm, normally a convex muscular sheath. Other palpable thoracic landmarks include the suprasternal notch found on the upper aspect of the sternum and the xiphoid process, which protrudes below the sternum. The clavicles and scapulae complete the bony structure of the chest (Figure 6-1).

The chest cavity consists of three potential spaces: the mediastinum and the right and left

FIGURE 6-1 ▲ Bony structure of the chest.

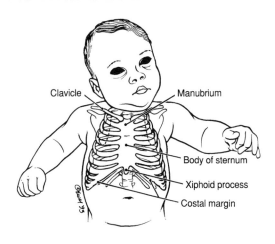

FIGURE 6-3 ▲ Reference lines.

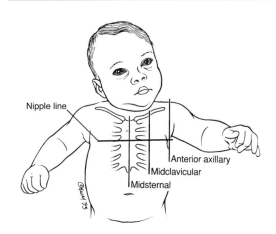

pleural cavities. The mediastinum contains the heart, esophagus, trachea, mainstem bronchi, thymus, and major blood vessels. The three lobes of the right lung and the two lobes of the left lung are encased in serous membranes, which make up the visceral and parietal pleura (Figure 6-2).

REFERENCE LINES

When describing the location of a physical finding in the chest and lung exam, use the following reference lines to aid accuracy (Figure 6-3):

FIGURE 6-2 ▲ Internal structure of the chest.

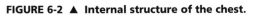
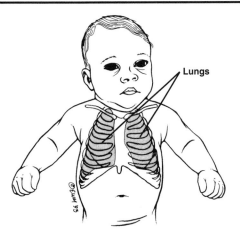

▶ Midsternal line: bisects the suprasternal notch
▶ Nipple line: horizontal line drawn through the nipples
▶ Midclavicular line: a vertical line drawn through the clavicle
▶ Anterior axillary line: extends from the anterior axillary fold

INSPECTION

GENERAL

Inspection should begin with an overall assessment of the infant's color, tone, and activity. These findings provide clues to oxygenation and respiratory status.

Color

Observe the color of the infant's skin and mucous membranes. In the normal neonate, the lips and mucous membranes are pink and well perfused. Acrocyanosis after birth is common and may persist during transition (up to 48 hours) following delivery.[1]

Color deviations might include cyanosis (either generalized or of the lips, tongue, and mucous membranes) and acrocyanosis or mottling in the infant beyond transition. Other abnormalities in color—such as ruddiness and paleness—are discussed in Chapter 7.

Tone and Activity

Observe the infant's tone and level and type of activity. Normal findings include flexed posture and active movement of all four limbs when awake. (Note that flexion is decreased with prematurity.) Deviations include hypotonia and inactivity.

RESPIRATIONS

Rate

Count the infant's respirations for one full minute. Normal findings are 40 to 60 breaths per minute, with wide variations. If the room is very warm or cool, the infant's respiratory rate may vary. Most infants experiencing temperature stress will be tachypneic, but occasionally, they may demonstrate bradypnea. Babies delivered by cesarean section generally have a more rapid respiratory rate in the first 12–24 hours than those delivered vaginally.

Although respiratory rates vary, persistent tachypnea (respirations greater than 60 breaths per minute) may indicate underlying lung pathology (transient tachypnea of the newborn, respiratory distress syndrome, meconium aspiration, pneumonia), hyperthermia, or pain.

Bradypnea (respirations less than 40 breaths per minute) or shallow respirations are associated with central nervous system depression secondary to factors such as maternal drug ingestion, asphyxia, or birth injury.

Quality

Observe the general appearance of the infant. Relaxed, symmetrical diaphragmatic respirations are normal. The newborn infant uses the diaphragm as the primary muscle of respiration.[2] As such, the lower thorax pulls in and the abdomen bulges with each respiration. Deviations include asymmetric chest movement and excessive thoracic expansion.

Nasal flaring and grunting may be noted immediately following birth. Mild nasal flar-

FIGURE 6-4 ▲ Retraction sites.

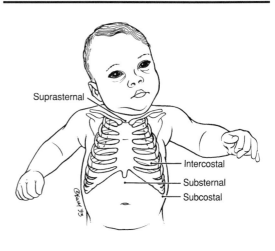

ing and substernal or intercostal retractions may be seen immediately after birth as the infant attempts to clear fetal lung fluid from the lungs. Beyond this period, flaring and retractions suggest respiratory problems (transient tachypnea of the newborn, respiratory distress syndrome, atelectasis, pneumonia). Suprasternal retraction, especially if accompanied by gasping or stridor, may indicate upper airway obstruction (laryngeal webs or cysts, tumors, vascular rings). Figure 6-4 shows the most common sites for retractions.

Expiratory grunting occurs as the infant closes the glottis in an attempt to increase intrathoracic pressure in response to alveolar collapse (respiratory distress syndrome).[3] In 1956, Silverman and Andersen developed a scoring system (upon which many of today's scoring systems are based) to measure respiratory distress objectively.[4] This scoring system, shown in Table 6-2, can be used to quantify the extent of respiratory distress experienced by the infant at the time of examination.

Asymmetric breathing may result from conditions such as diaphragmatic hernia, cardiac lesions inducing failure, pneumothorax, or phrenic nerve damage.

TABLE 6-2 ▲ Assessment of Respiratory Distress

Criterion	Score		
	0	1	2
Chest movement	Chest moves with abdomen	Chest sinks minimally as abdomen rises	See-saw respirations; chest sinks as abdomen rises
Intercostal retractions	None	Minimal	Marked
Xiphoid retractions	None	Just visible	Marked
Expiratory grunting	None	Heard only with stethoscope	Audible with naked ear
Nasal flaring	None	Minimal	Marked

Note: The distress score is calculated by adding the values (0,1,2) assigned to each category. A score of 10 indicates maximum distress.

Adapted from: Silverman WA, and Andersen DH. 1956. A controlled clinical trial of water mist on obstructive respiratory signs, death rate, and necropsy findings among premature infants. *Pediatrics* 17(1): 4. Reprinted by permission.

Pattern

While counting respirations, note the pattern (regularity) of inspiration. Normal newborns have an irregular pattern of respirations. The more preterm the infant, the more likely the presence of irregularities in the breathing pattern. Periodic breathing (vigorous breaths followed by up to a 20-second pause) is common in preterm infants and may persist for up to several days after birth in term infants. Periodic breathing persists in premature infants until they approach term.

A lapse of 15 to 20 seconds or more between respiratory cycles (one inspiration and expiration) accompanied by bradycardia or color changes indicates apnea.[5] This condition, associated with prematurity, is gradually outgrown as the infant approaches term. Apnea in the term or close-to-term infant should be considered abnormal and may indicate underlying illness (sepsis, hypoglycemia, central nervous system injury or abnormality, seizures) or factors such as maternal drug ingestion.

BONY STRUCTURE

Observe the infant's chest and measure its circumference. Normal findings include a symmetric, round shape with the anterior-posterior (AP) diameter approximately equal to the transverse diameter. The average chest circumference in term infants is 33 ± 3 cm or 2 cm less than the normal head circumference.[6]

Deviations include pigeon chest—protrusion of the sternum (Marfan syndrome, rickets); funnel chest—indented sternum (rickets, Marfan syndrome); and barrel chest—increased AP diameter (transient tachypnea of the newborn, meconium aspiration, hyperinflation) (Figure 6-5).

SOFT TISSUES

Muscle

Observe the chest for development, symmetry, and bulges or masses. The normal chest wall is symmetric and relatively smooth. Deviations include bulges or masses, atrophy, agenesis, or hypertrophy.

Nipples

Look at the placement, shape, and pigmentation of the nipples. Also inspect the nipples for fissures and secretions.

In the full-term infant, the areolae normally are raised and stippled, with 0.75 to 1 cm of palpable breast tissue. The distance from the outside of one areola to the outside of the other should be less than one-quarter of the chest circumference.[7] Breast size is also a useful indicator in gestational age assessment (Chapter 3).

In some infants, the influence of maternal estrogen results in breasts that are enlarged and

FIGURE 6-5 ▲ Different chest shapes.

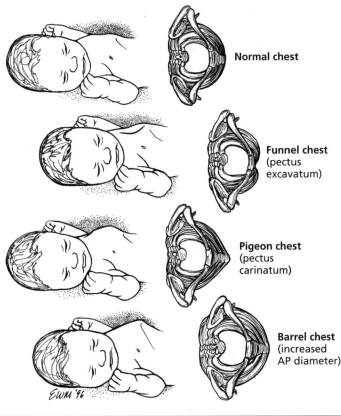

Normal chest

Funnel chest
(pectus
excavatum)

Pigeon chest
(pectus
carinatum)

Barrel chest
(increased
AP diameter)

sition, oral and nasal secretions reflect the lungs' attempt to clear themselves of fetal fluid. Normal secretions are usually clear to white frothy mucus. Oral secretions will also reflect the stomach contents swallowed during delivery and therefore may be yellow or green in the presence of meconium or blood tinged if maternal blood was swallowed.

Deviations include excessive frothy oral secretions, which may indicate the presence of an esophageal atresia. Nasal stuffiness is associated with maternal drug use.[9] Snuffles (rhinitis) may be found with congenital syphilis. Thick yellow secretions may be seen in the presence of a respiratory infection, and copious white nasal secretions are associated with respiratory syncytial virus (RSV) infection.[10]

AUSCULTATION

Breath sounds are louder and more coarse in the neonate than in the adult because the infant has less subcutaneous tissue to muffle transmission. Sounds are very readily referred in the neonate's chest due to its small size; therefore, localization of adventitious sounds is difficult. In addition, breath sounds may be decreased but are seldom absent, even over areas of atelectasis or pneumothorax. Breath sounds are less readily transmitted if (1) the pleural space contains fluid or air, (2) the bronchus contains secretions or foreign bodies, or (3) the lungs are hyperinflated. Sounds are more readily transmitted in the presence of consolidation—for example, with pneumonia.

To auscultate breath sounds, use the bell of a warmed neonatal stethoscope. Begin at the top of the chest and move systematically from side to side (Figure 6–6). Breath sounds in the lower lobes of the lung can be assessed

engorged with a milky secretion known as "witch's milk." The secretions may last one to two weeks and the enlargement, several months. Rarely, newborn infants may develop mastitis, characterized by redness, tenderness, breast enlargement, and discharge of pus.

Wide-spaced nipples may be indicative of a syndrome such as Turner.[8] Supernumerary (accessory) nipples are most commonly seen as raised or pigmented areas 5–6 cm below the normal nipple but can be located anywhere on a vertical line drawn through the true nipple. In Caucasian infants, supernumerary nipples may be associated with congenital anomalies.[1]

ORAL AND NASAL SECRETIONS

Observe the quantity and quality of the infant's oral and nasal secretions. During tran-

FIGURE 6-6 ▲ Sequence for breath sound auscultation: anterior and posterior chest.

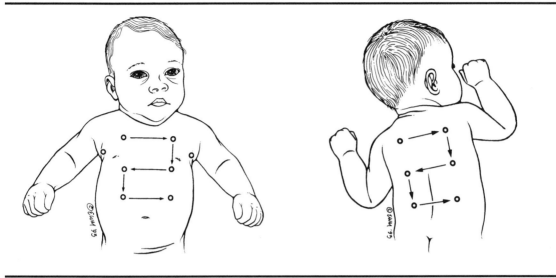

adequately only through the infant's back. Therefore, systematic auscultation of both the anterior and the posterior chest should be performed and one side of the chest compared with the other.

NORMAL BREATH SOUNDS

Breath sounds should be assessed for pitch, intensity, and duration. Normal breath sounds have been described in adults and older children according to their location in the chest. As previously noted, localization of breath sounds in the neonate is very difficult. The following terms are sometimes used, however, to describe normal sounds within the lungs.

Vesicular

Vesicular (from the Latin for "sac") breath sounds are soft, short, and low pitched during expiration and louder, longer, and higher pitched during inspiration. These sounds are normally found over the entire chest, except over the manubrium and trachea.

Bronchial

The loudest of the breath sounds, bronchial sounds are characterized by a short inspiration and a longer expiration. In adults, these sounds are found over the trachea, but are seldom heard in the neonate.

Bronchovesicular

Bronchovesicular sounds demonstrate an inspiration and an expiration that are equal in quality, intensity, pitch, and duration. Louder than vesicular but less intense than bronchial sounds, bronchovesicular sounds are normally found over the manubrium and intrascapular regions (Table 6-3).

ADVENTITIOUS SOUNDS

Adventitious (abnormal) breath sounds are usually a sign of disease and may be superimposed on normal breath sounds. Auscultation shortly after birth frequently demonstrates adventitious sounds due to the presence of fetal lung fluid. Care should be taken to distinguish sounds arising in the lungs from those in the upper airway. This may be achieved by placing the stethoscope over the infant's nose and mouth. Suctioning will often clear the upper airway and assist in identifying the presence of referred sounds.

Crackles

Crackles are defined as a series of brief crackling or bubbling sounds arising from a sudden

TABLE 6-3 ▲ Normal Breath Sounds

Sound	Characteristics	Findings
Vesicular	Heard over most of lung fields; low pitch; soft and short expirations	Low pitch, soft expirations
Bronchovesicular	Heard over main bronchus area and over upper right posterior lung field; medium pitch; expiration equals inspiration	Medium pitch, medium expirations
Bronchial	Heard only over trachea; high pitch; loud and long expirations	High pitch, loud expirations

From: Thompson JM, et al. 1993. *Mosby's Manual of Clinical Nursing*, 3rd ed. St. Louis: Mosby-Year Book, 136. Reprinted by permission.

release of energy—either an airway popping open or a liquid film breaking. In the past, this type of sound has also been referred to as *rales*. Currently, the preferred nomenclature is fine, medium, and coarse crackles.[11]

Fine crackles can be simulated by rubbing together a lock of hair. These sounds commonly originate in the alveoli in the dependent lobes of the lung and are usually heard at the end of inspiration. Frequently heard in the first few hours after birth, fine crackles are also associated with respiratory distress syndrome (RDS) and bronchopulmonary dysplasia (BPD).

Medium crackles can be compared to the fizz of a carbonated drink. Believed to originate in the bronchioles, these sounds are associated with the passage of air through sticky surfaces, such as those found with pneumonia, pulmonary congestion, or transient tachypnea of the newborn (TTN).

Coarse crackles are loud and bubbly. These sounds are associated with significant accumulations of mucus or fluid in the larger airways.

Rhonchi

When distinguished from wheezes, rhonchi are described as lower in pitch and more musical in quality than crackles. Rhonchi are seldom described in the neonate but may be heard when secretions or aspirated foreign matter is present in the large airways.[12]

Wheezes

Also referred to as high-pitched rhonchi, wheezes may be heard on inspiration or expiration but are usually louder on expiration. Seldom heard in the newborn, wheezes may be audible in the infant with BPD due to narrowing of the airways or presence of bronchospasm.

Rubs

Rubs may be simulated by holding a cupped hand to the ear and rubbing a finger over the cupped hand. Rubs are usually associated with inflammation of the pleura; however, in the neonate, this sound is frequently described during mechanical ventilation.

Stridor

Stridor is a high-pitched, hoarse sound produced during inspiration or expiration at the larynx or upper airways. This sound in a newborn indicates a partial obstruction of the airway and should be investigated promptly. Stridor may also be heard postextubation in infants with edema of the upper airway.

TABLE 6-4 ▲ Adventitious Breath Sounds

Sound/Characteristics	Simulation	Pictorial Findings
Crackles: discrete, noncontinuous sounds, sudden energy release		
Fine crackles (rales): high-pitched, discrete, noncontinuous crackling sounds heard during end of inspiration (indicates inflammation or congestion) (RDS)	Lock of hair	
Medium crackles (rales): lower, moister sound heard during mid-stage of inspiration; not cleared by a cough (edema, pneumonia)	Fizzy drink	
Course crackles (rales): loud, bubbly noise heard during inspiration; not cleared by a cough		
Rhonchi: loud, low, coarse sound like a snore heard at any point of inspiration or expiration; coughing may clear sound (usually means mucus or foreign body in trachea or large bronchi)		
Wheeze: musical noise sounding like a squeak; may be heard during inspiration or expiration; usually louder during expiration (BPD)		
Pleural friction rub: dry rubbing or grating sound, usually due to inflammation of pleural surfaces; heard during inspiration or expiration; loudest over lower lateral anterior surface (mechanical ventilation in RDS)	Rubbing cupped hand	

Adapted from: Thompson JM, et al. 1993. *Mosby's Manual of Clinical Nursing*, 3rd ed. St. Louis: Mosby-Year Book, 137. Reprinted by permission.

Table 6-4 summarizes adventitious breath sounds.

Bowel Sounds

Bowel sounds are occasionally auscultated over the lung fields. These may be referred sounds transmitted from the abdomen. If these sounds persist over the lung fields, especially on the left side, diaphragmatic hernia should be considered.

PERCUSSION

The small size of the neonatal chest relative to the examiner's hands makes percussion of limited value as a part of the neonatal physical examination. The infant's chest is normally hyper-resonant due to the thin chest wall. The experienced examiner may find percussion useful, however, in distinguishing between air and fluid or solid tissue in cases where the infant is in distress and a pneumothorax, pleural effusion, or diaphragmatic hernia is suspected.

The technique for percussion involves placing one finger firmly against the chest wall and tapping that finger with the index finger of the other hand. A change in resonance indicates a change in the consistency of the underlying tissue.

PALPATION

After a thorough inspection of the chest, auscultation of breath sounds, and percussion if necessary, the examiner next palpates certain areas of the infant's chest.

CLAVICLE

Palpate the entire length of the clavicles. Suspect fracture if crepitus, swelling, or both are present.

BREAST TISSUE

As indicated in the discussion of inspection, the breast buds should be gently palpated to determine the presence of hypertrophy, fissures, secretions, or masses.

TABLE 6-5 ▲ Common Findings and their Possible Causes in Infants Receiving Mechanical Ventilation

Finding	Possible Cause
Absence of air entry	Pneumothorax Blocked endotracheal tube (ETT) Accidental extubation Space-occupying lesion
Decreased or unequal air entry	Atelectasis Pneumothorax Intubation of right bronchus
Asymmetric chest movement	Pneumothorax Intubation of right bronchus
Increased chest excursion	Change in compliance resulting in overventilation
Decreased chest excursion	Underventilation Blocked ETT Accidental extubation Air leak

STERNUM AND RIBS

Palpate the sternum and the ribs for crepitus or masses. Crepitus may indicate subcutaneous air from an underlying pulmonary air leak. A lump or mass should be investigated for the presence of an underlying fracture. The tip of the xiphoid process often protrudes anteriorly and may be movable with slight pressure.

OVERALL STRUCTURE

The cartilages should be palpated to assess for hypertrophy. The costal cartilages enlarge in rickets and can be palpated as a series of small lumps down the side of the sternum. This phenomenon is known as the "rachitic rosary."

TRANSILLUMINATION

Transillumination is a useful adjunct to physical examination when a pneumothorax is suspected. A high-intensity fiberoptic light source is placed perpendicular to the neonate's chest. While moving the light source back and forth from side to side, compare the amount of transillumination between left and right and upper and lower aspects of the chest. In a darkened room, air pockets will present with hyperlucency or a lanternlike glow.[6,13]

Subcutaneous edema or air may result in a false positive reading. Chest wall edema, dark skin, tape, and equipment may obscure transillumination and result in a false negative finding.[14] Diagnoses obtained by transillumination should be confirmed by chest x-ray.

ASSESSMENT DURING MECHANICAL VENTILATION

CONVENTIONAL VENTILATION

The use of mechanical ventilation necessitates increased vigilance in all aspects of physical assessment. Particular attention should be given to assessing the adequacy and symmetry of chest expansion and to the auscultation of breath sounds. Care should be taken to eliminate water in the ventilator tubings before assessing chest sounds because gas bubbling through water produces referred sounds.

Breath sounds may be altered by the presence of an endotracheal tube, which effectively narrows the neonate's airway, and by the flow of gases from the ventilator, which may increase turbulence. Wheezes and rubs are more commonly heard in these cases. Harsh or sandpaper breath sounds are often described in infants receiving mechanical ventilation for RDS. These sounds may result from the forced opening of atelectatic alveoli. Harsh breath sounds may also result from air leaking around the endotracheal tube. Listening with the stethoscope over the infant's mouth may be useful in differentiating sounds produced at the larynx from those produced in the chest.

Table 6-5 outlines some common concerns in the neonate receiving mechanical ventilation.

HIGH-FREQUENCY VENTILATION

High-frequency ventilation techniques require several alterations in the traditional approach to physical assessment of the chest and lungs. The rapid rates used in high-frequency ventilation cause the infant to shake or vibrate, making it impractical to count respiratory rates. Many infants on high-frequency ventilation will be apneic; however, spontaneous respirations that do occur can be recorded in the usual fashion.

The chest should be both observed and palpated to assess the symmetry and quality of vibrations. Excessive movement of the chest or abdomen may indicate overventilation. Decreased or asymmetric movement may indicate complications such as air leak or airway obstruction.

Breath sounds during high-frequency ventilation will be high pitched, with a humming or jackhammer quality. Auscultation should be performed to assess changes in the pitch or quality of sound. Higher pitched or musical sounds may indicate the presence of secretions. Decreases in pitch may indicate the presence of a pneumothorax. Traditional breath sounds may be assessed during periods of manual ventilation or with sighs given during oscillation.

SUMMARY

The respiratory system undergoes rapid and significant changes during the transition to extrauterine life. These changes leave the lungs vulnerable to both transient and more life-threatening maladaptations. Careful scrutiny of the respiratory system is required to identify potential problems for treatment. Findings from the physical examination of the chest and lungs form the basis for further investigations. The findings should be documented using standard terms and reference points to permit comparison of findings with subsequent assessments.

REFERENCES

1. Seidel HM, et al. 1991. *Mosby's Guide to Physical Examination.* St. Louis: Mosby-Year Book, 293–295.
2. Hoekelman RA. 1991. The physical examination of infants and children. In *A Guide to Physical Examination,* Bates B, ed. Philadelphia: JB Lippincott, 606,607.
3. Turner B. 1991. Nursing procedures. In *Acute Respiratory Care of the Neonate,* Nugent J, ed. Petaluma, California: NICU Ink, 76.
4. Silverman WA, and Andersen DH. 1956. A controlled clinical trial of water mist on obstructive respiratory signs, death rate, and necropsy findings among premature infants. *Pediatrics* 17(1): 1–10.
5. Kenner CA. 1992. *Nurses Clinical Guide: Neonatal Care.* Springhouse, Pennsylvania: Springhouse, 40.
6. Scanlon JW, et al. 1979. *A System of Newborn Physical Examination.* Baltimore: University Park Press, 61, 64.
7. Alexander MM, and Brown MS. 1979. *Pediatric History Taking and Physical Diagnosis for Nurses,* 2nd ed. New York: McGraw-Hill, 164.
8. Goodman RM, and Gorlin RJ. 1983. *The Malformed Infant and Child.* New York: Oxford University Press, 128.
9. Nelson NM. 1985. *Current Therapies in Neonatal-Perinatal Medicine.* St. Louis: Mosby-Year Book, 265.
10. Christenson JC. 1992. Respiratory syncytial viral infection in the young infant: New developments in treatment and prevention. *Neonatal Pharmacology Quarterly* 1(1): 30–46.
11. Loudon RG. 1987. The lung exam. *Clinics in Chest Medicine* 8(2): 265–272.
12. Aloan CA. 1987. *Respiratory Care of the Newborn: A Clinical Manual.* Philadelphia: JB Lippincott, 56–59.
13. Brown-Gregory SW. 1987. Air leak syndromes. *Neonatal Network* 5(5): 40–46.
14. Fletcher MA, and MacDonald MG. 1993. *Atlas of Procedures in Neonatology.* Philadelphia: JB Lippincott, 313.

BIBLIOGRAPHY

- Bowers AC, and Thompson JM. 1992. *Clinical Manual of Health Assessment.* St. Louis: Mosby-Year Book, 226–262.
- Jarvis C. 1992. *Physical Examination and Health Assessment.* Philadelphia: WB Saunders.
- Karp TB, et al. 1986. High-frequency jet ventilation: A neonatal nursing perspective. *Neonatal Network* 4(5): 42–49.
- Nugent J, ed. 1991. *Acute Respiratory Care of the Neonate.* Petaluma, California: NICU Ink.
- Seidel HM, Rosenstein BJ, and Pathak A. 1992. *Primary Care of the Newborn.* St. Louis: Mosby-Year Book.

7 Cardiovascular Assessment of the Newborn

Lyn Vargo, RNC, MSN, NNP

Cardiovascular assessment of the newborn requires great skill with the techniques of inspection, palpation, and auscultation. Inspection of the general activity of the neonate, breathing patterns, presence or absence of cyanosis, and activity of the precordium are all important. Palpation of pulses, apical impulse, and thrills is also imperative. Auscultation, however, is the main focus of the cardiovascular exam. Through auscultation, the examiner assesses heart rate, rhythm, regularity, and heart sounds (especially murmurs). When auscultating, a pediatric or neonatal stethoscope with a diaphragm and bell is very helpful. The bell conducts sound without distortion (although it can be difficult to maintain an airtight seal). The bell is useful for low-pitched sounds. If properly sized, the diaphragm maintains its own seal and is useful for high-pitched sounds.

The dynamic properties of the newborn heart make cardiovascular assessment of the neonate challenging. The change from "fetal-placental" to "newborn-lung" circuitry means that the findings of the cardiovascular exam constantly change over the first few hours, days, and weeks of life. Practitioners performing cardiovascular assessments must be aware of these

changes and their timing and incorporate this knowledge into their examinations.

Because changes in ductal flow, decreasing pulmonary vascular resistance, and increasing systemic vascular resistance occur over the first few hours and days of life, cardiovascular assessments ideally should be done shortly after birth, at 6 to 12 hours of age, at one and three days of age, and at regular intervals thereafter. Because this is rarely possible in the normal newborn, it is recommended that, at a minimum, examinations be done shortly after birth, at one day of age, and at regular pediatric office visits thereafter.

REVIEWING MATERNAL, FAMILY, AND BIRTH HISTORIES

The first consideration in a complete cardiovascular assessment is a thorough maternal history. Several maternal conditions can affect the neonate's cardiovascular system. These include maternal diabetes, systemic lupus erythematosus, and a maternal history of congenital heart disease (CHD). Maternal diabetes can increase the risk of CHD in the neonate to three to four times that for the general population.[1] The incidence of CHD in the general

TABLE 7-1 ▲ Maternal Drugs Known To Cause Congenital Heart Defects

Causative Factor	Risk of CHD (Percent)	Defect
Drugs		
Diphenylhydantoin Fetal hydantoin syndrome	10	PS, AS
Trimethadione	50	VSD, TET
Thalidomide	20	TET, Truncus
Lithium	10	Ebstein's anomaly
Alcohol		
Fetal alcohol syndrome	30–40	VSD, ASD

Note: PS, pulmonary stenosis; AS, aortic stenosis; VSD, ventricular septal defect; TET, tetralogy of Fallot; ASD, atrial septal defect.

Adapted from: Garson A Jr, Bricker JT, and McNamara DG. 1990. *The Science and Practice of Pediatric Cardiology*. Philadelphia: Lea & Febiger, 676. Reprinted by permission.

population is 0.8 to 1 percent of all live births.[2] Ventricular septal defects and transposition of the great arteries are common defects seen in infants of diabetic mothers.[3]

Systemic lupus erythematosus in the mother has been shown to increase the incidence of congenital complete atrioventricular (AV) block in the neonate.[4] These infants will present with low resting heart rates, sometimes while *in utero*.

As women with CHD are living longer and reaching childbearing age, new information has become available. It has been documented that there is a 10 to 15 percent risk of CHD in the offspring of mothers with CHD.[3]

Even though only a small percentage of CHD can be related to environmental factors, a history of the pregnancy (especially of the first two months, when the heart is forming) is important. Drugs known to cause heart defects include lithium, phenytoin sodium, and alcohol (Table 7-1). Rubella during early pregnancy is also known to cause CHD, specifically pulmonary branch stenosis and patent ductus arteriosus. In addition, viral infections during the last two weeks of pregnancy may cause acute myocarditis in the neonate.

Due to the influence of genetic factors, family history is an important feature of a cardiovascular assessment. Details about other siblings with CHD should be identified. If one parent is affected or if an older sibling had a specific defect, there is a 1 to 5 percent risk of recurrence.[3] Also, several specific syndromes that might demonstrate dominant or recessive inheritance patterns are associated with specific congenital heart defects (Table 7-2). If any of these syndromes are identified in the family history, the neonatal assessment should be even more rigorous than usual.

Details of the labor and delivery history must be considered during the cardiovascular examination. Knowledge of any causal factors such as perinatal asphyxia, maternal infection, or drugs given to the mother during labor will help the examiner determine whether CHD is a likely explanation for abnormal physical findings.

Finally, birth weight, gestational age, and sex must be taken into consideration. There is an increased incidence of CHD in low birth weight infants, and premature infants have an increased risk of patent ductus arteriosus. Several congenital heart defects are more common in one sex than in the other.

OBSERVING APPEARANCE AND BEHAVIOR

Because of the central role the heart plays, a complete cardiovascular assessment encompasses most of the other systems. The cardiovascular exam cannot be considered in isolation from the neurologic, respiratory, abdominal, and skin examinations.

The initial cardiovascular assessment of the neonate should include general observation of the infant's overall appearance and behavior. A newborn with CHD may exhibit decreased activity and/or appear flaccid. Notation of extracardiac anomalies is important because CHD is associated with such anomalies in approximately 20 percent of infants.[5] Increased incidence of CHD is seen with gastrointestinal anomalies, tracheoesophageal fistulae, renal and urogenital anomalies, and diaphragmatic hernias.

INSPECTING SKIN AND MUCOUS MEMBRANES

The next step in the neonatal cardiovascular exam is inspection of the infant's color. Accurate assessment of skin color depends on the observer's astuteness and on ambient temperature and lighting conditions.[6] A cyanotic Caucasian infant may look pink under bright lighting, and a centrally pink infant may look cyanotic under dim lighting. In a well-lit room, the infant should be centrally pink—that is, not only should his general color appear pink, but his lips, tongue, earlobes, and (in males) scrotum should also appear pink.

POLYCYTHEMIA

Many infants appear pink at rest but become deep red to purplish with crying. This is usually related to polycythemia, a condition found when the infant's central hematocrit is greater than 65 percent. Although polycythemic/plethoric infants may appear cyanotic, as neonates they rarely are. The ruddy or reddish color may be mistaken for cyanosis simply because newborns who have increased amounts of hemoglobin usually have a larger percentage of that hemoglobin unsaturated. This unsaturated hemoglobin masks the satu-

TABLE 7-2 ▲ Congenital Heart Defects Associated with Syndromes

Syndrome	Frequency (Percent)	Type of Defect
Down	40	AV defect, VSD, PDA
Turner	40	Coarc, PS
Trisomy 13	80	VSD
Trisomy 18	90	VSD, PDA, DORV
Williams	90	Supravalvular aor stenosis
Marfan	80	Mit regurg, aor regurg, aor root dil
Pompe disease	100	Cardiomyopathy
VATER	20	VSD, TET
Cerebrohepatorenal		PDA, ± VSD/ASD
Holt Oram	20	ASD
Hurler	40	Cardiomyopathy, AV regurg
Ellis-van Creveld	20	ASD, single atrium, AV defect
Carpenter		Varies
Cornelia de Lange		Varies
Noonan	40	PS, ASD
Laurence Moon Biedl		TET
XXXXX		PDA
XXXXY		PDA
CHARGE association		TET, DORV, AV defect
Di George	80	Truncus, TET

Note: XXXXX, tentasomy X syndrome; XXXXY, Kleinfelter-like syndrome; AV, atrioventricular; PDA, patent ductus arteriosus; VSD, ventricular septal defect; coarc, coarctation of the aorta; PS, pulmonic stenosis; DORV, double outlet right ventricle; aor, aortic; mit, mitral; regurg, regurgitation; dil, dilitation; TET, tetralogy of Fallot; ASD, atrial septal defect.

Adapted from: Fanaroff A, and Martin RJ. 1992. *Neonatal-Perinatal Medicine.* St. Louis: Mosby-Year Book, 885. Reprinted by permission.

rated hemoglobin, and the infants appear purplish in color.

CYANOSIS

Central cyanosis refers to the bluish color of the skin, lips, tongue, earlobes, scrotum (in males), and nail beds seen in the neonate with significant arterial oxygen desaturation. Central cyanosis becomes visible when there are at least 5 gms of hemoglobin per 100 ml of blood not bound to oxygen.[7] Central cyanosis must be differentiated from peripheral cyanosis (acrocyanosis), which is blue color in the hands and feet, and circumoral cyanosis, which is blue color around the mouth. Peripheral cyanosis is normal in newborns until about two days of

FIGURE 7-1 ▲ Radial and brachial pulses.

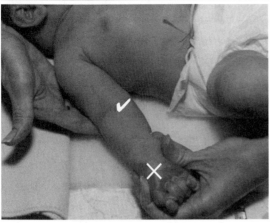

Demonstrates the location of radial pulse (✕), palpable on the flexor surface of the wrist just medial to the distal end of the radius. Demonstrates the location of the brachial pulse (✔) in and above the groove of the elbow, medial to the biceps muscle and tendon.

FIGURE 7-2 ▲ Femoral pulses.

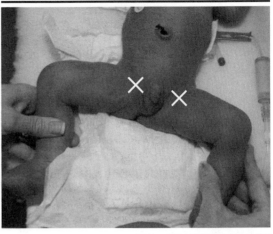

Demonstrates the location of the femoral pulses (✕), palpable just below the inguinal ligament, an equal distance between the pubic tubercle and the anterior superior iliac spine.

age and is thought to be due to vasomotor instability. No treatment is necessary for peripheral cyanosis.

Central cyanosis can be the result of many things: lung disease, sepsis, persistent pulmonary hypertension, or neurologic disease. Cyanosis is also one of the two best indicators of CHD. It is therefore important to carefully assess cyanosis and its response to oxygen. Cyanosis that does not improve upon administration of 100 percent oxygen is most likely due to cardiac causes, as is cyanosis that increases with crying.[7]

PALLOR/MOTTLING/PERFUSION

Pallor and mottling of the skin should also be considered in assessing cardiac status, as should the infant's general overall perfusion. Infants with compromised cardiac status may appear pale due to vasoconstriction and the shunting of blood away from the skin to more vital organs. Mottling may be a sign of cardiogenic shock.

Capillary filling time can give valuable information about the infant's cardiac perfusion to the skin and should be determined by pressing a finger against the infant's skin in both a central and a peripheral area. When blanching is noted, the examiner counts the seconds required for the color to return to the skin. Capillary filling time of greater than three to four seconds is usually considered abnormal.

EDEMA

In the infant, edema is rarely associated with cardiac problems, as it is in older patients. Isolated peripheral edema is a hallmark sign of Turner syndrome, however. Infants with this syndrome show a high incidence of coarctation of the aorta.

OBSERVING BREATHING PATTERNS

Respiratory activity must be observed in relation to the cardiac examination. Respiratory rate and effort should be documented (as addressed in Chapter 6). Signs of respiratory distress—such as grunting, flaring, retractions, tachypnea, and rales—may be signs of congestive heart failure. It is also important to keep in mind that an infant with nonlabored respiratory effort who is cyanotic is most likely cyanotic due to congenital heart disease.

FIGURE 7-3 ▲ Posterior tibial pulse.

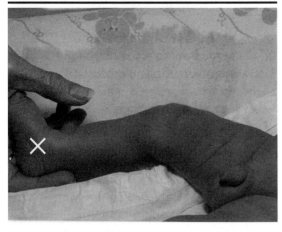

Demonstrates the location of the posterior tibial pulse (X), palpable just behind and slightly below the medial malleolus.

PALPATING PERIPHERAL PULSES

The character of the peripheral pulses should be assessed next. This is best done with the infant quiet. Pulse rate, rhythm, volume, and character should all be examined. Pulses represent an approximate determination of cardiac output. Using the index finger, the axillary, palmar, brachial, radial, femoral, popliteal, posterior tibial, and dorsalis pedis may be palpated (Figures 7-1 through 7-4). (Note that the dorsalis pedis may not be felt in newborns; this is considered normal.)

PULSE RATE

On initial palpation, the pulse rate should be noted. The significance of rate is discussed later in this chapter. After determining the rate, any irregularities in rhythm or skipped beats should be documented. A pulse deficit (a difference between the heart rate counted with a pulse and that counted by auscultation) is frequently seen with ectopic rhythms.

PULSE VOLUME/CHARACTER

Probably the most important determinations in neonatal pulse evaluation are those assessing volume and character. Volume of peripheral

FIGURE 7-4 ▲ Dorsalis pedis pulse.

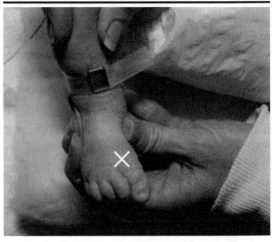

Demonstrates the location of the dorsalis pedis pulse (X), palpable on the dorsum of the foot by following an imaginary line that follows the groove between the first and second toes.

pulses is assessed on a scale of 0 to +4, with +4 being the strongest and 0 representing an absent or nonpalpable pulse (Table 7-3).[8] At a minimum, the femoral and brachial pulses should be palpated bilaterally, and then one femoral and the right brachial should be palpated simultaneously. (The right brachial should be palpated instead of the left because the right subclavian artery is always preductal, but the left subclavian artery may or may not be preductal.) Absent or weak femoral pulses—especially in comparison to the right brachial pulse—are abnormal and may indicate

TABLE 7-3 ▲ Grading of Pulses

Grade	Description
0	Not palpable
+1	Difficult to palpate, thready, weak, easily obliterated with pressure
+2	Difficult to palpate, may be obliterated with pressure
+3	Easy to palpate, not easily obliterated with pressure (normal)
+4	Strong, bounding, not obliterated with pressure

From: Wong DL. 1995. *Whaley & Wong's Nursing Care of Infants and Children,* 5th ed. St. Louis: Mosby-Year Book, 229. Reprinted by permission.

FIGURE 7-5 ▲ **Position of the heart within the chest cavity and base and apex of the heart.**

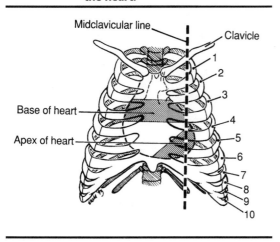

FIGURE 7-6 ▲ **Areas of cardiac inspection and palpation.**

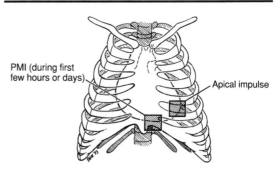

decreased aortic blood flow like that seen with coarctation of the aorta, aortic stenosis, and hypoplastic left heart syndrome.

Bounding pulses in any extremity should be noted. Bounding pulses are usually present with patent ductus arteriosus and other aortic-runoff lesions (truncus arteriosus, systemic arteriovenous fistula). Normal premature infants have prominent peripheral pulses, but strong palmar or digital pulses indicate a wide pulse pressure as that seen with patent ductus arteriosus.[9] Weak or absent peripheral pulses occur in the presence of low cardiac output from any cause, especially left heart obstructive lesions.

INSPECTING AND PALPATING THE CHEST

PRECORDIUM

In the cardiac exam, assessment of the chest should begin with inspection of the precordium, the area on the anterior chest under which the heart lies (Figure 7-5). Generally, except during the first few hours of life, the precordium of a full-term neonate should be quiet. Premature infants may have an active precordium due to their decreased subcutaneous tissue. When seen in the full-term neonate after the first hours of life, a bounding precordium is characteristic of heart disease, typically defects with increased ventricular volume work such as left-to-right shunt lesions (patent ductus arteriosus or ventricular septal defect).

APICAL IMPULSE

After general assessment of the precordium, the examiner should inspect for position and character of the apical impulse, the forward thrust of the left ventricle during systole. The apical impulse is usually seen in the neonate in the fourth intercostal space, either at or to the left of the midclavicular line (Figure 7-6). It can be further localized and examined with light palpation using the fingertips. An apical impulse placed downward and to the left suggests left ventricular dilatation. A very sharp apical impulse is found with high cardiac output or left ventricular hypertrophy.

The point of maximum impulse (PMI) and the apical impulse are usually the same, but this is not always true in neonates during the first few hours or days of life. During that time, an impulse stronger than the apical impulse can be found in the fifth intercostal space at the lower sternal border or even substernally. This then represents the PMI and is normal because of the right ventricular predominance found in the newborn (Figure 7-6). The PMI or the apical impulse may be displaced in several situations,

FIGURE 7-7 ▲ Four auscultatory areas of the heart.

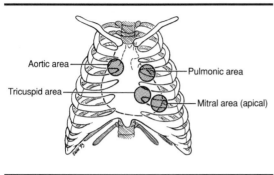

FIGURE 7-7 ▲ Four auscultatory areas of the heart.

Aortic area

Pulmonic area

Tricuspid area

Mitral area (apical)

such as dextrocardia, tension pneumothoraces, and diaphragmatic hernias.

HEAVES, TAPS, AND THRILLS

Further palpation of the precordium will yield other valuable information. Heaves, taps, and thrills can all be palpated. These findings are usually best felt by palpating with the portion of the palm at the base of the fingers rather than with the fingertips. This is because certain parts of the hand are more discriminatory than others for specific sensations. Vibratory sensations are best felt with the ulnar surface of the hand.

A heave (or lift) is a point of maximum impulse that is slow rising and diffuse. Heaves are associated with ventricular dilatation or volume overload.

A sharp, well-localized PMI is called a tap. Taps are usually associated with pressure overload or hypertrophy. A hypertrophied but not dilated right ventricle produces a distinct parasternal tap.[4]

Thrills are low-frequency, palpable murmurs that feel similar to touching a purring cat. In the neonate, thrills are not common. When present, they can provide useful information about cardiac problems. A thrill in the suprasternal notch and upper sternal border may be associated with pulmonary stenosis or tetralogy of Fallot. A thrill in the upper left sternal border noted after pulmonary vascular resis-

tance has fallen may be associated with patent ductus arteriosus.[10]

AUSCULTATING TO ASSESS CARDIOVASCULAR STATUS

Expert auscultation of the neonatal heart requires much practice over time. An experienced mentor can help the fledgling examiner learn to identify and distinguish heart sounds. The neonatal heart should be auscultated with the infant inactive and quiet.

At a minimum, the four traditional auscultatory areas should be examined. These are the aortic area (second intercostal space, right sternal angle), pulmonic area (second intercostal space, left sternal angle), tricuspid area (fourth intercostal space, left sternal angle), and mitral area (fourth intercostal space, left midclavicular line) (Figure 7-7). A more thorough examination is recommended, however. It should include right and left infraclavicular areas, both sides of the back, the right anterior chest, the anterior fontanel (examining for cerebral arteriovenous fistulas), and the liver (examining for hepatic arteriovenous fistulas).

HEART RATE

Heart rate should be auscultated first and counted. A full-term neonate's heart rate at rest should be 80–160 beats per minute (bpm). (Some healthy neonates in deep sleep will have heart rates as low as 70 bpm.) Premature infants have a slightly higher mean heart rate than that seen in term infants.

Sinus bradycardia, or a heart rate less than normal for age (usually less than 80 bpm) is a common transient finding in the full-term and premature infant. This is due to the predominance of the parasympathetic system. Any stimulus—such as yawning, stooling, or suctioning—may result in vagal stimulation and subsequent bradycardia. These episodes are usually transient, require no treatment, and are self-correcting. Some episodes, especially in

FIGURE 7-8 ▲ EKG rhythm strip of infant with supraventricular tachycardia with a ventricular rate of approximately 300 bpm.

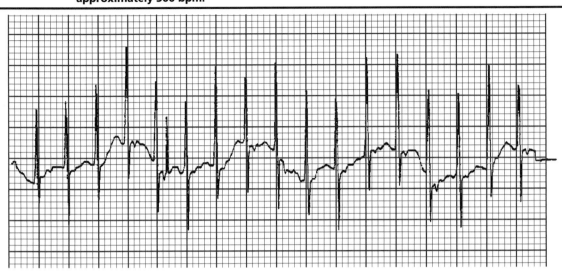

premature infants, may require stimulation or treatment of the underlying cause, such as treatment for apnea of prematurity with methylxanthines.

Sinus tachycardia is defined as a heart rate greater than normal for age (usually greater than 180–200 bpm). It is the most common form of rapid heart rate in the neonate.[11] It normally occurs with any stimulus—such as crying, feeding, fever, or activity—that causes increased demands on the heart. Normally, with removal of the stimulus, the heart rate slowly returns to baseline. Sinus tachycardia rarely requires treatment.

Variation in the heart rate is the norm among neonates and is seen as a positive sign of the infant's ability to react to the environment.[12] Infants who do not respond to stimuli are clearly abnormal and should be observed closely.

Although sinus tachycardia with rates up to 200 bpm can be tolerated by the neonate, heart rates greater than 200 bpm or supraventricular tachycardia (SVT) cannot. SVT encompasses paroxysmal atrial tachycardia and atrial flutter and fibrillation. Figure 7-8 is a rhythm strip of SVT. In the neonate, SVT represents a medical emergency and requires immediate intervention. At such rapid heart rates, cardiac output is extremely compromised due to short diastolic filling time. Without treatment, decreased cardiac output will cause congestive heart failure within 48 hours and possibly death. Treatment for SVT depends on the cause, but the condition may respond to cardioversion, drugs, or vagal stimulation (such as applying a cold washcloth or ice to the face).

CARDIAC RHYTHM AND REGULARITY

After assessing heart rate, evaluate cardiac rhythm and regularity. Carefully listen to the rhythm of the heart sounds and determine if there is any irregularity. Noting patterns and frequencies of the irregularity helps identify the type of arrhythmia. Whenever an arrhythmia is suspected, an EKG and/or continuous heart monitoring is indicated to establish a diagnosis. Arrhythmias are not uncommon in the neonate. Fortunately, they are usually benign and require no treatment. Those most commonly found in the neonate include the following:

▶ *Sinus arrhythmia.* A very common, normal variant in most newborns, this is characterized by irregularity of the R-R interval, with an otherwise normal cardiac cycle. No treatment is required for this rhythm.

▶ *Premature atrial beats.* This is an early beat arising from supraventricular focus. Ventricular conduction is usually normal. It is usually not serious and may be common in 30 percent of healthy term and premature infants. It is often seen with CHD, sepsis, hypoxia, maternal caffeine use, and severe respiratory distress.[12] If significant, the underlying cause may require treatment, but these beats are usually well tolerated.

▶ *Premature ventricular beats.* With this early beat arising from an irritable ventricular focus, ventricular conduction will be abnormal, giving rise to a wide and bizarre QRS complex. It may be due to hypoxia, irritation by an invasive catheter or surgical procedure, or CHD. Treatment is unnecessary if the phenomenon is infrequent.

HEART SOUNDS

Traditional cardiac physiology teaches that the first heart sound (S1) is produced by closure of the mitral and tricuspid valves, and the second heart sound (S2) is produced by closure of the aortic and pulmonic valves. More recent literature debates this, however, and the true origin of heart sounds remains unclear. Despite this uncertainty, the traditional concept can be helpful in conceptualizing and learning to recognize heart sounds and therefore continues to be used.[3]

S1

The first heart sound, if thought of as representing closure of the mitral and tricuspid valves at the onset of ventricular systole, should be heard loudest at the apex of the heart. (See Figure 7-5 for location of the apex and base of the heart.) Indeed, S1 is best heard at the mitral or tricuspid area. The first heart sound is usually loud at birth, decreasing in intensity during the first 48 hours of life. Also, any factor that increases cardiac output also increases the intensity of S1.

Splitting is defined as hearing two distinct components of a heart sound. It is caused by the asynchronous closure of the two valves that create the heart sound. The neonate's rapid heart rate usually makes splitting difficult to distinguish. Although some studies have documented splitting of S1 in the newborn, splitting is not commonly heard; S1 is usually described as being single.

S2

The second heart sound, if thought of as representing closure of the aortic and pulmonic valves, should be heard loudest at the base of the heart. Indeed, S2 is best heard at the aortic or pulmonic area. S2 is usually single at birth, but it is split in two-thirds of infants by 16 hours of age and in 80 percent of infants by 48 hours of age.[3] With practice, the trained examiner should be able to recognize the splitting of S2 despite the infant's rapid heart rate.

Wide splitting of the heart sound S2 should be considered abnormal in newborns. It can occur with pulmonary stenosis, Ebstein's anomaly, total anomalous pulmonary venous return, and tetralogy of Fallot.[13]

S3

In addition to S1 and S2, extra heart sounds can potentially be heard in the neonate. Again, due to the infant's rapid rate, they may be difficult to distinguish. A third heart sound (S3) can occasionally be heard in infancy; if present, it is best heard at the apex of the heart during early diastole. S3 most often signifies rapid or increased flow across the atrioventricular valves (rapid ventricular filling) and is commonly heard in premature infants with patent ductus arteriosus. Rarely is it heard in the newborn with overt congestive heart failure.[13]

S4

A fourth heart sound (S4) should rarely be heard in neonates. If present, it is heard at the apex of the heart. An S4 is almost always pathologic and is seen with conditions characterized by decreased compliance (especially cardiomyopathy).

Ejection Clicks

Ejection clicks (snappy, high-frequency sounds) can, if they are present, best be heard just after the first heart sound. Ejection clicks occur at the time of ventricular ejection and resemble in timing, but not in quality, a widely split first heart sound. Ejection clicks are commonly heard during the first 24 hours of life and are usually normal during that time. Anytime after the first 24 hours of life, ejection clicks are always considered abnormal. The most frequent findings associated with these clicks are aortic or pulmonic stenosis, truncus arteriosus, or tetralogy of Fallot (often with pulmonary atresia).[9]

Murmurs

Murmurs are caused by turbulent blood flow. They are often described as prolonged heart sounds. There are two kinds of murmurs: innocent and pathologic. Pathologic murmurs are due to underlying cardiovascular disease; innocent murmurs are not.

Whenever an examiner detects a murmur, the question of its origin arises. The murmur must therefore be fully evaluated as to its timing, location, intensity, radiation, quality, and pitch. The neonate's age in hours and days is also especially significant because of the dynamic properties of the newborn heart. Putting all this information together with the other findings of the physical examination should help the examiner determine the significance of the murmur.

The *timing* of the murmur is the first quality the examiner must listen for. Does it occur in systole or diastole? Is it early, mid, or late in systole or diastole? Does it occur throughout systole (holosystolic or pansystolic) or during midsystolic ejection? Continuous murmurs are heard through both systole and diastole.

Loudness, or intensity, of the murmur should be determined next. Murmurs are graded from I to VI, as follows:

Grade I: Barely audible, audible only after a period of careful auscultation

Grade II: Soft, but audible immediately

Grade III: Of moderate intensity (but not associated with a thrill)

Grade IV: Louder (may be associated with a thrill)

Grade V: Very loud, can be heard with the stethoscope rim barely on the chest (may be associated with a thrill)

Grade VI: Extremely loud, can be heard with the stethoscope just slightly removed from the chest (may be associated with a thrill)

Sometimes the intensity of a murmur will change from exam to exam. This may be due to changing pulmonary vascular resistance or to anything else that changes the status of cardiac output, such as anemia, activity, or changing ventilatory requirements.

Location of the maximum intensity of the murmur is another important feature to evaluate. Location is usually described in terms of the interspace and the midsternal, midclavicular, or axillary lines (Figure 6-3) because the anatomic site of most murmurs is usually found at the location below where they are best heard. Describing murmurs in terms of aortic, pulmonary, tricuspid, or mitral areas is not recommended in neonates because malposition of valves and vessels may be found in CHD.

Other locations where a murmur is heard should also be documented. This is described as *radiation* or transmission of the murmur. Radiation from the normally positioned pulmonary outflow tract is to the left upper back;

radiation from the normally positioned aortic outflow tract is to the carotid arteries.

Quality and *pitch* of the murmur are the final two features that should be assessed. Pitch is described as high, medium, or low. High-pitched murmurs occur when there is turbulence from a high-pressure to a low-pressure area.[9] An example of this is aortic or mitral insufficiency. Low-pitched murmurs occur when there is a low pressure difference in the turbulent flow. An example of this is mitral stenosis. Identifying the quality of a murmur (terms include harsh, rumbling, or musical) also helps to describe it.

Innocent murmurs. As stated earlier, there are two types of murmurs, innocent and pathologic. During the first 48 hours of life, many normal newborns have murmurs, the majority of which are innocent. They are usually associated with the decreasing pulmonary vascular resistance occurring at this time and with the gradual closure of the patent ductus arteriosus. Innocent murmurs are most often Grade I or II, are associated with normal EKG and chest x-ray findings, are usually systolic murmurs, and are not associated with any symptoms. Some of the more common innocent murmurs heard during the first 48 hours of life include the following:

▶ *Systolic ejection murmur.* Most common innocent murmur (heard in up to 56 percent of newborns).[9] Usually Grade I–II/VI. Best heard along the mid- and upper left sternal border and described as vibratory. Presents within the first day of life and may last as long as one week. Most likely due to the significant increase in flow across the pulmonary valve associated with rapidly decreasing pulmonary vascular resistance.[13]

▶ *Continuous systolic or crescendo systolic murmur.* Occurs in up to 15 percent of normal infants. Intensity is usually Grade I–II/VI. Best heard in upper left sternal border. Pre-

sents within the first eight hours of life. Caused by the transient left-to-right flow through the ductus arteriosus during the period when pulmonary vascular resistance is falling but ductal closure has not yet been accomplished.[13]

▶ *Early soft midsystolic ejection murmur.* Also called peripheral pulmonic stenosis or pulmonary branch murmur. Heard often in newborns, especially premature infants. Intensity is usually Grade I–II/VI and is medium to high pitched. Best heard in upper left sternal border, with wide radiation to both lung fields and back. Presents within the first week or two of life. Generally disappears by one to eight weeks of age.[14] Due to turbulence produced at the relatively acute angle of the bifurcation of the pulmonary artery.[15]

Pathologic murmurs. Pathologic murmurs in the neonate occur at varying times, depending on the anatomic abnormality causing them and on normal changes associated with transitional circulation. Many specific defects do not present with a murmur until three days, one week, or four to six weeks of age, when the pulmonary vascular resistance has fallen sufficiently. Atrial septal defects sometimes do not present until one year of age. The absence of a murmur does not rule out the potential for serious CHD. As many as 20 percent of infants who died from congenital heart defects during the first month of life did not have heart murmurs.[13] In fact, the absence of a murmur may be an ominous sign in both acyanotic and ductal-dependent lesions.

The examiner should approach all murmurs cautiously. Soft murmurs heard in otherwise asymptomatic infants can be observed carefully by the experienced practitioner for the first 48 hours of life. But any murmur that persists beyond this time, is louder than a Grade I or II, or occurs in a symptomatic neonate requires

FIGURE 7-9 ▲ Diagram showing how to select accurate BP cuff size.

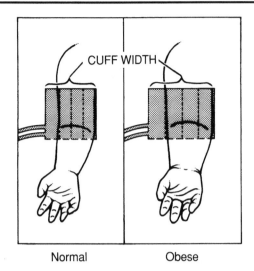

CUFF WIDTH

Normal   Obese

The end of the cuff is at the top. Note that the end is 20–25% wider than the diameter of the limb being measured.

further investigation. The cardiovascular workup should include a chest x-ray, an EKG, an echocardiogram, and a consultation with a cardiologist.

Pathologic murmurs are more difficult to categorize than innocent murmurs. The following commonly occur in the immediate neonatal period:

▶ *Loud systolic ejection murmur.* Usually Grade II or III. Appears within hours of birth and is almost always the result of aortic or pulmonary stenosis or coarctation of the aorta.

▶ *Continuous murmur.* Appears in one-third of premature infants with a patent ductus arteriosus. This type of murmur is also heard in infants with arteriovenous fistulas regardless of gestational age.

In addition, pathologic systolic murmurs may occasionally be heard with mitral and tricuspid insufficiency of various causes (especially with left ventricular failure in infants with critical left ventricular outlet obstruction and tetralogy of Fallot). Pathologic murmurs associated with ventricular septal defect and patent duc-

tus arteriosus in full-term neonates do not present until pulmonary vascular resistance has fallen—often not until after discharge from the nursery or at several weeks of age.

PALPATING THE LIVER

Palpation of the liver (described in Chapter 8) is a significant part of the cardiovascular assessment. The liver becomes engorged when central venous pressure increases. A liver located more than 3 cm below the right costal margin (RCM) is a good indicator of right-sided heart failure in a term infant.

EVALUATING BLOOD PRESSURE

Evaluation of the neonate's blood pressure (BP) should be done with the infant quiet. This assessment should be left until the end of the examination because the pressure of the cuff inflating may make the infant cry. Systemic BP should be measured in every neonate.

The proper size cuff must be used when obtaining BP. Indeed, the most frequent reason for a hypertensive BP is the use of a BP cuff that is too small for the infant. Using limb length as the sole criterion for establishing cuff size for BP monitoring can be misleading. This method does not take into consideration large-for-gestational-age infants with excessive subcutaneous fat. These infants will show falsely elevated BPs if cuff size is inappropriate. It is therefore recommended that the cuff width (not the cuff length) should be 20–25 percent wider than the diameter of the limb being measured (Figure 7-9). In addition, the inflatable bladder should entirely encircle the extremity without overlapping.[8]

MONITORING METHODS

There are several methods for monitoring systemic BP in neonates: flush, palpation, ultrasound doppler, and oscillometric measurements. BP obtained by auscultation is not appropriate for neonates.

FIGURE 7-10 ▲ Systolic, diastolic, mean, and pulse pressures for newborns (based on birth weight) during the first 12 hours of life.

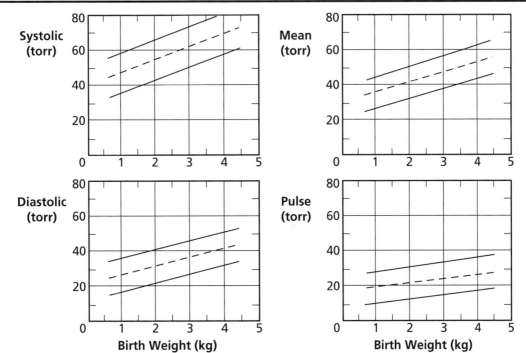

Linear regressions (broken lines) and 95 percent confidence limits (solid lines) of systolic (top left) and diastolic (bottom left) aortic blood pressures and mean pressure (top right) and pulse pressure (bottom right) on birth weight in healthy newborn infants during the first 12 hours after birth.

Adapted from: Versmold HT, et al. 1981. Aortic blood pressure during the first 12 hours of life in infants 610 to 4,220 grams. *Pediatrics* 67(5): 611. Reprinted by permission.

Flush Method

The flush method, now rarely used, is simple to do and can be useful in certain situations. With this method, the hand or foot is squeezed to blanch it, and the BP cuff is rapidly inflated. The pressure in the cuff is released, and the pressure point at which the extremity suddenly flushes is documented. The pressure obtained by this method represents the mean arterial pressure.

Palpation

BP can also be obtained by palpatory methods in infants. While releasing the pressure in the cuff, the examiner palpates the pulse distal to the cuff. The pressure point at which the pulse reappears upon deflation approximates the systolic blood pressure.

Ultrasonic Doppler

A more accurate method, similar to the palpatory method of BP measurement, is done with an ultrasonic doppler. A transducer is placed over the artery distal to the BP cuff after a conductive gel is applied, and an audible pulse is listened for as the BP cuff is deflated. The pressure point at which the pulse is heard is documented. This method also approximates the systolic BP.

Oscillometric Measurement

Most recently, centers have begun using oscillometric methods to document BP in neonates. Systolic, diastolic, mean arterial BP, and heart rate are all digitally recorded using special cuffs and these systems. These systems have been found to be fairly reliable, with the mean arterial BP being the most accurate.

Catheter

Finally, indwelling arterial catheters also provide systolic and diastolic blood pressures. These catheters provide minute-by-minute readings of blood pressure values. Accuracy of this type of monitoring requires a knowledge of the system and the variables that will affect it. Some of these variables include transducer position, air bubbles in the system, and equipment calibration.

Normal Values

Blood pressure norms for newborns vary, depending on body weight and postnatal age. In the first few hours of life, BP can be significantly affected by type of delivery, birth asphyxia, and placental transfusion. The newborn's initial BP decreases during the first 3 to 4 hours of life, presumably due to fluid shifts into and out of the vascular space.[13] The systolic pressure reaches a minimum at 3 to 4 hours of age and then gradually increases to reach a plateau at about four to six days of age to a level closer to the initial postpartum level.[16] Blood pressures in neonates are also affected by activity, temperature, and behavioral state. Figure 7-10 documents confidence limits for newborns (based on birth weight) during the first 12 hours of life.

Whenever there is any concern of CHD, there are difficulties obtaining blood pressures, a murmur is heard, or there is an absence of femoral pulses on the physical exam, four extremity blood pressures must be obtained. Pressures obtained in the leg are often slightly higher than those in the arm, but they can be equal or slightly lower. A systolic blood pressure in the upper extremities greater than 20 mmHg higher than that in the lower extremities strongly suggests coarctation of the aorta.[13] This pressure difference can sometimes be masked in the left arm by a patent ductus arteriosus that allows blood to pass around the restricted area; therefore, the right arm will yield the most valuable information because it is always preductal.

In addition to systolic, diastolic, and mean BP readings, the pulse pressure can provide valuable information. The pulse pressure is defined as the difference between the systolic and the diastolic blood pressures. Averages for term neonates are between 25 and 30 mmHg; for premature infants, they are between 15 and 25 mmHg.[13] Wide pulse pressures may be a sign of a large aortic runoff, as seen with patent ductus arteriosus. Narrow pulse pressures are documented in neonates with peripheral vasoconstriction, heart failure, or low cardiac output.

Summary

Properly executed, the cardiovascular assessment provides a great deal of information about the overall health of the newborn, as well as valuable information about congenital heart defects that might be present. Time, patience, and experience with inspection, palpation, and auscultation are all necessary to develop the skills essential to a thorough cardiac examination.

References

1. Nora JJ, and Nora AH. 1978. The evolution of specific genetic and environmental counseling in CHD. *Circulation* 57(2): 205–213.
2. Kannell WB, and Thom TJ. 1994. Incidence, prevalence and mortality of cardiovascular diseases. In *The Heart, Arteries and Veins*, Schlant RC, et al., eds. New York: McGraw-Hill, 185–197.
3. Duff DF, and McNamara DG. 1990. History and physical examination of the cardiovascular system. In *Science and Practice of Pediatric Cardiology*, Garson A, et al., eds. Philadelphia: Lea & Febiger, 671–690.
4. Hull D, Binns BA, and Joyce D. 1966. Congenital heart block and widespread fibrosis due to maternal lupus erythematosus. *Archives of Disease in Childhood* 41(220): 688–690.
5. Hazinski MF. 1983. Congenital heart disease in the neonate. Part I: Epidemiology, cardiac development, and fetal circulation. *Neonatal Network* 1(4): 29–43.
6. Hazinski MF. 1984. Congenital heart disease in the neonate. Part VII: Common congenital heart defects producing hypoxemia and cyanosis. *Neonatal Network* 2(6): 36–51.

7. Hazinski MF. 1983. Congenital heart disease in the neonate. Part IV: Cyanotic heart disease. *Neonatal Network* 2(1): 12–24.

8. Monett ZJ, and Moynihan PJ. 1991. Cardiovascular assessment of the neonatal heart. *Journal of Perinatal and Neonatal Nursing* 5(2): 50–59.

9. Moller JH. 1990. Physical examination. In *Fetal, Neonatal, and Infant Cardiac Disease.* Moller JH, et al., eds. Norwalk, Connecticut: Appleton & Lange, 167–177.

10. Fanaroff AA, and Martin RJ. 1992. The cardiovascular system. In *Neonatal-Perinatal Medicine: Diseases of the Fetus and Infant,* 5th ed. St. Louis: Mosby-Year Book, 884–893.

11. Fuller R. 1989. Cardiac function and the neonatal EKG. Part III: Tachycardia. *Neonatal Network* 7(6): 65–67.

12. Kombol P. 1988. Dysrhythmias in infancy. *Neonatal Network* 6(5): 41–52.

13. Johnson GL. 1990. Clinical examination. In *Fetal and Neonatal Cardiology,* Long WA, ed. Philadelphia: WB Saunders, 223–235.

14. Danford DA, and McNamara DG. 1990. Innocent heart murmurs and heart sounds. In *Science and Practice of Pediatric Cardiology,* Garson A, et al., eds. Philadelphia: Lea & Febiger, 1919–1928.

15. Danilowicz DA, et al. 1972. Physiologic pressure differences between main and branch pulmonary arteries in children. *Circulation* 45(2): 410–419.

16. Scanlon JW, et al. 1979. Examination of the cardiovascular system. In *A System of Newborn Physical Examination.* Baltimore: University Park Press, 67–73.

NOTES

NOTES

8 Abdomen Assessment

Garris Keels Conner, RN, DNS

Techniques for assessing the newborn's abdomen include inspection, palpation, auscultation, and rarely, percussion. Occasionally, transillumination is used to determine the presence of an abdominal mass, fluid, or air. The abdominal assessment should proceed in an orderly fashion, beginning with the least intrusive technique. Examiners sometimes combine two techniques during the physical assessment. For example, if the examiner observes a suspicious bulge, the area will be palpated to determine the cause. Rigid rectus abdominis muscles and a distended abdomen will hinder the examination. If the infant is active or fussy, use calming methods, such as offering a pacifier or holding the infant, before beginning the examination.

INSPECTING THE ABDOMEN

MOVEMENT

Inspect the abdomen for movement patterns and shape. Normal abdominal movements are synchronous with chest movements. Dichotomous movements suggest respiratory distress, central nervous system disease, or peritoneal irritation. Intermittent peristaltic movements become visible after the first hour of life. Persistent peristaltic movements may be signs of intestinal obstruction.

SHAPE

The examiner determines if the abdomen is symmetric, asymmetric, distended, or scaphoid. The normal full-term infant has a slightly rounded, soft, and symmetric abdomen. The preterm infant's abdomen appears slightly distended due to poor muscle tone. An asymmetrically shaped abdomen may indicate an abdominal mass, organomegaly, or intestinal obstruction. Abdominal distention may be a nonspecific sign of obstruction, a ruptured viscus with resultant free air in the peritoneal cavity (pneumoperitoneum), ascites, or infection or can be secondary to an air-filled bowel after vigorous resuscitation measures with bag/mask ventilation. If epigastric distention and visible peristalsis (classic signs of pyloric stenosis) are observed, they may indicate duodenal or jejunal obstruction because pyloric stenosis does not usually present in the newborn period. When distention is present, the examiner should institute serial abdominal measurements to detect change in girth. A tape measure is placed

FIGURE 8-1 ▲ Congenital deficiency of the abdominal musculature, showing typical "prune" (wrinkled) belly appearance.

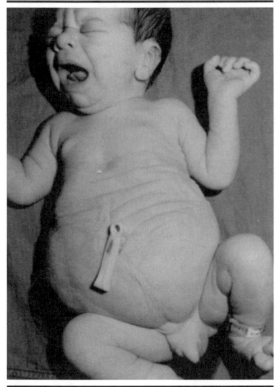

Courtesy of David A. Clark, MD, Louisiana State University.

around the abdomen at the level of the umbilicus. Sometimes marking the border of the tape measure on the skin helps ensure that all examiners are positioning the tape in the same place.

FIGURE 8-2 ▲ Omphalocele.

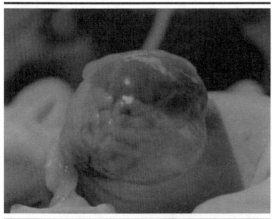

Courtesy of David A. Clark, MD, Louisiana State University.

FIGURE 8-3 ▲ Gastroschisis.

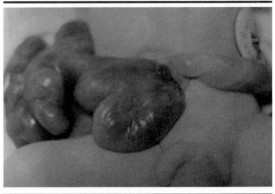

Courtesy of David A. Clark, MD, Louisiana State University.

A scaphoid abdomen may indicate a diaphragmatic hernia or extreme malnutrition.

A flat, flabby abdomen indicates decreased muscle tone, which can be drug induced (maternal or neonatal) or can result from neurologic depression. Prune belly syndrome (Figure 8-1) is a congenital deficiency of the abdominal muscles.[1] The cause of this muscular deficiency (hypoplasia) is uncertain. Two possibilities exist. The deficiency of the abdominal muscles results either from failure of the muscle cells to develop or from an intrauterine insult affecting the muscles or their innervation.[2] This rare syndrome occurs almost exclusively in males and is associated with renal and urinary tract abnormalities.

Skin

In the term infant, the skin covering the abdomen is pink in color, smooth, and opaque, with a medium-thick texture. A few large blood vessels may be visible. Thin, translucent skin is one indication of prematurity. The preterm infant has visible veins and tributaries in the trunk area. Postterm infants have thick, parchment-like skin with superficial or deep cracking. Vessels are not seen over the trunk of the postterm infant. During inspection, all rashes and cutaneous lesions should be noted and follow-up assessment done on a regular basis.

FIGURE 8-4 ▲ Exstrophy of the urinary bladder.

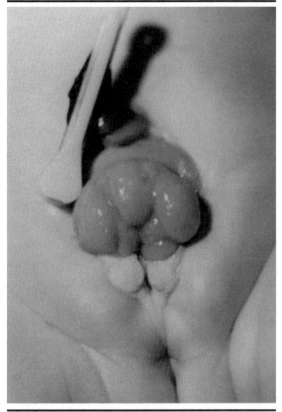

Courtesy of David A. Clark, MD, Louisiana State University.

FIGURE 8-5 ▲ Umbilical hernia.

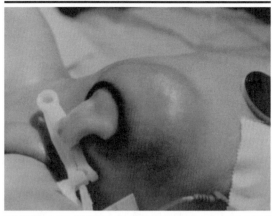

Courtesy of David A. Clark, MD, Louisiana State University.

MIDLINE DEFECTS

Three of the midline defects observable in the infant are omphalocele, gastroschisis, and exstrophy of the bladder. Fetal ultrasound is a useful assessment tool for detection of these abdominal defects. Infants with these defects are at additional risk for infection, hypothermia, and fluid and electrolyte loss and therefore require immediate surgical intervention. Other defects are also discussed below.

Omphalocele

An omphalocele (Figure 8-2) is the herniation of the umbilicus through which abdominal contents and occasionally other organs protrude.[3] A translucent membranous sac covers the defect. Occasionally, this sac will rupture during delivery. In infants with an omphalocele, there is a high occurrence of other

life-threatening congenital malformations, such as trisomies 13–15, 18, and 21; Beckwith-Wiedemann syndrome; and congenital heart disease.[4] There is a higher incidence of the defect in premature infants and in males.

Gastroschisis

Gastroschisis (Figure 8-3) is also a herniation through which abdominal contents and other organs protrude. This defect is distinguished from an omphalocele by location. The gastroschisis is usually located to the right of the midline without involvement of the umbilicus.[3] In addition, there is no membranous covering of the eviscerated contents.[1] Fewer congenital malformations are associated with gastroschisis than with an omphalocele.

Exstrophy of the Bladder

Exstrophy of the bladder (Figure 8-4) is a fissure between the anterior abdominal wall and the urinary bladder.[5] The defect is readily visible over the bladder area. Epispadias is a common finding with bladder exstrophy in male infants.

Diastasis Recti

The midline of the abdomen is normally closed, but diastasis recti (a gap between the rectus muscles) is a common finding in otherwise healthy infants. Signs of diastasis recti

FIGURE 8-6 ▲ Malformations of the urachus.

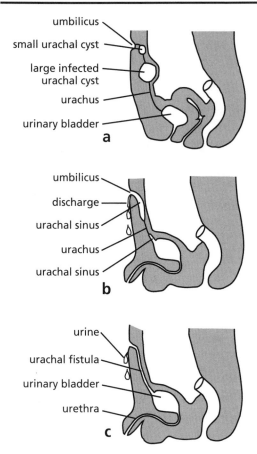

(a) Urachal cysts. The most common site is in the super-ior end of the urachus, just inferior to the umbilicus. (b) Two types of urachal sinus are illustrated: One is continuous with the bladder; the other opens at the umbilicus. (c) Patent urachus or urachal fistula, con-necting the bladder and umbilicus.

From: Moore KL, and Persaud TVN. 1993. The urogeni-tal system. In *The Developing Human*, 5th ed. Philadelphia: WB Saunders, 277. Reprinted by per-mission.

are a palpable midline gap and visible bulging at the site in the crying infant. This is a benign finding in the absence of a hernia.

Umbilical Hernia

An umbilical hernia is a common finding in low birth weight and African American male infants (Figure 8-5). Non–African American infants with hypothyroidism often have umbil-ical hernias.[6] Palpation confirms the diagnosis.

The examiner notes the size of the herniation as well as protrusion of abdominal contents into the herniated area. Umbilical hernias usually reduce spontaneously within the first two years of life. A large hernia or strangulation of abdom-inal contents requires surgical intervention.

Epigastric Hernia

A less common finding in the newborn is an epigastric hernia.[7] In epigastric hernia, there is a protrusion of fat through the defect. This must be distinguished from diastasis recti and umbilical hernia. A firm palpable mass is felt between the umbilicus and the inferior end of the sternum. Very often palpation elicits a pain response from the infant. Surgical inter-vention is necessary.

UMBILICAL CORD

Inspect the umbilical cord for number of ves-sels, color, odor, drainage, and thickness. Nor-mally, the umbilical cord is bluish white and gelatinous at birth. The cord darkens and shriv-els as it dries, falling off within 10 to 14 days. There are two ventrally placed, thick-walled arteries and one dorsally placed, thin-walled vein visible on the umbilical stump. Deter-mine the number of umbilical vessels as soon after birth as possible. Cord drying hinders detection of umbilical vessels. One percent of infants will have only one umbilical artery.[5,8] This condition may be associated with con-genital anomalies of the cardiovascular or renal systems.[9,10]

Unusual cord color or the presence of drainage from the cord is generally indicative of neonatal compromise or disease. A meconi-um-stained green or yellow cord indicates intra-uterine compromise. Suspect infection with the presence of a red, oozing, or foul-smelling cord. A clear discharge from the umbilical stump sug-gests a patent urachus or an omphalomesen-teric duct. A patent urachus (Figure 8-6) is the persistence of an embryologic communication

FIGURE 8-7 ▲ Imperforate anus.

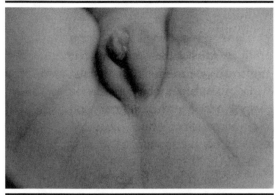

Courtesy of David A. Clark, MD, Louisiana State University.

FIGURE 8-8 ▲ Rectovaginal fistula.

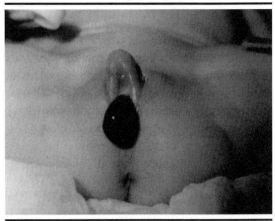

Courtesy of David A. Clark, MD, Louisiana State University.

between the urinary bladder and the umbilicus.[1] Urine passes from the bladder through the umbilicus, making the umbilicus constantly wet. Infants with a patent urachus are at risk for urinary tract infection, often the first sign of a patent urachus.[1] Pustular drainage may indicate a urachal cyst or abscess. An omphalomesenteric duct is the persistence of an embryologic tract connecting the ileum to the umbilicus. Ileal liquid content seeps out of this duct.[1] Presence of fecal drainage indicates that a fistula between the omphalomesenteric duct and colon has developed. Serous or serosanguineous discharge after cord separation indicates the formation of a granuloma, a red solid mass deep in the umbilicus. The granuloma may be cauterized to stop the oozing and to eliminate a possible site of infection.

The thickness of the cord relates to the quantity of Wharton's jelly. Large-for-gestational-age infants have thick, gelatinous cords. Infants with congenital syphilis may also have thick umbilical cords. A small, thin cord suggests intrauterine growth retardation.

PERIANAL AREA

Inspect the perianal area for sphincter tone, fistulae, and the presence of an anus (Figure 8-7). Determine sphincter tone and placement of the anal sphincter by gently stroking the anal area. An anal wink will occur. The presence of meconium in the vaginal or urethral orifice suggests a rectovaginal or rectourethral fistula (Figure 8-8).[4]

The presence of an anal orifice and passage of meconium determines anal patency. The single finding of an anal orifice does not confirm anal patency. Anal stenosis or atresia may occur anywhere along the anorectal canal. With anal atresia, there is no passage of stools. Small, thin stools suggest anal stenosis. There is progressive abdominal distention with both anal atresia and stenosis. Vomiting eventually ensues.

A rectal examination is not performed unless clinically indicated. Ninety-four percent of all

FIGURE 8-9 ▲ Obstruction causing abdominal distention.

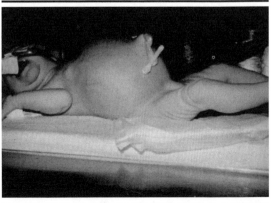

Courtesy of David A. Clark, MD, Louisiana State University.

term infants pass meconium within 24 hours after birth, with the majority doing so by 12 hours after birth.[4] No passage of meconium in conjunction with abdominal distention indicates mechanical or functional obstruction of the gastrointestinal tract (Figure 8-9). A history of maternal polyhydramnios or maternal diabetes, hypotonia, prematurity, Hirschsprung's disease, or cystic fibrosis places the infant at risk for intestinal obstruction.

AUSCULTATION

Auscultation is the next step in the physical examination of the infant's abdomen because palpation and percussion may alter normal sounds in the abdomen. The examiner uses a stethoscope to listen to all four abdominal quadrants. Breath sounds are often heard in the upper abdominal region. Bowel sounds are absent immediately after birth. With crying and sucking, the abdomen begins to fill with air. Bowel sounds become audible within the first 15 minutes after birth.[2] The sounds have a metallic, tinkling quality and are usually heard every 15 to 20 seconds. Absent or hyperactive bowel sounds may suggest obstruction or hypermotility of the gastrointestinal tract, or, depending on the time of the last feeding, they may be normal. Hyperactive sounds heard immediately after feedings in the infant with a soft abdomen, with the sounds diminishing in intensity prior to the next feeding, are normal. Friction rubs may be present with peritoneal irritation.

Also auscultate for vascular sounds. Bruits—sounds similar to a systolic murmur—are heard with dilated, tortuous, or constricted vessels. When bruits are heard, change the infant's position to determine if the sound continues. Bruits that continue despite position changes may indicate abnormalities of the umbilical vein and the hepatic vascular system, as well as renal artery stenosis and hepatic hemangiomas.

FIGURE 8-10 ▲ Abdominal organs of infant.

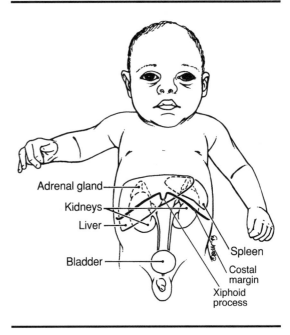

Adrenal gland
Kidneys
Liver
Bladder
Spleen
Costal margin
Xiphoid process

PALPATION

Gently palpate the infant's abdomen with warm hands. Observe the infant for pain responses during this part of the examination. To facilitate palpation, flex the infant's knees and hips with one hand, or lift the hip off the bed slightly, and use the free hand to palpate the abdomen. This maneuver relaxes the abdominal musculature.

TONE

Tense, rigid tone suggests peritoneal irritation. (This muscular rigidity is not always present in the infant with peritoneal irritation because of the normally limited muscular control in newborns.) Flaccid tone suggests neuromuscular disease, perinatal compromise, or maternal medication causing neonatal depression.

Assess skin turgor by gently pinching a small piece of skin and then releasing it. The skin should quickly return to the original position. A slow response indicates dehydration.

LIVER AND SPLEEN

Next palpate the liver to define its margins (Figure 8-10). Care must be used when palpating the liver. Because it is a superficial organ, deep probing is unnecessary. Place the index finger just above the groin parallel to the right costal margin, and with a gentle, compressing motion, gradually move the finger upward until the liver edge is felt. It is important to begin palpation at the groin because an enlarged liver can be missed if the examiner begins palpation where he or she thinks the liver should be. Normally, the liver edge is felt 1 to 2 cm below the right costal margin at the midclavicular line. A liver that is palpated beyond the midpoint between the xiphoid process and the umbilicus is considered enlarged. A hyperexpanded chest will cause the liver to be lower than expected. Hepatomegaly may be present with perinatal infection and blood group incompatibilities.

The normal liver is smooth and firm with a sharp and well-defined edge. A rounded liver edge suggests congestion, an early sign of congestive heart failure. A hard, nodular liver is abnormal.

Use a similar maneuver on the left side of the abdomen to palpate the spleen. Normally, the spleen is not felt. A spleen tip felt 1 cm or more below the left costal margin is an indication of disease processes seen with hepatosplenomegaly. Such disease processes include intrauterine infections and erythroblastosis fetalis.

The examiner should be aware of the possibility of a ruptured liver or spleen with traumatic deliveries or aggressive resuscitative measures. With a ruptured liver, the infant will appear well for the first 24 to 48 hours. A mass in the liver region may be palpable. Abdominal distention ensues, with free blood filling the peritoneal cavity.[4] A ruptured spleen is suspected in a breech delivered infant who presents with anemia not associated with jaundice in the first 24 to 72 hours of life.

MASSES

Use a systematic approach covering all four quadrants to palpate the abdomen for the presence of masses. With the pads of the fingertips, and the fingers together, begin a shallow, smooth, gentle pressure; then proceed with deeper palpation. Do not use jabbing movements. The meconium-filled descending colon, located in the lower quadrants, has a sausage shape. Intussusception presents as a sausagelike mass in the right or left upper quadrant. Although pyloric stenosis rarely presents in the newborn period, an ovoid mass between the umbilicus and the right lower costal margin is palpable in the majority of infants with a pyloric stenosis. The mass is easily detected immediately after feeding or vomiting. Solid or cystic masses are usually renal in origin.

KIDNEYS

Normal kidneys are sometimes difficult to palpate.[2,7] The left kidney is more easily palpated than the right kidney, unless the descending colon is filled with meconium. Usually, the right kidney is covered by the liver, impeding successful palpation. The ideal time to palpate normal kidneys is immediately after birth, before the abdominal cavity begins to fill with air. The maneuvers employed to palpate the kidneys will disturb the infant. It is therefore best to wait until the end of the physical examination to examine the kidneys.

Use the following technique to palpate the kidneys. Place the fingers of both hands under the infant, with the thumbs adjacent to the umbilicus. Gently compress the thumbs; then palpate the kidney regions. Deep palpation with a smooth, firm pressure is used. Another method is to place one hand under the infant's flank and press downward with the other hand

FIGURE 8-11 ▲ Technique for palpating the kidneys.

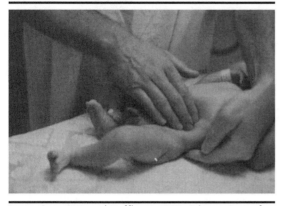

From: Coen RW, and Koffler H. 1987. *Primary Care of the Newborn.* Boston: Little, Brown, 30. Reprinted by permission.

FIGURE 8-12 ▲ Inguinal hernia.

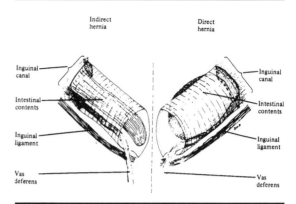

From: Alexander MM, and Brown MS. 1979. *Pediatric History Taking and Physical Diagnosis for Nurses,* 2nd ed. New York: McGraw-Hill, 223. Reprinted by permission of the authors.

(Figure 8-11). Nodular or enlarged kidneys are reasons for concern.

BLADDER

The bladder is palpated 1–4 cm above the symphysis pubis. A frequently or continuously distended bladder occurs with central nervous system defects or urethral obstruction.[9]

GROIN

The groin area is examined by both inspection and palpation. The groin is flat in the quiet infant. Visible femoral pulsations in the preterm or thin term infant are common. Any swelling in the groin area is suspicious. Bulging in the groin area is most likely an inguinal hernia or undescended testis. An inguinal hernia (Figure 8-12) is a muscle wall defect that allows bowel loops to enter the scrotal sac in the male or soft tissues in the female. Inguinal hernias occur more often in males than in females. A bulge in the labia majora may be an inguinal hernia or abnormal gonad. The examiner is unlikely to see or feel an inguinal hernia in the quiet, relaxed infant. Determine if bowel or gonads are reducible and able to be returned to their proper positions. Surgery is indicated when herniated organs are strangulated. Hydrocele and undescended testes are discussed in Chapter 9.

FEMORAL AREA

The femoral area (Figure 8-13) is examined for the presence of bulges and pulses. A femoral hernia may be observed as a small bulge adjacent and medial to the femoral artery.[4] This finding is more common in females than in males.

The femoral pulses are palpated to determine quality and rate. Both right and left pulses are palpated simultaneously. The examiner decides if the arterial pulses are present, equal, weak, thready, irregular, or bounding. If suspicious characteristics are present, palpate the femoral pulse simultaneously with the brachial pulse. Significant differences between the upper and lower pulses, along with decreased femoral pulse intensity, indicate coarctation of the aorta. Absence of femoral pulses also suggests coarctation of the aorta.[11] If coarctation is suspected, obtain blood pressure readings in both upper and lower extremities. Normally, lower extremity blood pressure is higher than upper extremity pressure. With coarctation, lower extremity pressure is lower than upper extremity pressure. Bounding femoral pulses may be indicative of a patent ductus arteriosus.

FIGURE 8-13 ▲ The femoral triangle.

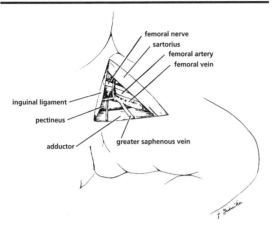

femoral nerve
sartorius
femoral artery
femoral vein

inguinal ligament

pectineus

adductor

greater saphenous vein

From: Short BL, and Avery GB. 1983. Arterial puncture. In *Atlas of Procedures in Neonatology*, Fletcher MA, MacDonald MG, and Avery GB, eds. Philadelphia: JB Lippincott, 60. (Adapted from Plaxico DT, and Bucciarelli RL. 1978. Greater saphenous vein venipuncture in the neonate. *Journal of Pediatrics* 93[6]: 1025.) Reprinted by permission.

PERCUSSION

Percussion of the abdomen is not usually performed in the newborn. If suspect findings are present during the examination, the examiner may want to consider percussion as a technique to add to the scope of the data already collected. Percuss the abdomen to distinguish between tympany and dullness. Tympanic sounds are present over the organs that contain air. Increased tympany suggests abnormal amounts of air. If tympany is not present just below the left costal margin over the stomach, suspect esophageal obstruction or stomach deformity. Dull sounds are percussed over the liver, spleen, and bladder. (Respiratory movements change liver position; the examiner must be aware of these movements when percussing the liver.) Increased areas of dullness suggest organ enlargement. Hepatic and splenic enlargements produce dull sounds extending below the costal margin. If the bladder is full, dullness will extend toward the umbilicus. Reexamine after the infant voids. Dull sounds in other areas of the abdomen suggest masses. Shifting dullness is common with ascites.

SUMMARY

The infant's abdomen is examined beginning with inspection, proceeding to palpation and auscultation. Transillumination is a helpful noninvasive technique used to determine the presence of a mass, fluid, or air in the abdominal cavity. An orderly, logical assessment approach will ensure a thorough examination covering all abdomen quadrants. The examination is best accomplished with a quiet, calm infant.

REFERENCES

1. Guzzetta PC, et al. 1987. Surgery of the neonate. In *Neonatology: Pathophysiology and Management of the Newborn*, 3rd ed., Avery GB, ed. Philadelphia: JB Lippincott, 974–977.

2. Coen RW, and Koffler H. 1987. *Primary Care of the Newborn*. Boston: Little, Brown, 20, 28.

3. Kenner C, Harjo J, and Brueggemeyer A, eds. 1988. *Neonatal Surgery: A Nursing Perspective*. Orlando, Florida: Grune & Stratton, 129–130.

4. Gryboski J, and Walker WA. 1983. *Gastrointestinal Problems in the Infant*, 2nd ed. Philadelphia: WB Saunders, 7, 287, 369, 492.

5. Moore KL. 1989. *Before We Are Born: Basic Embryology and Birth Defects*, 3rd ed. Philadelphia: WB Saunders, 100, 185.

6. DiGeorge AM. 1992. The endocrine system. In *Textbook of Pediatrics*, 14th ed., Behrman RE, et al, eds. Philadelphia: WB Saunders, 1196.

7. Scanlon JW, et al. 1979. *A System of Newborn Physical Examination*. Baltimore: University Park Press, 76–77, 79.

8. Blackburn ST, and Loper DL. 1992. The perinatal period and placental physiology. In *Maternal, Fetal, and Neonatal Physiology: A Clinical Perspective*. Philadelphia: WB Saunders, 94.

9. Page EW, Villee CA, and Villee DB. 1981. *Human Reproduction: Essentials of Reproductive and Perinatal Medicine*. Philadelphia: WB Saunders, 175–207.

10. Belman B. 1987. Abnormalities of the genitourinary system. In *Neonatology: Pathophysiology and Management of the Newborn*, 3rd ed., Avery GB, ed. Philadelphia: JB Lippincott, 1006, 1008.

11. Merenstein GB, and Gardner SL. 1989. *Handbook of Neonatal Intensive Care*, 2nd ed. St. Louis: Mosby-Year Book, 441.

NOTES

9 Genitourinary Assessment

Terri A. Cavaliere, RNC, MS, NNP

A comprehensive physical assessment of the newborn includes evaluation of the genitourinary (GU) system, which consists of the kidneys, the urinary tract, and the reproductive tract. Because these organs are closely related both anatomically and embryologically, they are discussed together. This chapter focuses on examination of the GU system in the neonate using the techniques of inspection, palpation, and occasionally, percussion. Normal newborn characteristics and simple variations from normal are presented first, followed by a discussion of abnormalities and malformations.

HISTORY REVIEW

A review of the prenatal history is part of any neonatal physical examination. A history of polyhydramnios or oligohydramnios during pregnancy should alert the examiner to the possibility of abnormalities of the GU tract or renal impairment.[1,2] Antenatal sonography often assists in the diagnosis of disorders before the onset of signs and symptoms in the neonate. Disturbances in the amount of amniotic fluid and structural abnormalities may have been detected by ultrasound.

Family history is an important consideration because certain GU anomalies are associated with a genetic predisposition.[1,2] Parents of newborns with GU disorders should be questioned as to the occurrence of anomalies in other family members. Genetic counseling may be appropriate in some instances.

RELATED FINDINGS

Even without a documented history of oligohydramnios, physical signs of intrauterine compression in the newborn, such as flattened facies, malformed ears, and contraction deformities of the limbs (Figure 9-1), suggest urogenital defects. Pulmonary hypoplasia, presenting as respiratory distress, may occur secondary to oligohydramnios or to limited excursion of the diaphragm caused by an intra-abdominal mass.[1]

There is a well-established association between GU anomalies and abnormalities of other systems: cardiovascular, neurologic, gastrointestinal, and musculoskeletal, as well as those that are genetic in origin. Careful evaluation of the GU system is warranted in neonates with other congenital anomalies such as myelomeningocele, complex congenital heart

FIGURE 9-1 ▲ Compression effects of oligohydramnios, which may signal possible GU or renal abnormalities.

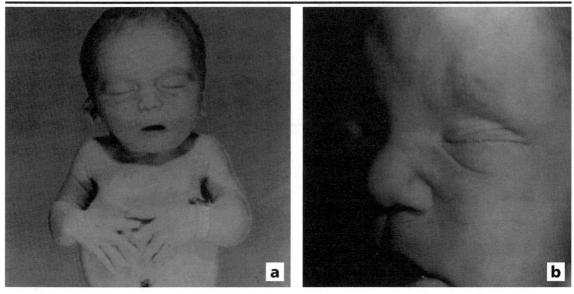

(a) Joint contractures, narrow thorax, malformed ear. (b) Typical facies: flattened nose, epicanthal fold, furrowed brow.

Courtesy of J. Hernandez, MD, The Children's Hospital, Denver, Colorado.

disease, and VACTERL association (**v**ertebral anomalies, **a**nal atresia, **c**ardiac abnormalities, **t**racheoesophageal abnormalities, **r**enal abnormalities, and **l**imb anomalies).

The presence of oliguria and anuria may indicate underlying urologic disease. Ninety-two percent of healthy neonates void within the first 24 hours of life. Many times the first void occurs in the delivery room, and the event may go unnoticed. By 48 hours of age, 99 percent of all newborns will have voided for the first time.[3] If a neonate has not passed any urine by 36 hours of age, the possibility of renal disease, obstructive uropathy, or renovascular accident should be considered.[3] Oliguria can also be a sign of malformation or obstruction of the urinary tract.

Urine output is normally low during the first two days of life: 15–60 ml total output in 24 hours. The amount subsequently increases to 100 to 300 ml total output in 24 hours from the third to tenth days.[1] Documentation of ade-

quate urinary output is important, especially with early hospital discharge of newborns. Parent counseling and adequate follow-up care are essential.

NORMAL PHYSICAL EXAMINATION

ABDOMEN

A comprehensive abdominal examination is described in Chapter 8. Those details pertinent to the GU system are presented here.

On inspection, the abdomen of a term neonate is rounded and symmetric, with smooth, opaque skin. A preterm newborn has a more protuberant abdomen due to immature muscle development, and the skin covering the abdomen may be thinner, with more prominent blood vessels.

At birth, the umbilical cord is gelatinous and bluish white in color. It contains three vessels: two arteries and one vein. There should be no exudate or discharge from the umbilicus.

FIGURE 9-2 ▲ One technique for palpating the kidneys.

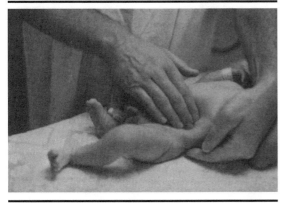

From: Coen RW, and Koffler H. 1987. *Primary Care of the Newborn.* Boston: Little, Brown, 30. Reprinted by permission.

FIGURE 9-3 ▲ Alternate method for palpating the kidneys.

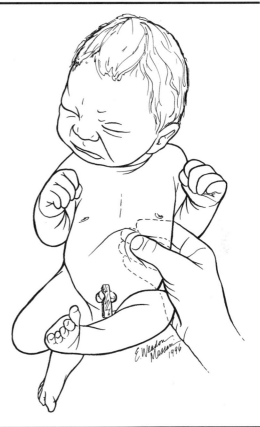

Palpation of the abdomen is easiest in the first 24 hours of life, before air fills the entire gastrointestinal tract and before abdominal tone increases.[3,4] It is best performed on a quiet neonate lying in a supine position with knees and hips maintained in flexion by the examiner's hand. Providing a pacifier to evoke the sucking reflex may help to relax the abdominal musculature.

All four quadrants should be examined to detect any masses. The neonate's kidneys are in a lower position in the abdomen than they will be later in life. Normally, the inferior poles of both kidneys can be felt; the right kidney is usually lower than the left.[3] Kidneys should be approximately equal in size and smooth to the touch. Ureters are not palpable.

The presence of stool-filled intestines or a fussy, crying baby may make this portion of the exam somewhat difficult. If the examiner is unable to palpate the kidneys, the fact that the neonate has voided ensures the presence of some renal tissue. Enlarged kidneys are easy to detect; this finding should prompt further investigation.

Figure 9-2 illustrates one technique for palpating the kidneys. The upper hand palpates the upper and lower quadrants while the other hand supports the flank. The process is repeat-ed on the opposite side. An alternate method is depicted in Figure 9-3: Place the fingers of one hand under the infant, with the thumb on the abdomen. To palpate the kidneys, compress your fingers against your thumb; the fingers support the flank while the thumb explores the area.[2,4]

The bladder can either be percussed or it can be palpated between the umbilicus and the symphysis pubis. A distended bladder may be palpated as a subumbilical fullness or mass. Because the bladder wall is thin, this organ may be difficult to palpate. Percussion may then be helpful to detect a full bladder over the symphysis pubis.[4]

MALE GENITALIA

Inspect the urogenital area with the male infant in the supine position. Figure 9-4 is a

FIGURE 9-4 ▲ **Normal newborn genitalia (male).**

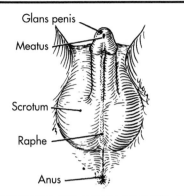

From: Grumbach MM, and Conte FA. 1992. Disorders of sexual differentiation. In *William's Textbook of Endocrinology*, 8th ed., Wilson JD, and Foster DW, eds. Philadelphia: WB Saunders, 331. Reprinted by permission.

FIGURE 9-5 ▲ **Appearance of genitalia in (a) preterm, (b) term, and (c) postterm male neonates.**

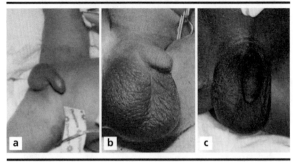

Term infant is from: Lepley CJ, Gardner SL, and Lubchenco LO. 1989. Initial nursery care. In *Handbook of Neonatal Intensive Care*, 2nd ed., Merenstein GB, and Gardner SL, eds. St. Louis: Mosby-Year Book, 88. Reprinted by permission.

diagram of normal male genitalia. Gestational age has a great impact on the appearance of the external genitalia. Figure 9-5 illustrates the changes in external genitalia with advancing gestation. Rugae (wrinkles or creases) begin to form on the ventral surface of the scrotum at approximately 36 weeks gestation. At term, the scrotum is fully rugated and more deeply pigmented than the surrounding skin.

Palpate the scrotal sac and inguinal canal to locate the testes and to detect any masses. Prior to 28 weeks gestation, the testes are abdominal organs; at 28 to 30 weeks, they begin to descend into the inguinal canal. By term, the testes should be well situated in the scrotum.[1,5,6] When palpated, normal testes are firm and smooth and comparatively equal in size.

Newborn males may have edema of the genitalia due to the effects of transplacentally acquired maternal hormones. Trauma may occur during breech delivery (Figure 9-6) or in very large babies. Ecchymosis, edema, or even hematoma may be seen. These findings are transient and should begin to dissipate after a few days.

The prepuce, or foreskin, covers the entire head of the penis in an uncircumcised male neonate. Normally, the prepuce is tight, with a tiny orifice. Physiologic phimosis, a nonretractable foreskin, is normal in young males. Usually, the opening in the prepuce is adequate to allow urination; forceful retraction of the foreskin should be avoided.[1,7] Gentle traction is applied on the foreskin to visualize the urethral meatus at the

FIGURE 9-6 ▲ **Genital bruising with breech presentation.**

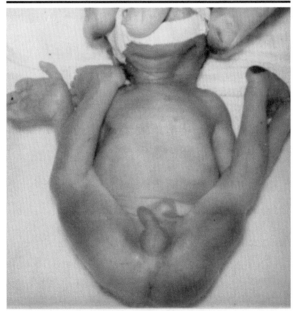

Courtesy of David A. Clark, MD, Louisiana State University Medical Center and Wyeth-Ayerst Laboratories, Philadelphia, Pennsylvania.

FIGURE 9-7 ▲ **Technique for measuring penile length.**

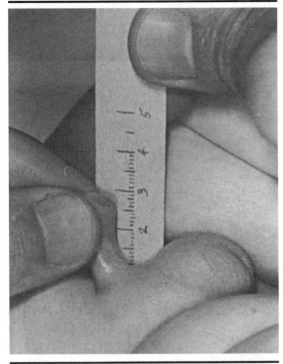

central tip of the penis. The penis should be straight; erections are commonly seen in neonates. Observation and documentation of the force and direction of the urine stream while voiding are important. The urine stream should be forceful, straight, and continuous.[1,7]

Penile length should be assessed. The average length of the penis in a term neonate is 3.5 ± 0.4 cm, measured from the pubic bone to the tip of the glans (omitting excess foreskin). Some neonates have a large deposit of adipose tissue overlying the pubic bone, giving the illusion of a small penis. In such cases, it is important to depress the fat pad while stretching the shaft for assessment of length. Comparative nomograms are available to document an abnormally sized penis.[8] Figure 9-7 demonstrates a measurement technique for penile length.

FIGURE 9-8 ▲ **Normal newborn genitalia (female).**

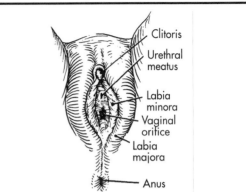

- Clitoris
- Urethral meatus
- Labia minora
- Vaginal orifice
- Labia majora
- Anus

FEMALE GENITALIA

The female genitalia are also inspected with the newborn in the supine position. An illustration of the normal external female anatomy is provided in Figure 9-8. For the first eight weeks of life, the term female neonate may have prominent labia, a large clitoris, and a urethral meatus that is difficult to visualize because of the influence of maternal estrogen.[9] Maternal hormone exposure can stimulate a white, mucoid vaginal discharge and/or bleeding (pseudomenses). These findings may persist for up to ten days. The genitalia of breech-positioned and large babies may be edematous and ecchymotic for several days after delivery.

FIGURE 9-9 ▲ **Appearance of genitalia in (a) preterm and (b) term female neonates.**

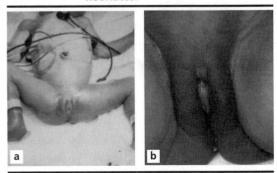

FIGURE 9-10 ▲ Hymenal tag in a neonate.

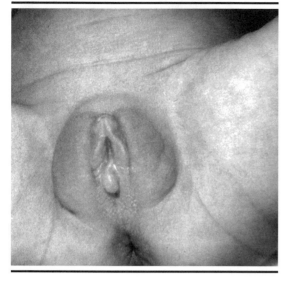

FIGURE 9-11 ▲ Congenital deficiency of the abdominal musculature: prune belly syndrome.

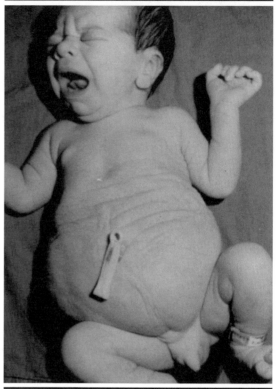

Courtesy of David A. Clark, MD, Louisiana State University.

Gestational age influences the appearance of the female genitalia (Figure 9-9). In preterm females, the labia minora and clitoris are very prominent, and the labia majora are small due to a lack of adipose tissue. The labia majora are larger in more mature neonates; in full-term females, they usually cover the clitoris and labia minora.

The labia and the inguinal and suprapubic areas are inspected and palpated to detect any masses, bulges, or swelling. The labia are then separated with gentle lateral and downward traction of the examiner's fingers. The clitoris is the uppermost structure, located at the junction of the labia minora. Directly below the clitoris and above the vaginal opening is the urethral meatus. The perineum is the area between the vaginal opening and the anus; it should be smooth, without dimpling or fistulae. Normally, in the term female, the perineum is as wide as a fingertip. Abnormal length of the perineum with abnormal spacing between the vaginal, urethral, and anal orifices are occasionally associated with GU anomalies.[1,7] The hymen is a thickened avascular membrane with a central orifice. A hymenal tag (Figure 9-10) is a common neonatal variation that usually disappears in a few weeks.

ABNORMAL FINDINGS ON ABDOMINAL EXAMINATION

ABDOMINAL DISTENTION

Abdominal distention is a frequent finding in the neonate because of poorly developed abdominal musculature. Masses, or less commonly ascites, can be causes of abdominal distention. Most palpable abdominal masses in newborns are of renal origin.[4] Causes of renal masses in neonates are multicystic renal dysplasia, hydronephrosis, polycystic kidneys, and venous thrombosis.[1,3] Dilated, enlarged ureters caused by urinary tract obstruction can present as an abdominal mass.

FIGURE 9-12 ▲ Exstrophy of the bladder.

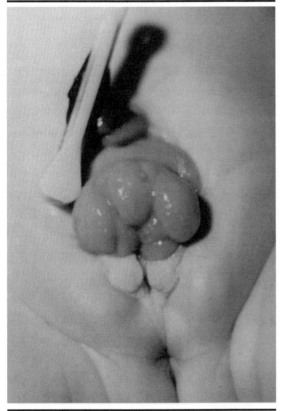

Courtesy of David A. Clark, MD, Louisiana State University.

FIGURE 9-13 ▲ Exstrophy of the bladder with epispadias.

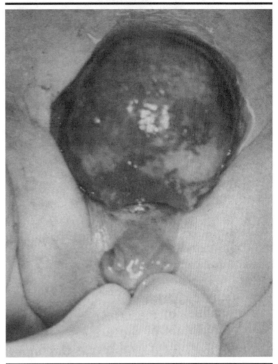

From: Belman B. 1987. Abnormalities of the genitourinary system. In *Neonatology: Pathophysiology and Management of the Newborn,* 3rd ed., Avery GB, ed. Philadelphia: JB Lippincott, 996. Reprinted by permission.

Because the urinary bladder is higher in the abdomen in the neonate than in the older infant, bladder distention is a frequent cause of abdominal distention and the most common midline abdominal mass. Persistent bladder distention might signify structural urethral defects, bladder obstruction, or neuromuscular disease.[7] An abdominal mass is a cause for concern and warrants further investigation.

Ascites is an intra-abdominal collection of fluid. Percussion reveals its presence. Lower urinary tract obstruction, particularly posterior urethral valves, can be a cause of ascites. In these cases, ascitic fluid is composed of urine that has either escaped through a frank rupture in the collecting system or leaked through a renal calyx into the peritoneal cavity.[1,3]

ABDOMINAL WALL DEFECTS

Prune belly syndrome, or congenital deficiency of the abdominal musculature, is readily apparent at birth (Figure 9-11). Its characteristics are a large, flaccid, wrinkled abdominal wall, undescended testes, and various genitourinary malformations, such as hydroureter, hydronephrosis, and renal dysplasia. Occasionally, imperforate anus, intestinal malrotation, rib cage anomalies, cardiovascular abnormalities, and lower limb defects are also present. This syndrome is seen almost exclusively in males; reports of affected females are rare.[2,3,10]

Exstrophy of the bladder is a part of a spectrum of malformations involving defects of the urinary and genital tracts, musculoskeletal system, and sometimes the intestinal tract.[11] As the result of an embryologic defect, there is an

FIGURE 9-14 ▲ Balanic (or glanular) hypospadias.

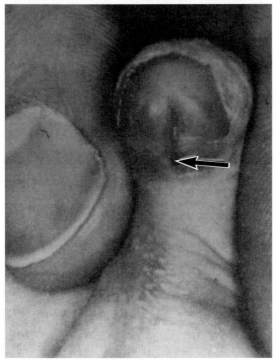

This is the most common form of hypospadias. The external urethral orifice is indicated by the arrow. There is a shallow pit at the usual site of the orifice. Note the moderate degree of chordee, causing the penis to curve ventrally.

From: Moore KL, and Persaud TVN. 1993. *Before We Are Born: Essentials of Embryology and Birth Defects*, 4th ed. Philadelphia: WB Saunders, 223. (Jolly H. 1968. *Diseases of Children*, 2nd ed. Oxford: Blackwell Scientific Publications.) Reprinted by permission.

absence of muscle and connective tissue in the anterior abdominal wall over the bladder.[12] This presents as eversion and protrusion of the bladder through the abdominal wall defect (Figure 9-12). Complete exstrophy of the bladder is associated with epispadias in some male infants (Figure 9-13).

UMBILICAL CORD ANOMALIES

A single umbilical artery is found in 1 percent of neonates. This finding is sometimes associated with urogenital defects, and some experts recommend a screening renal/abdominal ultrasound be done in these newborns.[1]

The urachus is an embryologic structure that connects the fetal bladder with the umbilicus. Postnatal patency of the urachal remnant can result in a clear discharge (urine) from an otherwise normal appearing umbilical cord. The discharge of urine may be intermittent or minimal. Obtaining the specific gravity of the discharge may confirm it to be urine. A large, edematous umbilical cord that does not separate in the normal amount of time may be the only sign of a patent urachus or of a urachal cyst.[4,10,12]

ABNORMALITIES OF THE MALE GENITALIA

THE PENIS

Hypospadias is the abnormal location of the urethral meatus on the ventral surface of the penis. It is a common abnormality and results from the incomplete development of the anterior urethra. Failure of the urethra to develop inhibits proper development of the prepuce. Most neonates with hypospadias also have a hooded or malformed prepuce.[13,14] It is important to locate the urethral meatus in a neonate with a malformed or hypoplastic prepuce and not simply to dismiss the malformation as a "natural circumcision."

Classification of hypospadias is based on meatal position: (1) Balanic (glanular) hypospadias exists when the urethral opening is ventrally situated at the base of the glans (Figure 9-14); (2) Penile hypospadias occurs when the meatus is found between the glans and scrotum (Figure 9-15); (3) Penoscrotal (Figure 9-16) or perineal hypospadias is defined as the urethral opening at the penoscrotal junction or on the perineum, respectively.[13,14]

Mild hypospadias (types 1 and 2) without other genital abnormalities or dysmorphic features is rarely associated with chromosomal or endocrine disorders, or with problems of sexual differentiation. Infants with penoscrotal or perineal hypospadias have a higher risk of

FIGURE 9-15 ▲ Penile hypospadias.

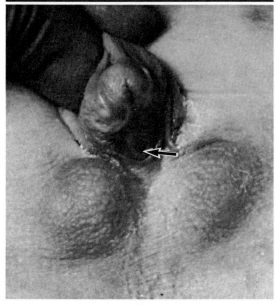

The penis is short and curved (chordee). The external urethral orifice (arrow) is **near** the penoscrotal junction.

From: Moore KL, and Persaud TVN. 1993. *Before We Are Born: Essentials of Embryology and Birth Defects,* 4th ed. Philadelphia: WB Saunders, 223. Reprinted by permission.

these problems. Also, in infants with hypospadias and additional genital anomalies, such as cryptorchidism or micropenis, the risk of endocrine imbalance or problems with sexual differentiation rises.[4,8] Further investigation is warranted in these cases.

Chordee is curvature of the penis caused by fibrous tissue growth in an area of failed urethral development or by skin traction from skin deficiency as seen in hypospadias or epispadias.[8] Ventral chordee frequently, but not always, accompanies hypospadias (Figure 9-14).

Epispadias, the location of the urethral meatus on the dorsal aspect of the penis, varies in severity from a glanular defect (Figure 9-17) to the complete version seen in exstrophy of the bladder (Figure 9-13). All forms of epispadias are associated with differing degrees of dorsal chordee.[11]

FIGURE 9-16 ▲ Penoscrotal hypospadias.

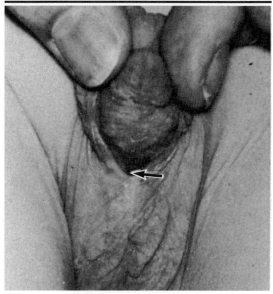

The external urethral orifice (arrow) is located **at** the penoscrotal junction.

From: Moore KL, and Persaud TVN. 1993. *Before We Are Born: Essentials of Embryology and Birth Defects,* 4th ed. Philadelphia: WB Saunders, 223. Reprinted by permission.

FIGURE 9-17 ▲ Epispadias.

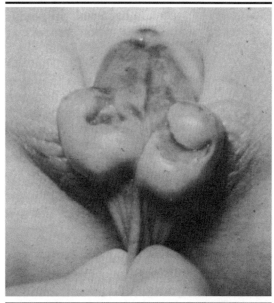

From: Belman B. 1987. Abnormalities of the genitourinary system. In *Neonatology: Pathophysiology and Management of the Newborn,* 3rd ed., Avery GB, ed. Philadelphia: JB Lippincott, 1006. Reprinted by permission.

FIGURE 9-18 ▲ Hydrocele.

A. Cyst that arose from an unobliterated portion of the processus vaginalis. This condition is called a hydrocele of the spermatic cord. B. Hydrocele of the testis and spermatic cord resulting from peritoneal fluid passing into an unclosed processus vaginalis.

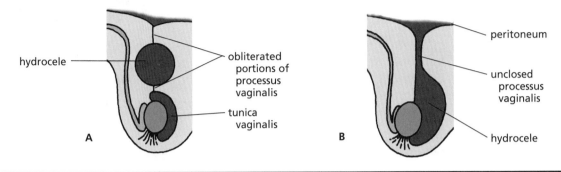

From: Moore KL. 1993. The urogenital system. In *The Developing Human*, 5th ed. Philadelphia: WB Saunders, 299. Reprinted by permission.

Circumcision should not be performed on neonates with hypospadias or epispadias because the foreskin is often used in the repair of these defects. Parents should be instructed that reconstructive surgery by a pediatric urologist may be required.

Hypospadias or epispadias can cause abnormalities in voiding. A weak urine stream, especially in the presence of a distended bladder, suggests the possibility of lower urinary tract obstruction. Neonates with sacral lipomas, spinal cord tethering, caudal regression syndrome, or myelomeningocele may also have abnormalities in voiding due to neurogenic bladders. In these newborns, lesions of the nervous system interrupt the conduction of impulses from the brain to the bladder, preventing normal micturition. Evaluation by a nephrologist and urodynamic studies are commonly obtained in these neonates.

A *micropenis* is abnormally short or thin, that is, greater than two standard deviations below the mean of length and width for age using standard charts. Penis width is measured midshaft on a stretched penis.[8] Normal width is 0.9–1.3 cm at midshaft.[8] The evaluation and management of a newborn with a micropenis frequently requires an endocrinologist and a geneticist. (See Abnormal Sexual Differentiation/Ambiguous Genitalia later in this chapter.)

Priapism, a constantly erect penis, is an abnormal finding in the neonate; its presence should be noted.

THE SCROTUM

Cryptorchidism—literally, hidden testis—refers to a testis or testes that assume an extrascrotal location. The condition occurs when one or both testes fail to descend completely into the scrotum and is detected by inability to palpate one or both testes in the scrotal sac. Cryptorchidism is seen in 33 percent of premature and 3 percent of full-term males. A unilateral undescended testis is more commonly seen than is bilateral cryptorchidism.

A retractile testis is a normally descended organ that recedes into the inguinal canal because of activity of the cremasteric muscle. Because this muscle is inactive in newborns, retractile testes do not occur in this age group. Thus, an empty or a hypoplastic scrotal sac in a neonate, when detected by inspection and palpation, indicates truly undescended testes, ectopic testes (outside the external inguinal ring), or anorchia (absent testes).[1]

FIGURE 9-19 ▲ **Inguinal hernia.**

A. Incomplete congenital inguinal hernia resulting from persistence of the proximal part of the processus vaginalis.
B. Complete congenital inguinal hernia into the scrotum resulting from persistence of the processus vaginalis. Cryptorchidism, a commonly associated malformation, is also illustrated.

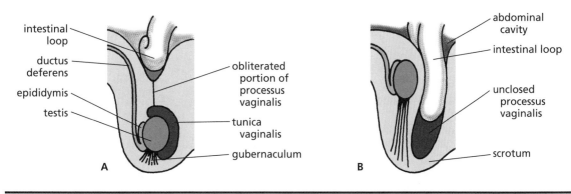

From: Moore KL. 1993. The urogenital system. In *The Developing Human*, 5th ed. Philadelphia: WB Saunders, 299. Reprinted by permission.

Most undescended testes will descend by three months of age.[6] Spontaneous descent rarely occurs after nine months of age. There is an associated risk of infertility and malignancy in the cryptorchid testis. Corrective surgery, called orchiopexy, is currently recommended between the ages of one and two years. Progressive histologic deterioration occurs in the undescended testis after this time.[6,15]

Cryptorchidism is a coincidental finding in many malformations and syndromes. Neonates with undescended testes and other abnormal features, such as micropenis, bifid scrotum, and hypospadias, should be evaluated for endocrine problems and gender ambiguity.[15]

A *hydrocele* is a nontender, fluid-filled scrotal mass overlying the testis and spermatic cord. It presents as a scrotal swelling and is caused by the passage of peritoneal fluid through a patent processus vaginalis into the scrotum or by the persistence of peritoneal fluid that has not been reabsorbed (Figure 9-18). Upon examination, the entire circumference of the testis can be palpated.[16]

Actual or potential indirect *inguinal hernia* is often associated with hydrocele. Loops of intestine can herniate through a persistent processus vaginalis into the scrotum (Figure 9-19).

The presence of intestine in the scrotal sac renders the entire circumference of the testis impalpable. A scrotal mass or swelling from a hydrocele may be further distinguished from that caused by a hernia in that a hydrocele appears translucent on transillumination (Figure 9-20). Because the bowel contains air, hernias may also transilluminate;[17] however, hernias are reducible.

Bowel incarceration and ischemic injury to the testis are potential complications of inguinal hernias. Redness, pain, symptoms of intestinal

FIGURE 9-20 ▲ **Transillumination of a scrotal hydrocele.**

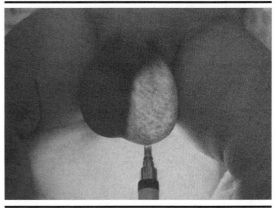

From: Coen RW, and Koffler H. 1987. *Primary Care of the Newborn.* Boston: Little, Brown, 33. Reprinted by permission.

FIGURE 9-21 ▲ Hydrometrocolpos.

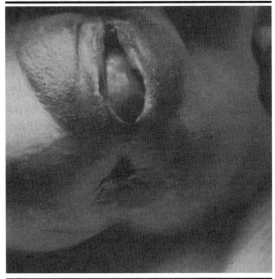

From: Coen RW, and Koffler H. 1987. *Primary Care of the Newborn.* Boston: Little, Brown, 90. Reprinted by permission.

FIGURE 9-22 ▲ Newborn male infant (46,XY) with ambiguous genitalia.

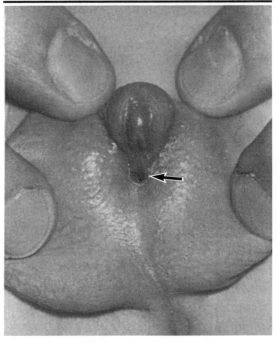

Note penoscrotal hypospadias (arrow). Testes are palpable in the scrotum.

From: Danish RK. 1992. Abnormalities of sexual differentiation. In *Neonatal-Perinatal Medicine: Diseases of the Fetus and Infant*, 5th ed., Fanaroff AA, and Martin RJ, eds. St. Louis: Mosby-Year Book, 1249. Reprinted by permission.

obstruction, and difficulty in reduction are evidence of incarceration.[18]

Hernia repair can be deferred if the hernia is easily reducible and there are no signs of incarceration, but surgery should be scheduled as soon as possible. Most hydroceles resolve in the first year of life. Because communicating hydroceles are, in reality, indirect inguinal hernias, repair is recommended if they persist after two years of age or intermittently change in size.[18]

Testicular torsion, or twisting of the testis on its spermatic cord, may occur prenatally and is usually unilateral. The neonate presents with a swollen scrotum that is red to bluish red in color. This condition compromises blood supply to the testis; therefore, it requires urgent evaluation and possibly emergency management.[19] With prenatal torsion, the duration of the torsion is unknown; by birth, irreversible ischemic damage to the testis may have occurred. Surgical intervention involves removal of the involved testis and prophylactic orchiopexy of the remaining testis in the scrotum.[18] Testicular torsion may be painful, but this is

not a universal finding in neonates.[3,5] Therefore, one should not be misled into discounting the possibility of testicular torsion in the case of a newborn male with a *nontender,* red, swollen scrotum.

ABNORMALITIES OF THE FEMALE GENITALIA

Hydrocolpos (distention of the vagina) and *hydrometrocolpos* (distention of the vagina and the uterus) (Figure 9-21) are the result of either incomplete canalization of the vagina during gestation or an imperforate hymen. These anomalies present in the newborn as a lower abdominal mass and frequently as a urinary tract obstruction.[20] When the hymen is imperforate, it may bulge secondary to accumulation

FIGURE 9-23 ▲ Newborn female with ambiguous genitalia: clitoral enlargement and fusion of labia majora.

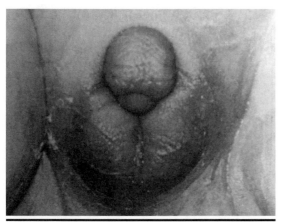

From: Moore KL, and Persaud TVN. 1993. *Before We Are Born: Essentials of Embryology and Birth Defects,* 4th ed. Philadelphia: WB Saunders, 222. Reprinted by permission.

of vaginal secretions, creating the appearance of a cystic mass between the labia.

The urethral meatus should be just ventral to the vaginal opening. Deviation from this position may indicate a urogenital sinus or ambiguous genitalia.[20]

Inguinal hernias occur less frequently in females than in males.[17,21] When they do occur, they may present as a reducible swelling of the labia. Occasionally, a gonad may be palpated in the suprapubic area. The question then arises whether the infant is a female with a prolapsed ovary or a genotypic male with ambiguous genitalia. Commonly, health care providers obtain a buccal smear for Barr body analysis and chromosomes as initial screening tools to rule out gender ambiguity.

ABNORMAL SEXUAL DIFFERENTIATION/ AMBIGUOUS GENITALIA

Ambiguous genitalia (Figures 9-22 and 9-23) may be defined as the presence of a phallic structure that is not discretely male or female, an abnormally located urethral meatus, and the

inability to palpate one or both gonads in males.[1] One should suspect problems of sexual differentiation in phenotypic males with bilateral impalpable testes, perineal hypospadias, or unilateral undescended testis with hypospadias. Similarly, phenotypic females with clitoral hypertrophy, a palpable gonad, inseparably fused labia, or abnormal openings or dimpling on the perineum should be evaluated.[1,22]

The association of ambiguous genitalia with serious underlying endocrine disorders and the understandable distress of the parents mandate rapid identification and evaluation of these newborns. It is imperative that an endocrinologist, a genetic specialist, a urologist, and a psychologist/social worker be included on the evaluation team. The infant should be referred to simply as "baby" until the appropriate sex of rearing is determined.

SUMMARY

Evaluation of the GU tract in the newborn is important to ensure rapid detection and treatment of abnormalities. Too frequently, this examination is cursory, and abnormalities, both major and minor, go unnoticed. Identification of problems in the neonatal period may preserve organ function and prevent mortality and morbidity in the future.

REFERENCES

1. Walker RD. 1992. Presentation of genitourinary disease and abdominal masses. In *Clinical Pediatric Urology,* vol. 1, 3rd ed., Kelalis PP, King LR, and Belman AB, eds. Philadelphia: WB Saunders, 218–243.
2. Kenner C, and Brueggemeyer A. 1993. Assessment and management of genitourinary dysfunction. In *Comprehensive Neonatal Nursing: A Physiologic Perspective,* Kenner C, Brueggemeyer A, and Gunderson LP, eds. Philadelphia: WB Saunders, 706–741.
3. Spitzer A, et al. 1992. Kidney and urinary tract. In *Neonatal-Perinatal Medicine: Diseases of the Fetus and Infant,* 5th ed., Fanaroff AA, and Martin RJ, eds. St. Louis: Mosby-Year Book, 1293–1327.
4. Grupe WE. 1993. The kidney. In *Care of the High-Risk Neonate,* 4th ed., Klaus MH, and Fanaroff AA, eds. Philadelphia: WB Saunders, 374–396.
5. Fonkalsrud EW. 1987. Testicular undescent and torsion. *Pediatric Clinics of North America* 34(5): 1305–1318.

6. Rozanski TA, and Bloom DA. 1985. The undescended testis: Theory and management. *Urologic Clinics of North America* 22(1): 107–118.

7. Connor GK. 1993. Genitourinary assessment. In *Physical Assessment of the Newborn: A Comprehensive Approach to the Art of Physical Examination,* Tappero EP, and Honeyfield ME, eds. Petaluma, California: NICU Ink, 91–100.

8. Danish RK. 1992. Abnormalities of sexual differentiation. In *Neonatal-Perinatal Medicine: Diseases of the Fetus and Infant,* 5th ed., Fanaroff AA, and Martin RJ, eds. St. Louis: Mosby-Year Book, 1222–1292.

9. Baldwin DD, and Landa HM. 1995. Common problems in pediatric gynecology. *Urologic Clinics of North America* 22(1): 161–176.

10. Skoog SJ. 1992. Prune-belly syndrome. In *Clinical Pediatric Urology,* vol. 2, 3rd ed., Kelalis PP, King LR, and Belman AB, eds. Philadelphia: WB Saunders, 943–972.

11. Gearhart JP. 1992. Bladder and urachal abnormalities: The exstrophy-epispadias complex. In *Clinical Pediatric Urology,* vol. 1, 3rd ed., Kelalis PP, King LR, and Belman AB, eds. Philadelphia: WB Saunders, 579–618.

12. Moore KL, and Persaud TVN. 1993. *Before We Are Born: Essentials of Embryology and Birth Defects,* 4th ed. Philadelphia: WB Saunders.

13. Stock JA, Scherz HC, and Kaplan GW. 1995. Distal hypospadias. *Urologic Clinics of North America* 22(1): 131–138.

14. Belman AB. 1992. Hypospadias and other urethral abnormalities. In *Clinical Pediatric Urology,* vol. 1, 3rd ed., Kelalis PP, King LR, and Belman AB, eds. Philadelphia: WB Saunders, 619–663.

15. Kogan SJ. 1992. Cryptorchidism. In *Clinical Pediatric Urology,* vol. 2, 3rd ed., Kelalis PP, King LR, and Belman AB, eds. Philadelphia: WB Saunders, 1050–1083.

16. Bates B. 1995. *A Guide to Physical Examination and History Taking.* Philadelphia: JB Lippincott.

17. Skoog SJ, and Colin MJ. 1995. Pediatric hernias and hydroceles: The urologist's perspective. *Urologic Clinics of North America* 22(1): 119–130.

18. Bloom DA, Wan J, and Key DW. 1992. Disorders of the male external genitalia and inguinal canal. In *Clinical Pediatric Urology,* vol. 2, 3rd ed., Kelalis PP, King LR, and Belman AB, eds. Philadelphia: WB Saunders, 1015–1049.

19. Rabinowitz R, and Hulbert WC. 1995. Acute scrotal swelling. *Urologic Clinics of North America* 22(1): 101–106.

20. Merguerian PA, and McLorie GA. 1992. Disorders of the female genitalia. In *Clinical Pediatric Urology,* vol. 2, 3rd ed., Kelalis PP, King LR, and Belman AB, eds. Philadelphia: WB Saunders, 1084–1105.

21. Shandling B. 1992. Indirect inguinal hernias. In *Nelson's Textbook of Pediatrics,* 14th ed., Behrman R, ed. Philadelphia: WB Saunders, 995, 996.

22. Aaronson IA. 1992. Sexual differentiation and intersexuality. In *Clinical Pediatric Urology,* vol. 2, 3rd ed., Kelalis PP, King LR, and Belman AB, eds. Philadelphia: WB Saunders, 977–1014.

NOTES

10 Musculoskeletal System Assessment

Ellen P. Tappero, RNC, MN, NNP

Careful scrutiny of the musculoskeletal system during the newborn's physical examination is imperative because the information recorded during the first exam forms the database for all future examinations. The musculoskeletal system provides stability and mobility for all physical activity. It consists of the body's bones (Figure 10-1), joints, and their supporting and connecting tissue. In addition to allowing movement and providing structure, the musculoskeletal system protects vital organs (brain, spinal cord), stores minerals (calcium, phosphorus), and produces red blood cells.

The bones of the newborn are soft because they are composed mostly of cartilage, which contains only a small amount of calcium. Compared with the skeleton of an adult or a child, the newborn's skeleton is flexible, and the joints are elastic. This elasticity is necessary to enable the infant to pass through the birth canal.

A thorough evaluation of the musculoskeletal system involves the techniques of inspection, palpation, and, on some occasions, listening. It includes an appraisal of (1) posture, position, and gross anomalies; (2) discomfort from bone or joint movement; (3) range of joint motion; (4) muscle size, symmetry, and strength; and (5) the configuration and motility of the back. Normal variations in shape, size, contour, or movement may be due to position *in utero* or genetic factors. These normal variations should be distinguished

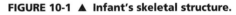

FIGURE 10-1 ▲ Infant's skeletal structure.

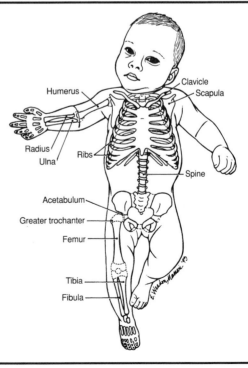

from congenital anomalies and birth trauma. Early diagnosis of musculoskeletal disorders and early intervention often preempt the need for complex medical treatment and lead to more favorable outcomes.[1,2]

Disorders that affect the musculoskeletal system may also originate from the neurologic system. An asymmetric Moro reflex, for example, may be caused by pain from a broken bone or a muscle injury, or it may be the result of a neurologic defect. Because there is some overlap between the musculoskeletal and neurologic examinations, assessment of muscle strength and motor activity are discussed with other neurologic assessments in Chapter 11.

PRENATAL HISTORY

Obtaining a comprehensive prenatal history is vital to the musculoskeletal assessment because a normal uterine environment is essential to the development of the fetus. Any event or condition that changes the intrauterine environment can alter fetal growth, movement, or position. Such prenatal factors as oligohydramnios, breech presentation, abnormal growth patterns, and exposure to teratogenic agents may adversely affect the development and maturation of the musculoskeletal system *in utero*. The perinatal history should be reviewed for possible birth trauma or neurologic insult. The practitioner must note such factors as duration of labor, signs of fetal distress, and the type of delivery (vaginal or cesarean). These factors may have a bearing on conditions such as cerebral palsy, brachial palsy, and torticollis. In multiple gestations, the birth order is also worth noting because there is a higher incidence of congenital hip dysplasia in firstborn children.[3] An accurate gestational age assessment or estimated date of confinement from the obstetrical record is necessary for accurate assessment of the infant's posture and muscle tone.

GENERAL SURVEY

Ideally, a thorough physical examination should be done within the first 24 hours after delivery. Because it is difficult to find a totally motionless, cooperative newborn, much of the musculoskeletal examination must be done while watching the newborn or while examining other systems. The practitioner must compile all the information produced by the exam and record all findings concerning the musculoskeletal system in a systematic manner.

For examination, the infant should be completely undressed and positioned initially on the back. The examination area should be well lit, warm, and free of drafts. A radiant warmer or other heat source is necessary to prevent loss of body heat. The practitioner should develop a routine for examining the newborn so that no part of the musculoskeletal system is overlooked. The examination routine varies from practitioner to practitioner. Most proceed from head to toe.

Examination of the bony structures is important in a newborn examination because it is one of the first opportunities to assess intrauterine development. Deviations from the norm may be the first indicator of a genetic abnormality or disease.[4]

The best instrument for measuring an infant's length, head circumference, and chest circumference is a narrow steel measuring tape. However, most nurseries provide paper tapes. These tapes may be inaccurate, and one must pay particular attention to being precise. Folding the paper tape in half lengthwise may add strength as well as decrease slippage when measuring rounded contours such as the head.[5]

MEASUREMENTS

"Growth, reflected in increased body weight and length along expected pathways and within certain limits, is probably the best indicator of health."[4] Measurements taken soon after birth demand careful attention to detail because they will act as a baseline for subsequent assessments of growth and development. All measurements are plotted on a growth chart and correlated with gestational age (Chapter 3).

Weight

Infants should be weighed without clothing or diaper and at approximately the same time each day. Using a balance scale rather than a spring scale, put a protective cloth or paper liner in place, and then place the infant on the scale.[6] Newborn weight varies with gestational age. Average weight for a term newborn is between 2,500 and 4,000 gm (5 lb 8 oz to 8 lb 13 oz).[7] Newborns initially lose weight, with a loss of 10 percent or less considered acceptable. Birth weight should be regained within the first two weeks.

Length

The infant's recumbent length is measured from the heel to the crown (top of the head). The infant should be placed supine, with legs extended and the head flat. Make a mark on the bed to indicate the crown and a mark at the heel of the infant. Measure the distance between those two marks. Direct measurement of the infant is difficult because of head molding and incomplete extension of the knees. An alternate method for measuring length is to hold the zero point of the tape at the heel and to run the tape along the surface of the bed to the top of the head. Mark the spot on the tape with a finger, remove the tape, and read the measurement. Average length for a full-term infant is 50 cm (20 in), with a range of 45 to 55 cm (18 to 22 in).[7]

Head Circumference

The head should be measured over the occipital, parietal, and frontal prominence, avoiding the ears. The average findings in a full-term infant are 33 to 35.5 cm (13 to 14 in), with normal variations of 31 to 38 cm (12.25 to 15 in).[6,7] As a general rule, the head circum-

ference in centimeters is equal to one-half the length in centimeters plus ten.[8]

Chest Circumference

Measurement of chest circumference is no longer a routine part of newborn physical examination in many hospitals. If it is measured, the chest circumference should be measured at the nipple line during expiration. In term infants, the average chest circumference is approximately 2 cm smaller than the head circumference, with the average 33 ± 3 cm.[7] The head and chest circumferences may be about the same for the first one to two days after birth. The more immature the infant, the greater the difference between the head and chest circumferences.[6]

TERMINOLOGY

The following terms are used to accurately and consistently describe skeletal positions and muscle movements observed during examination:

Flexion: bending a limb at a joint

Extension: straightening a limb at a joint

Abduction: moving a limb away from the midline of the body

Adduction: moving a limb toward or past the midline of the body

Pronation: turning the face down

Supination: turning the face up

Dorsiflexion: flexion toward the back, as in flexion of the foot so that the forefoot is higher than the ankle

Plantar flexion: as in extension of the foot so that the forefoot is lower than the ankle

Rotation (neck): as in turning the face to the side

Valgus: bent outward or twisted away from the midline of the body

Varus: turned inward

Everted: turning out and away from the midline of the body

Inverted: turning inward toward the midline of the body

FIGURE 10-2 ▲ Posture of a term newborn.

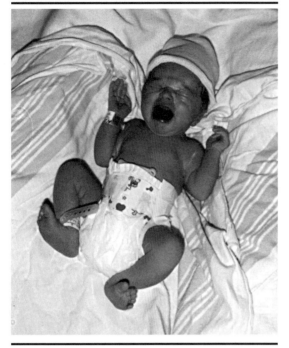

FIGURE 10-3 ▲ Posture of the preterm infant.

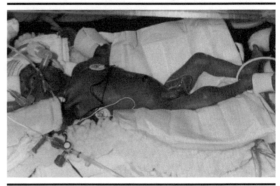

GENERAL INSPECTION

Inspection should proceed from the general to the specific. General inspection includes observation for symmetry of movement, as well as size, shape, general alignment, position, and symmetry of different parts of the body. Soft tissues and muscles should be observed for swelling, muscle wasting, and symmetry.

In the extremities, no asymmetry of length or circumference, constrictive bands, or length deformities should be noted. Unequal length or circumference has been associated with intraabdominal neoplasms.[6]

The ratio of extremity length to body length is also observed. If a discrepancy is seen, measurements of thoracic length and extremities should be recorded. The gestational age of the newborn determines the normal values for these measurements. In the full-term newborn, the ratio of the upper body length to the lower body segment should not exceed 1.7:1.[8] A higher ratio suggests congenitally shortened lower extremities, as in achondroplasia.

Term newborns lie in a symmetric position with the limbs flexed, the legs partially abducted at the hips so that the soles of the feet may nearly touch each other (Figure 10-2). The head is slightly flexed and positioned in the midline or turned to one side. The resting position of the newborn is often that of the tonic neck reflex (Figure 11-6). Spontaneous motor activity of flexion and extension, alternating between the arms and legs, is random and uncoordinated. The fingers are usually flexed in a fist, with the thumb under the fingers. Slight tremors may be seen in the arms and legs with vigorous crying during the first 48 hours of life. Any tremors noted after four days of age while the infant is at rest are considered abnormal and signal a neurologic problem.[4] The resting posture of the preterm infant is one of extension and is discussed in Chapter 11 (Figure 10-3).

The position and appearance of the extremities at birth can reflect intrauterine position. Because the lower extremities of the fetus have been folded on the abdomen, the newborn's lower extremities often appear externally rotated and bowed, with everted feet. The infant delivered in a breech presentation often has flexed, abducted hips and extended knees (Figures 10-4 and 10-5). These positional deformities can usually be corrected by passive joint manipulation and should not be confused with congenital malformations.

FIGURE 10-4 ▲ Breech presentation showing flexed, abducted hips and extended knees.

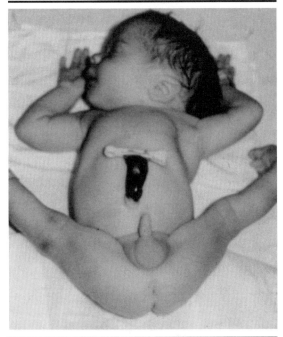

Courtesy of David A. Clark, MD, Louisiana State University Medical Center and Wyeth-Ayerst Laboratories, Philadelphia, Pennsylvania.

FIGURE 10-5 ▲ Breech presentation showing flexed, abducted hips and extended knees.

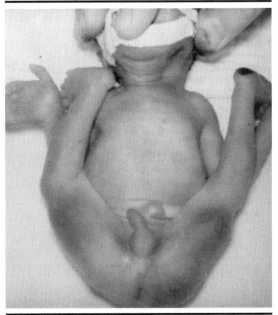

Courtesy of David A. Clark, MD, Louisiana State University Medical Center and Wyeth-Ayerst Laboratories, Philadelphia, Pennsylvania.

PALPATION

Palpation is the next important technique used in the examination of the newborn's musculoskeletal system. This technique, along with inspection, is used on each extremity to identify component parts (for example, the two bones in the forearm), function, and normal range of motion. Some aspects of this assessment are shared with the gestational age assessment. Muscular contour in the term infant is smooth, and despite lack of strength, the infant's muscles should feel firm and slightly resist pressure. If an infant feels limp, the condition should never be mistaken for a mere characteristic of immaturity. Further assessment is necessary to rule out a neurologic defect. When testing range of motion, note any asymmetry, tightness, or contractures. Range of motion of all joints is greatest in infancy, gradually less-

ening as the infant matures. As with posture and muscle tone, the range of joint motion varies with gestational age. It is not necessary to assess the exact number of degrees of range of motion, but only whether the range of movement is less than normal or significantly beyond normal findings. Never use excessive force to assess range of motion.

NECK

The neck is passively examined for rotation and for anterior and lateral flexion and extension. Rotation of 80 degrees and lateral flexion of 40 degrees to both the right and left sides is considered normal. In anterior flexion, the chin should touch or almost touch the chest, and on extension, the occipital part of the head should touch or almost touch the back of the neck. When there is asymmetric rotation or lateral flexion or when range of motion is limited, x-rays of the neck should be taken.

TABLE 10-1 ▲ Normal Neonatal Range of Motion in Upper Extremities

Joint or Bony Unit	Flexion	Extension	External Abduction	Internal Rotation	Rotation
Shoulder	Close to 180°	≥25°	Close to 180°	≥45°	≥80°
Elbow	145°	165°–170°			
Forearm				Supination* ≥80°	Pronation* ≥80°
Wrist	75°–80°	65°–75°			
Digits	Able to clench	Full extension			
Metacarpal-phalangeal		0°			
Interphalangeal		0° → 5°–15°			

*These maneuvers are done while the humerus is held immobile and elbow is at 90 degrees.

From: Scanlon JW, et al. 1979. *A System of Newborn Physical Examination*. Baltimore: University Park Press, 40. Reprinted by permission of the author.

UPPER EXTREMITIES

Skeletal examination of the upper extremities includes the bones of the shoulder girdle (the clavicle and scapula) as well as the humerus, elbow, forearm, and hand. Normal ranges for joint movements of the upper extremities are listed in Table 10-1. Asymmetry in range of motion may indicate weakness, paralysis, fractures, or infection. Failure to move an extremity may indicate a spinal cord injury or brachial plexus palsy.

Clavicles

The clavicles are inspected and palpated for size, contour, and crepitance (grating that can be felt or heard on movement of ends of a broken bone). A fractured clavicle should be suspected when there is a history of a difficult delivery, irregularity in contour, shortening, tenderness, or crepitance on palpation. A broken clavicle is one of the most common birth injuries in newborns.[9]

Humerus

Length and contour of each humerus should also be noted. A fractured humerus should be suspected if there is a history of difficult delivery, one feels a mass due to hematoma formation, or there are signs of pain during palpation. After the clavicle, the humerus is the bone most often fractured during the birth process.[10]

Elbow, Forearm, and Wrist

The elbow, forearm, and wrist are examined for size, shape, and number of bones, as well as for range of joint motion. It is sometimes difficult to evaluate the elbow in infants because the normal neonate has a mild flexion contracture that doesn't disappear until a few weeks after birth. Wrist flexion varies with the infant's gestational age, with greater wrist flexion seen in the full-term than in the preterm infant.

FIGURE 10-6 ▲ Single palmar crease (simian crease).

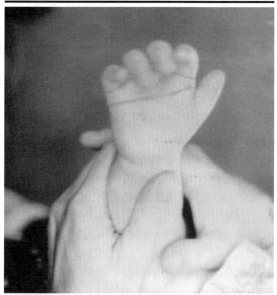

Courtesy of Eva Sujansky, MD, Associate Professor of Pediatrics, University of Colorado Health Sciences Center.

FIGURE 10-7 ▲ Landmarks used in measuring palm and finger length.

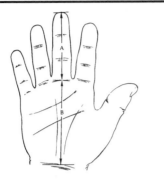

From: Avery GB. 1987. *Neonatology: Pathophysiology and Management of the Newborn*, 3rd ed. Philadelphia: JB Lippincott, 1051. Reprinted by permission.

Hand

The hand should be examined for shape, size, and posture while the fingers are examined for number, shape, and length. Inspection of palm creases should also be included. Although a simian crease across the palm (Figure 10-6) is usually associated with Down syndrome, it is often found in normal infants. However, a combination of short fingers, an incurved little finger, a low-set thumb, and a simian crease should lead the examiner to investigate the possibility of Down syndrome. In full-term infants, the distance from the tip of the middle finger to

FIGURE 10-8 ▲ Macrodactyly.

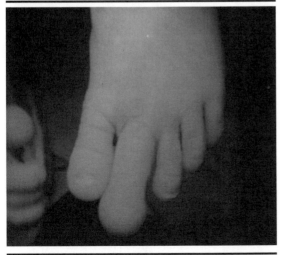

Courtesy of David A. Clark, MD, Louisiana State University.

FIGURE 10-9 ▲ Finger position in an infant with trisomy 18.

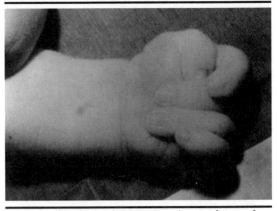

Courtesy of Eva Sujansky, MD, Associate Professor of Pediatrics, University of Colorado Health Sciences Center.

the base of the palm is 6.75 ± 1.25 cm. Middle finger length to total hand length is usually 0.38 to 0.48:1 (Figure 10-7).[8] *Macrodactyly*, an enlarged finger or toe, may be normal, or it may be a sign of neurofibromatosis (Figure 10-8). Overlapping of the second and third fingers (Figure 10-9) should lead one to investigate the possibility of trisomy 18.[9]

Examine the nails for size and shape. The nails are usually smooth and soft and extend to the fingertips. They may be long in postterm infants or may be absent or spoon shaped in the presence of some syndromes. Nails may appear hypoplastic if the infant's hands are edematous. A detailed discussion of nail examination is found in Chapter 4.

SPINE

The back is examined with the infant lying prone or held suspended with the examiner's hand under the chest. First inspect the spine from the base of the skull to the coccyx, noting any skin disruption, tufts of hair, soft or cystic masses, hemangiomas, a pilonidal dimple (Figure 10-10), cysts, or sinus tracts. Such pathologic conditions may be signs of a congenital spinal or neurologic anomaly. The position of the scapula should also be noted while the infant is

FIGURE 10-10 ▲ Pilonidal dimple.

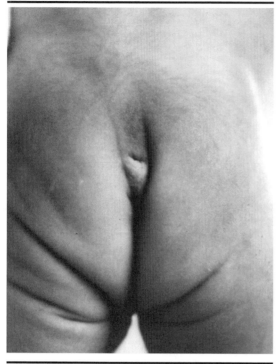

Courtesy of David A. Clark, MD, Louisiana State University.

FIGURE 10-11 ▲ Scoliosis.

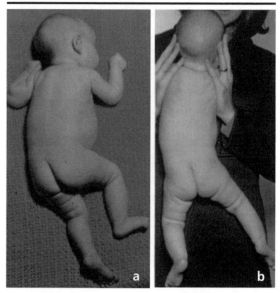

Scoliosis denotes spinal curvature convex to the right or left. Scoliosis in the newborn is rare but when it occurs, it is usually associated with a structural anomaly of the vertebral column. Infants with scoliosis are usually female, and the condition may be familial. (a) Inspection of the infant in the supine position may lead to equivocal signs. But when the baby is lifted by the armpits (b), the scoliosis becomes obvious.

From: Milner RDG, and Herber SM. 1984. *Color Atlas of the Newborn*. Oradell, New Jersey: Medical Economics, 88. Reprinted by permission of Blackwell Science, Inc.

FIGURE 10-12 ▲ Convex curvature of the thoracic and lumbar spine.

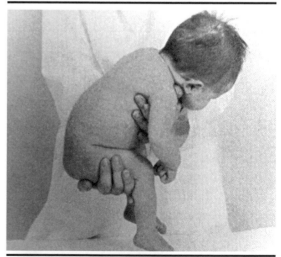

From: Jarvis C. 1992. *Physical Examination and Health Assessment*. Philadelphia: WB Saunders, 705. Reprinted by permission.

in the prone position to rule out Sprengel deformity, a winged or elevated scapula.

The entire length of the spine should be palpated to determine the presence of dorsal spinal processes and any abnormal curvatures. Gross abnormalities such as scoliosis (Figure 10-11), lordosis, and kyphosis are easily observed. A lateral curvature, however, is usually secondary to *in utero* position. A convex curvature of the thoracic and lumbar spine will be apparent when the infant is in a sitting position (Figure 10-12). The lumbar and sacral curves that are seen in adults develop later, when the infant sits up and begins to stand (Figure 10-13).[5] Extension and lateral bending of the spine can be noted by passive flexion. Flexion and extension should be smooth and rhythmic, without muscle spasm. A neurologic evaluation is necessary to complete the examination of the spine. Techniques are explained in Chapter 11.

TABLE 10-2 ▲ Normal Neonatal Range of Motion in Lower Extremities

Joint or Extremity	Flexion	Extension	Abduction	Adduction	Internal Rotation	Rotation
Hip	145°		90°	10°–20°	40°	80°
Knee	120°–145°	90°				
Ankle	Dorsiflexion: above resting position Plantar flexion: >10° from resting position					
Forefoot			≥10°–15°	≥10°–15°		
Hindfoot			Valgus ≥10°	Varus ≥5°		

From: Scanlon JW, et al. 1979. *A System of Newborn Physical Examination.* Baltimore: University Park Press, 42. Reprinted by permission of the author.

LOWER EXTREMITIES

Examination of the lower extremities includes the hip, femur, tibia, fibula, knee, ankle, and foot. Normal ranges for joint movement in the lower extremities are listed in Table 10-2.

Hips

The hips of a newborn generally have a flexion contracture. When the pelvis is stabilized and the lumbar spine is flattened out by flexing one hip, a flexion contracture of the contralateral hip can be detected. The degree of flexion contracture on the extended leg is the angle that is measured between the thigh and the horizontal plane of the bed or examining table.[11] This is usually 25 to 30 degrees in a normal newborn.

The stability of the hip must also be evaluated to rule out congenital hip dysplasia (CHD). Asymmetry of skin folds in the gluteal and femoral regions suggest dislocation (Figure 10-14).

The Ortolani and Barlow maneuvers are the most reliable screening tests for evaluating hip stability (Figure 10-15). Although they are described as separate tests, in clinical practice,

FIGURE 10-13 ▲ Spinal curves of the adult (left) and infant (right).

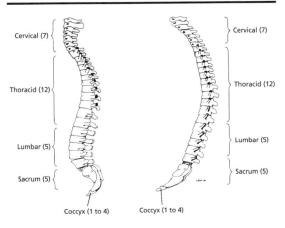

From: Alexander MM, and Brown MS. 1979. *Pediatric History Taking and Physical Diagnosis for Nurses*, 2nd ed. St. Louis: Mosby-Year Book, 292. Reprinted by permission of the authors.

FIGURE 10-14 ▲ Asymmetric gluteal folds.

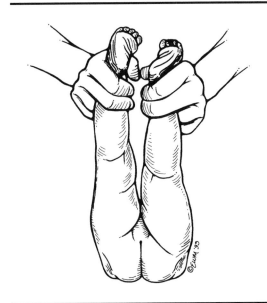

FIGURE 10-15 ▲ Ortolani and Barlow maneuvers.

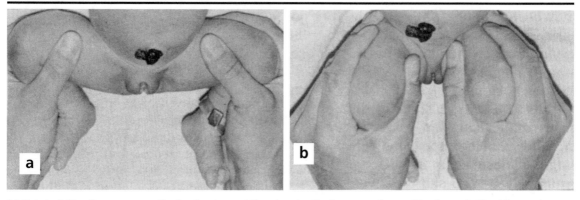

(a) Ortolani: The fingers are on the trochanter and thumb grips the femur as shown. The femur is lifted forward as the thighs are abducted. If the femur head was dislocated, it can be felt to reduce. (b) Barlow: The thighs are adducted, and if the femur head dislocates, it will be both felt and seen as it suddenly jerks over the acetabulum.

From: Avery GB. 1994. *Neonatology: Pathophysiology and Management of the Newborn*, 4th ed. Philadelphia: JB Lippincott, 1180. Reprinted by permission.

both maneuvers are done in a sequence, not as separate examinations. The infant must be relaxed and on a relatively firm surface.[12] These are not forceful examinations; a forceful exam only makes the infant cry and yields unreliable results. A crying, kicking infant can generate enough muscle strength by tightening the adductors and hamstrings to create a false result.[2,13] Accuracy of the examination is affected by the cooperation of the infant and the patience of the practitioner.

The Ortolani maneuver is a test of hip reduction. It produces the reduction of the dislocated femoral head into the acetabulum by abduction. With the infant positioned supine, the practitioner flexes the infant's knee and hip, then grasps the thigh with the thumb positioned medially and the third or fourth finger placed over the greater trochanter laterally. While simultaneously abducting the hips, the practitioner's finger on the greater trochanter presses up against the head of the femur and the hand presses the shaft of the femur toward the mattress. A positive Ortolani test is produced when a palpable "clunk" is noted, indicating that the femoral head has slipped from

a dislocated position into the acetabulum. Higher-pitched clicks and snaps can be heard and felt but are not associated with hip pathology and are usually due to movement of the tendons, ligaments, or fluid in the hip joint.[12,13]

The Barlow maneuver determines whether the femoral head can be dislocated and is the opposite of the Ortolani maneuver. The practitioner's hand position is the same as for the Ortolani maneuver with the infant's hips and legs flexed. As the knees are brought together (adducted) from the abducted position, the practitioner's thumb pushes laterally on the upper inner thigh. A "clunk" indicates that the femoral head has slipped over the lateral edge of the acetabulum and demonstrates an unstable hip joint that is dislocatable. The amount of force needed to push the femoral head out or into the acetabulum is minimal.

A variation of the Barlow maneuver is to stabilize the pelvis with one hand while the other hand attempts to move the thigh anteriorly and posteriorly (upward and downward) without flexing the hip. This maneuver enables the practitioner to determine if the femoral head can be displaced posteriorly out of the acetabulum.

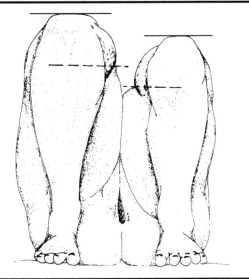

From: Alexander MM, and Brown MS. 1979. *Pediatric History Taking and Physical Diagnosis for Nurses*, 2nd ed. St. Louis: Mosby-Year Book, 301. Reprinted by permission of the authors.

FIGURE 10-17 ▲ **Examination for tibial torsion.**

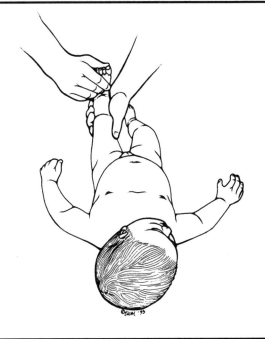

Legs

Palpate the legs to confirm the presence of the femur, tibia, and fibula. Fractures should be suspected when there is a history of difficult delivery or palpation reveals irregularities in contour, crepitance, or masses due to hematoma formation. Although birth trauma rarely causes a fracture of the femur, avulsion of the femoral epiphysis may occur and should be suspected if there is pain on passive movement or little spontaneous movement of the leg.[5] Femoral length can be observed by testing for the Galeazzi or Allis's sign (Figure 10-16). Keeping the feet flat on the bed and the femurs aligned, flex both of the infant's knees. With the tips of the big toes in the same horizontal plane, face the feet and observe the height of the knees.[6] It will be apparent if one knee is higher than the other, a positive Allis's sign. A discrepancy in knee height should also lead one to investigate for CHD.

The lower extremities are examined for length and shape. With the infant supine, draw an imaginary line connecting the anterior-superior iliac spine with the midpatella, and continue down to the foot. If the line falls medial to the big toe, external tibial torsion is present. If the line falls lateral to the second toe, internal tibial torsion (a slight varus curvature) is present (Figure 10-17). The normal newborn has between 0 and 20 degrees of internal tibial torsion; this gradually changes to external tibial torsion by childhood.[3] Although lateral tibial bowing without a significant shortening of the extremity is considered normal in the newborn, anterior bowing is an abnormal finding, and an orthopedic consultation should be sought.

Ankles and Feet

Examination of the ankles and feet includes observation of the resting position and stimulation for active motion. To stimulate for motion, stroke the sole as well as the dorsal, medial, and lateral sides of the foot. Passive motion of the ankle in dorsiflexion and plantar flexion varies, depending on the infant's position *in utero.* For example, ankle and fore-foot adduction, a positional deformity, can be differentiated from congenital equinovarus (clubfoot) malformation by passively positioning the foot in the midline and dorsiflexing it. A clubfoot or other structurally abnormal foot and ankle will not have a full range of motion and will resist dorsiflexion.

The toes should be examined for number, position, and spacing between them. Overlapping toes in infancy is usually a hereditary condition; correction may involve only stabilizing the toe in the correct position with an adhesive bandage for approximately six weeks.[9] The soles of the feet should be inspected as part of the gestational age assessment. Most newborns are flat footed due to a plantar fat pad (a pad of fat in the longitudinal arch of the foot), which gradually disappears during the first year of life.

MUSCULOSKELETAL ANOMALIES

Congenital anomalies of the musculoskeletal system may be evident as the absence of a part, extra parts, or malformed or malfunctioning tissue. Congenital anomalies usually affect the infant's movement, muscle tone, or posture. It is not within the scope of this chapter to discuss all the musculoskeletal anomalies encountered by the practitioner. However, many of the common problems and other special conditions seen in neonates are included in this section.

ANOMALIES OF THE NECK

Klippel-Feil Syndrome

This is a defect of the cervical vertebrae in which there is both a decrease in the number of vertebrae and a fusion of two or more vertebrae. The neonate's neck appears shorter than normal, and motion is limited in all directions. There is usually asymmetry in both rotation and lateral flexion. The asymmetric motion may be confused with torticollis (see following

FIGURE 10-18 ▲ Myelomeningocele.

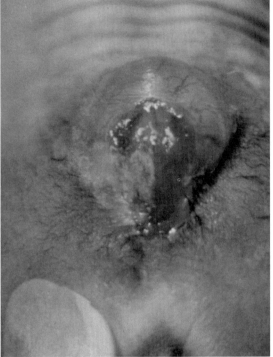

Courtesy of David A. Clark, MD, Louisiana State University.

section), but an x-ray of the neck will confirm the presence of the Klippel-Feil deformity.

Torticollis

Congenital torticollis, or wry neck, "a spasmodic, unilateral contraction of the neck muscles,"[8] is thought to be the result of birth trauma or ischemia due to *in utero* position.[13] This anomaly is not usually seen in the immediate newborn period, but a hematoma may sometimes be palpated shortly after birth. Torticollis usually appears as a firm, fibrous mass or tightness in the sternocleidomastoid muscle at approximately two weeks of age. The mass is 1 to 2 cm in diameter, hard, immobile, and felt in the midportion of the sternocleidomastoid muscle.[10] The right side is more commonly involved than the left.[3] In this condition, the infant's head will be tilted laterally toward one shoulder with the chin rotated away from the affected shoulder.[13] If the mass goes unnoticed, the torticollis may not be detected until there is facial asymmetry and limited rotation of the neck toward the side of the lesion. If the torticollis persists, there is a flattening of the occiput on the opposite side and a flattening of the frontal bones on the side of the lesion. These are most likely caused by the infant's head position while sleeping.[3]

SPINAL DEFORMITIES

Congenital Scoliosis

Scoliosis in the neonate may range from undetectable to very severe. It is not chromosomal or inherited, but rather an embryonic defect. The structural basis for congenital scoliosis is a failure of vertebral formation, segmentation, or a variety of both. The failures can be in any area of the vertebral body. If undetected, severe deformities can develop and affect neurologic function as well as cosmetic appearance. Upon diagnosis, the infant should also be evaluated for genitourinary tract anomalies (unilateral renal agenesis being the most common) because there is an increased incidence (20–30 percent) with congenital vertebral anomalies.[2,13] Klippel-Feil syndrome and Sprengel deformity of the scapula are also seen with congenital scoliosis.[2,14]

Myelomeningocele

This anomaly is a congenital neural tube defect that usually presents as a failure of closure at the caudal (tail) end of the vertebral column, permitting the meninges and sometimes the spinal cord to protrude into a saclike structure (Figure 10-18). Skin disruption is not always present, however, so any soft mass noted over the spine or just off the midline must be examined closely to rule out myelomeningocele. Because the functional deficit of the lower extremities is linked to the level of involvement of the myelomeningocele, it is important

FIGURE 10-19 ▲ Cleidocranial dysostosis.

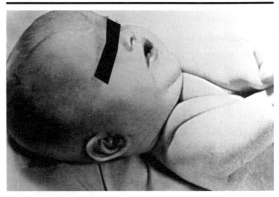

Infant showing marked adduction of the shoulders
resulting from absence of the clavicles.

From: Swaiman KF, and Wright FS. 1982. *The Practice of Pediatric Neurology.* St. Louis: Mosby-Year Book, 441. Reprinted by permission.

to examine muscle function of the lower extremities. This examination is discussed in Chapter 11.

UPPER EXTREMITY ANOMALIES

Sprengel Deformity (Congenital Elevated Scapula)

Sprengel deformity is one of the more common congenital anomalies of the shoulder girdle. The elevation may be unilateral or, in one-third of cases, bilateral.[3,14] The asymmetry of the shoulder seen with unilateral involvement makes diagnosis relatively easy. The scapula is somewhat hypoplastic and malrotated so that, when palpated, the vertebral border lies superiorly and more horizontal than normal.[1,2] There is some limitation of shoulder abduction and flexion. Internal and external shoulder rotation may be only slightly affected. Sprengel deformity is frequently associated with congenital spinal problems, renal anomalies, and Klippel-Feil syndrome.[2,3,13]

Cleidocranial Dysostosis

Cleidocranial dysostosis is a defect in which there is the complete or partial absence of the clavicles (Figure 10-19). This skeletal dysplasia is inherited as an autosomal dominant trait.

It is recognized by palpation and by the presence of excessive scapulothoracic motion. Complete absence of the clavicle is usually accompanied by defective ossification of the cranium, large fontanels, and delayed closure of the sutures.[6] Although the deformities may not be cosmetically pleasing, there is usually little functional disability, and therefore no treatment is required.

Brachial Palsy

Brachial palsy results from a prolonged and difficult labor ending in a traumatic delivery. It is seen most often in large babies who are therefore vulnerable to stretching injuries to the components of the brachial plexus. The infant with an upper arm paralysis holds the affected arm adducted and internally rotated, with extension at the elbow, pronation of the forearm, and flexion of the wrist (Figure 10-20). Paralysis of the upper arm is more common than paralysis of the lower arm or of the entire arm.[3] The grasp reflex remains intact, but the Moro reflex is absent on the affected side. In cases where the nerve roots are not disrupted, infants regain neurologic function within several days as the hemorrhage and edema in the area resolve. Although most infants gain significant functional improvement, by three months of age close examination usually reveals tightness of the shoulder on internal rotation, difficulties in supination of the forearm, and abduction of the shoulder.[10]

Congenital Absence of the Radius

In this anomaly, the hand and wrist are deviated 90 degrees or more. Congenital absence of the radius (Figure 10-21) is easily recognized. It may be unilateral but is bilateral in 50 percent of infants who exhibit it.[2,3] The clinical presentation is shortened forearm with bowing of the ulna. The thumb is usually absent or hypoplastic. The elbow has limited movement. A consultation with a pediatric hand surgeon is required.

FIGURE 10-20 ▲ Brachial palsy.

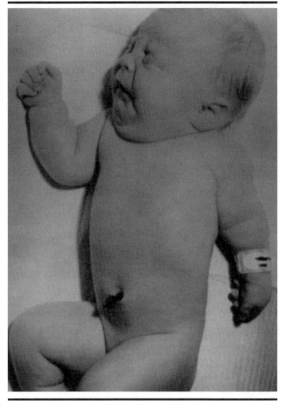

Courtesy of David A. Clark, MD, Louisiana State University.

LOWER EXTREMITY ANOMALIES

Congenital Hip Dysplasia

Congenital hip dysplasia is one of the most significant deformities of the newborn period. It covers a spectrum of conditions that arise from abnormal development of the hip joint. These conditions range from minimal instability (in which the femoral head remains in the acetabulum) to irreducible dislocation (where the femoral head loses contact completely with the acetabular capsule and is displaced over the fibrocartilaginous rim).[3,6] CHD is thought to be caused by lack of acetabular depth, ligamentous laxity, and/or intrauterine breech position. Approximately 17 to 50 percent of all CHD occurs in infants born after breech presentation.[2,3] The incidence of detectable dysplasia overall is approximately 1 in every 1,000 live births.[13] However, the incidence does vary by

FIGURE 10-21 ▲ Congenital absence of the radius.

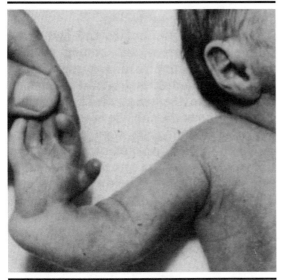

From: Avery GB. 1994. *Neonatology: Pathophysiology and Management of the Newborn,* 4th ed. Philadelphia: JB Lippincott, 1183. Reprinted by permission.

FIGURE 10-22 ▲ Genu recurvatum.

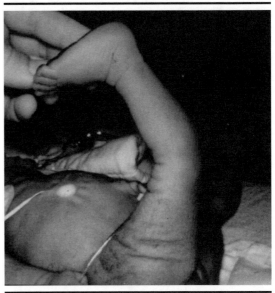

Courtesy of David A. Clark, MD, Louisiana State University Medical Center and Wyeth-Ayerst Laboratories, Philadelphia, Pennsylvania.

race. In Caucasian infants, the incidence of detectable instability of the hip at birth is 1 in 60; the incidence of complete dislocation is 1 in 500.[3] For unknown reasons, African American and Asian infants are less likely to develop CHD.[3] Females are more prone to the condition than males, and the left hip is more frequently affected than the right.[1,2] If a family history reveals that the mother had a dislocated hip as a child or an older female sibling has hip dysplasia, the risk for dislocated hip in the infant is increased. CHD is also more common in infants with other orthopedic conditions, such as torticollis (10–20 percent), and with congenital foot deformities, such as clubfoot and metatarsus adductus (1 percent).[2,3,15] Early diagnosis and treatment appropriate to the specific anomaly are important for normal hip anatomy and function. The longer the dislocation remains untreated, the greater the chance of problems in returning the femoral head to its normal position and the less satisfactory the results.[2,13] Assessment techniques and signs of CHD were discussed earlier in this chapter.

Congenital Absence of the Tibia or Fibula

Although congenital absence of a long bone is unusual, when it does occur, the bone most frequently affected is the fibula.[3] These deformities are easily recognized. Tibia or fibula absence may be partial or complete. When a portion of the bone is present, the deformity is likely to be less severe. In absence of the tibia, the clinical presentation is mild to marked shortening of the lower leg. The knee is unstable and has a flexion contracture. The foot may be normal or fixed in a mild to severe varus position. Approximately 20 percent of the cases are bilateral.[3] In absence of the fibula, the clinical presentation is shortening of the involved leg with bowing of the tibia anteriorly and medially. The foot deformity is often severe, with a valgus position.[1] Treatment depends upon the severity of the condition and focuses on the problems of foot deformity and leg length discrepancy. These deformities should be seen by an orthopedist early in the neonatal period.

FIGURE 10-23 ▲ Metatarsus adductus.

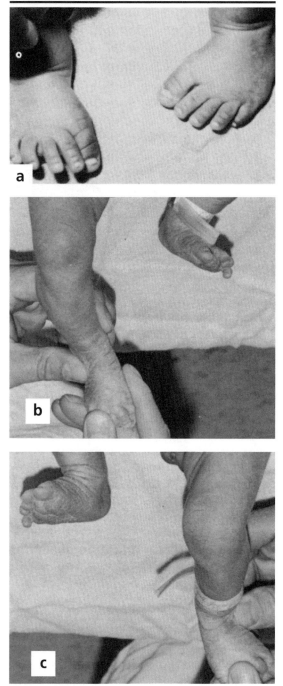

(a) Structural metatarsus adductus. (b) Structural
metatarsus adductus. The forefoot does not abduct
beyond neutral. (c) Positional metatarsus adductus.
The forefoot abducts beyond the midline.

From: Avery GB. 1994. *Neonatology: Pathophysiology
and Management of the Newborn,* 4th ed. Philadelphia: JB Lippincott, 1186. Reprinted by permission.

FIGURE 10-24 ▲ Clubfoot.

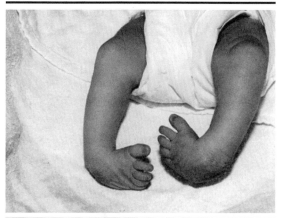

Courtesy of Carol Trotter, St. John's Mercy Medical
Center, St. Louis, Missouri.

Genu Recurvatum

This rare anomaly is a congenital dislocation
or hyperextension of the knee (Figure 10-22).
It is thought to be due to a frank breech position *in utero* or a prenatal developmental defect.
It may be associated with oligohydramnios,
congenital absence of the quadriceps muscle,
or a syndrome such as sacral agenesis.[3] More
common in females, it is usually seen bilaterally. Because early treatment prevents further
deformity or interference with normal function, an orthopedic consultation should be initiated on the day of birth.

Metatarsus Adductus

The most common congenital foot anoma-
ly, metatarsus adductus is caused by intrauterine
positioning.[6] It may be a positional (flexible)
deformity with no bony abnormality involved
or a structural (fixed) deformity (Figure 10-23).
In a structural deformity, the arch appears to
be greater than normal, and there may be a
medial crease at the middle portion of the arch.
The forefoot usually cannot be abducted
beyond the midline (neutral position). In a
positional deformity, the forefoot is very mobile
and can be easily abducted. In infants with
severe structural anomaly, the heel (hindfoot)
is in a valgus position. In a positional metatarsal

FIGURE 10-25 ▲ **Congenital constricting bands (amniotic bands).**

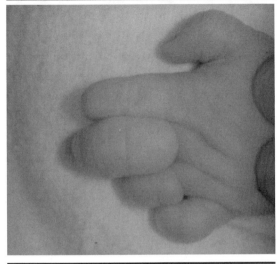

Courtesy of David A. Clark, MD, Louisiana State University.

adductus, the heel is likely to be in a varus or neutral position. A positional deformity of the involved foot will correct without treatment. In a rigid foot, an orthopedic consultation is necessary for early treatment.

FIGURE 10-26 ▲ **Congenital constricting bands (amniotic bands).**

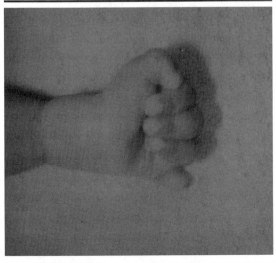

Courtesy of David A. Clark, MD, Louisiana State University Medical Center and Wyeth-Ayerst Laboratories, Philadelphia, Pennsylvania.

FIGURE 10-27 ▲ **Congenital constricting bands (amniotic bands).**

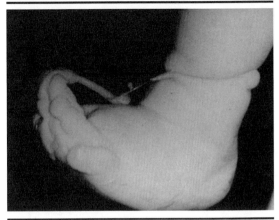

Courtesy of David A. Clark, MD, Louisiana State University Medical Center and Wyeth-Ayerst Laboratories, Philadelphia, Pennsylvania.

Clubfoot (Talipes Equinovarus)

Clubfoot (Figure 10-24) is a complex foot deformity that is readily apparent at birth. It is one of the most common congenital anomalies, whose incidence varies with race and sex. In Caucasians, the birth frequency is approximately 1 per 1,000 live births, with males affected twice as often as females.[3,16] The highest incidence is seen in Polynesians and South African blacks at a rate of 6.8 and 3.5 per thousand births. Asian infants are the least likely to

FIGURE 10-28 ▲ **Amniotic bands resulting in finger amputation.**

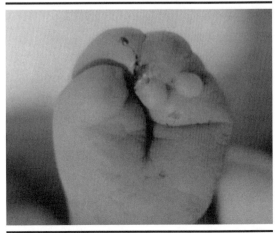

Courtesy of David A. Clark, MD, Louisiana State University.

FIGURE 10-29 ▲ Syndactyly of the fingers.

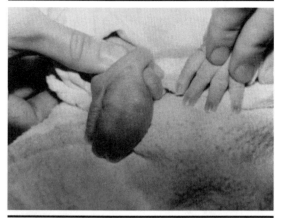

Courtesy of Carol Trotter, St. John's Mercy Medical Center, St. Louis, Missouri.

FIGURE 10-30 ▲ Polydactyly of the toes.

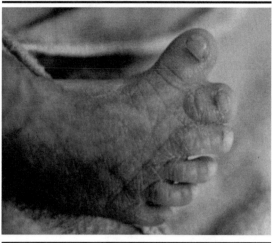

Courtesy of David A. Clark, MD, Louisiana State University.

present with clubfoot.[16] Clinical presentation is adduction of the forefoot (points medially), pronounced varus of the heel, and downward pointing of the foot and toes (equinus positioning). If the condition is unilateral, the affected foot is smaller, with the ankle and foot joints contracted and thickened, inhibiting function. The right is affected more often than the left in unilateral cases, and involvement is bilateral in about 50 percent of the cases.[16] There are variations in the severity of clubfoot. Some are relatively flexible and correctable with serial exercises and casting. Treatment can often be started in the nursery; an orthopedic consultation should be initiated on the day of birth.

CONDITIONS AFFECTING UPPER AND/OR LOWER EXTREMITIES

Congenital Constricting Bands (Streeter Dysplasia)

Presenting as a band encircling the arms, legs, fingers, or toes, this deformity can vary from mild, shallow indentations of the soft tissue to severe constrictions causing partial or complete amputation (Figures 10-25 through 10-28). Occasionally, craniofacial structures are affected. The etiology is unknown, but the most widely accepted theory is that of amniotic bands or other abnormalities of the intrauterine environment. Treatment depends upon the severity of the condition. Severe bands may need to be treated as an emergency, especially if there is evidence of vascular or lymphatic obstruction. A surgical consultation is needed for these cases.

Syndactyly

Congenital webbing of the fingers or toes—syndactyly—is one of the most common congenital anomalies (Figure 10-29). Syndactyly is frequently a familial tendency.[1] The severity of involvement varies from minimal "bridging" between adjacent fingers/toes to complete webbing of the hand/foot. The more severe the syndactyly, the greater the likelihood of bony abnormalities as well. Syndactyly of the toes does not interfere with function but may be unacceptable cosmetically. Surgical treatment is not required but may be requested by the parents. Treatment for syndactyly of the fingers depends on the severity of the webbing and the presence or absence of bony abnormalities. When multiple fingers are involved, function may deteriorate as the fingers grow. Early correction should therefore be considered. An orthopedic consultation is needed.

FIGURE 10-31 ▲ Polydactyly of the fingers.

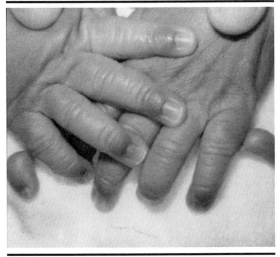

Courtesy of David A. Clark, MD, Louisiana State University Medical Center and Wyeth-Ayerst Laboratories, Philadelphia, Pennsylvania.

Polydactyly

Extra digits are common abnormalities affecting both the hands and the feet (Figures 10-30 and 10-31). Polydactyly is seen more commonly in African American than in Caucasian infants, and there is a familial tendency.[3] The most common type of polydactyly is a floppy digit or skin tag on either the radial or the ulnar side of the hand. Polydactyly may, however, involve the duplication of a normal-looking digit, giving the infant a functional six-fingered hand or a foot with six toes. Treatment depends on the extent of the anomaly. Consultation is required so that therapeutic decisions can be based on function as well as cosmetic considerations.

SUMMARY

The examination of the musculoskeletal system provides a wealth of information about the overall development of the infant *in utero*, as well as the potential for normal development and function. Many of the common congenital anomalies of infancy are found in the musculoskeletal system. Although these anomalies may not interfere with vital functions (as do anomalies of the respiratory, cardiovascular, or other systems), they are a frequent cause of parental anxiety. The more accomplished the examiner becomes at performing the musculoskeletal exam, the easier it is to recognize deviations from normal, potential problems, and the necessity to initiate early interventions.

REFERENCES

1. Griffin P. 1994. Orthopedics. In *Neonatology: Pathophysiology and Management of the Newborn*, 4th ed., Avery GB, Fletcher MA, and MacDonald MG, eds. Philadelphia: JB Lippincott, 1179–1194.
2. Hensinger RN, and Jones E. 1992. Orthopedic problems in the newborn. In *Textbook of Neonatology*, 2nd ed., Robertson NR, ed. New York: Churchill Livingstone, 889–914.
3. Renshaw TS. 1986. *Pediatric Orthopedics*. Philadelphia: WB Saunders, 1–10, 39–43, 63–74, 91–92.
4. Hoekelman RA. 1995. The physical examination of infants and children. In *A Guide to Physical Examination*, 6th ed., Bates B, ed. Philadelphia: JB Lippincott, 565, 573, 578.
5. Lawrence RA. 1984. Physical examination. In *Assessment of the Newborn, A Guide for the Practitioner*, Ziai M, Clark T, and Merritt TA, eds. Boston: Little, Brown, 99–101.
6. Seidel HM, et al. 1991. *Mosby's Guide to Physical Examination*, 2nd ed. St. Louis: Mosby-Year Book, 599–603.
7. Perry S. 1991. Normal newborn. In *Essentials of Maternity Nursing*, 3rd ed., Bobak IM, and Jensen MD, eds. St. Louis: Mosby-Year Book, 441–481.
8. Scanlon JW, et al. 1979. *A System of Newborn Physical Examination*. Baltimore: University Park Press, 39–43.
9. Alexander MM, and Brown MS. 1979. *Pediatric History Taking and Physical Diagnosis for Nurses*, 2nd ed. New York: McGraw-Hill, 283–305.
10. Mangurten HH. 1992. Birth injuries. In *Neonatal-Perinatal Medicine: Diseases of the Fetus and Infant*, 5th ed., Fanaroff AA, and Martin RJ, eds. St. Louis: Mosby-Year Book, 346–371.
11. Davidson RS. 1992. Orthopedic examination of the newborn. In *Fetal and Neonatal Physiology*, Polin RA, and Fox WW, eds. Philadelphia: WB Saunders, 1685.
12. Coen RW, and Koffler H. 1987. The physical examination. In *Primary Care of the Newborn*. Boston: Little, Brown, 33–38.
13. Tolo VT, and Wood B. 1993. *Pediatric Orthopaedics in Primary Care*. Baltimore: Williams & Wilkins, 16–21, 30–33, 92–93, 143–154.
14. Bayne LG, and Costas BL. 1990. Malformations of the upper limb. In *Pediatric Orthopedics*, 3rd ed., Morrissy RT, ed. Philadelphia: JB Lippincott, 563–610.
15. Herring JA. 1990. Congenital dislocation of the hip. In *Pediatric Orthopedics*, 3rd ed., Morrissy RT, ed. Philadelphia: JB Lippincott, 815–830.
16. Tachdjian MO. 1990. The foot and leg. In *Pediatric Orthopedics*, 2nd ed., Tachdjian MO, ed. Philadelphia: WB Saunders, 2428–2440.

BIBLIOGRAPHY

- Balsan MJ, and Holzman IR. 1992. Neonatology. In *Atlas of Pediatric Physical Diagnosis*, 2nd ed., Zitelli BJ, and Oski FA, eds. Philadelphia: JB Lippincott, 2.1–2.19.
- Barkauskas VH, et al. 1994. *Health and Physical Assessment.* St. Louis: Mosby-Year Book, 801–805.
- Lieber MT, and Taub AS. 1988. Common foot deformities and what they mean for parents. *MCN: American Journal of Maternal Child Nursing* 13(1): 47–50.

- Milner RDG, and Herber SM. 1984. *Color Atlas of the Newborn.* Oradell, New Jersey: Medical Economics.
- Sterk L. 1993. Neonatal orthopedic conditions. In *Core Curriculum for Neonatal Intensive Care Nursing*, Beachy P, and Deacon J, eds. Philadelphia: WB Saunders, 462–470.
- Swaiman KF, and Wright FS. 1982. *The Practice of Pediatric Neurology,* 2nd ed. St. Louis: Mosby-Year Book, 441.
- Tachdjian MO. 1990. *Pediatric Orthopedics*, 2nd ed. Philadelphia: WB Saunders, 112–116, 128–138, 302–317.

NOTES

11 Neurologic Assessment

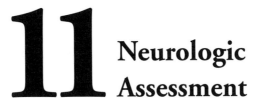

Barbara E. Carey, RNC, MN, NNP, CPNP

The neurologic evaluation is a critical part of neonatal assessment. A single examination may verify the presence of normal neurologic responses and status. It may also indicate a low risk of subsequent abnormal neurologic development related to perinatal causes. An abnormal or suspect examination should be followed by repeat examinations to validate abnormalities identified on the first examination and to document their changes or disappearance over time. Steady improvement in responses and disappearance of abnormal responses during the neonatal period offer a better prognosis than static abnormal responses.

A traditional and simple approach to assessment of neurologic status is through the systematic testing of specific functions of the nervous system, including the motor system, reflexes, sensory system, and the cranial nerves. This approach is followed here. More formal neurologic assessments, designed as clinical and research tools, are available. The neurologic evaluation developed by Amiel-Tison is designed to evaluate neonates at term or corrected term age during the first year of life and emphasizes neuromotor function.[1] Prechtl has also developed and validated a neurologic exam-

ination for the full-term neonate.[2] Another comprehensive neurologic examination has been designed by Lilly and Victor Dubowitz and is applicable to both term and preterm neonates.[3] The Dubowitz exam places heavy emphasis on evaluation of movement and tone. It also includes some behavioral items which are evaluated on the Brazelton assessment.

MATERNAL AND FAMILY HISTORY

Before performing the neurologic examination, the examiner should thoroughly review the history for genetic or neurologic problems of the family, maternal medical problems, problems arising during the pregnancy, as well as the use of medication, alcohol, or drugs. Any test results of chromosome analysis, fetal well-being, and maturity should be reviewed. The intrapartum course is reviewed for abnormal presentation, prolonged labor, precipitous delivery, fetal distress, and difficult extraction. Anesthetic agents and medications administered around the time of delivery may also affect the neurologic examination and should be noted. The history is also reviewed for Apgar scores, the presence of neonatal depression, difficulties in transition, medical problems, and feed-

FIGURE 11-1 ▲ Posture and passive tone. Increase of tone with maturity showing the ascending direction of tone.

Gestational age	28 wk	30 wk	32 wk	34 wk	36 wk	38 wk	40 wk
Posture	Completely hypotonic	Beginning of flexion of the thigh at the hip	Stronger flexion	Froglike attitude	Flexion of the 4 limbs	Hypertonic	Very hypertonic
Heel to ear maneuver							
Popliteal angle	150°	130°	110°	100°	100°	90°	80°
Dorsiflexion angle of the foot			40–50°		20–30°		Premature reached 40 weeks 40° / Full term
Scarf sign	Scarf sign complete with no resistance		Scarf sign more limited		Elbow slightly passes the midline		Elbow does not reach the midline
Return to flexion of forearm	Absent (upper limbs very hypotonic lying in extension)			Absent (flexion of forearms begins to appear when awake)	Present but weak, inhibited	Present, brisk, inhibited	Present, very strong, not inhibited

From: Amiel-Tison C. 1991. Newborn neurologic examination. In *Rudolph's Pediatrics,* 19th ed., Rudolph AM, and Hoffman J, eds. Stamford, Connecticut: Appleton & Lange, 178. Reprinted by permission.

ing ability. The gestational age is noted. An accurate assessment of gestational age is essential for appropriate interpretation of posture, tone, and reflexes. Neurologic response varies predictably at different stages of maturity.

GENERAL INSPECTION

Before disturbing the neonate, evaluate for the presence of dysmorphic features, evidence of birth trauma, skin lesions, posture, and activity.

Evidence of *birth trauma* may include cephalhematoma, a depressed area of the skull, forceps marks, lacerations, abrasions, bruising, petechiae, and localized swelling. If evidence of trauma is found on the face or limbs, spontaneous movement and symmetry of movement should be evaluated to identify possible underlying damage to the nerves.

Certain types of *skin lesions* may be significant in the assessment of neurologic abnormality. Café au lait spots of 1.5 cm or larger or six or more in number may indicate the presence of neurofibromatosis, one of the more common autosomal dominant genetic disorders. In this disease, dysplastic tumors occur along nerves and sometimes in the eyes and/or meninges as well as at other sites in the body and on the skin.[4] Port wine facial hemangiomas involving both eyelids, with bilateral distribution, or those that are unilateral but involve all three branches of the trigeminal nerve are associated with a significantly higher incidence of eye and central nervous system abnormalities.[5] They may indicate the presence of Sturge-Weber syndrome with underlying arteriovenous malformations. Macrocephaly is also a common finding in affected neonates. Glaucoma and leptomeningeal vessels in the brain that can lead to seizures are other abnormalities. Areas of skin depigmentation may be significant; they may be the earliest manifestation of tuberous sclerosis, a progressive degenerative neurologic disease in which collections of abnormal neurons and glia occur in the subependymal and cortical areas of the brain. The skin lesion is white, macular, and has irregular leaflike borders. One or several lesions may be present.

If the neonate is awake and crying, attention should be paid to the *quality of the cry*, symmetry of movement, and facial expression. A loud, lusty cry is usual in the term neonate. A weaker, more feeble cry may be present in the premature, depressed, or ill neonate. A high-pitched cry may be present in infants with neurologic disturbances, metabolic abnormalities, and drug withdrawal. Neonates with high-pitched, incessant, or easily stimulated crying and who are also hyperirritable should raise the concern of possible drug withdrawal. A catlike cry may be heard with cri du chat syndrome, deletion of the short arm of the fifth chromosome. Stridor should raise the concern of partial vocal cord paralysis related to cervical nerve damage or to partial webs, stenosis, or malacia of the airway. Lack of movement of an extremity may indicate trauma and nerve damage. Lack of movement of one arm may indicate brachial plexus injury, Erb's palsy (damage to the upper spinal roots C-5 and C-6), and/or Klumpke's palsy (damage to the lower spinal roots C-8 and T-1). If respiratory distress or sustained tachypnea is present in the neonate with a brachial plexus injury, the possibility of phrenic nerve damage and resultant diaphragm

paralysis should be considered. According to Volpe, approximately 5 percent of brachial plexus injuries have phrenic nerve injury.[6] Facial asymmetry or lack of expression is seen in infants with facial weakness due to Bell's palsy.

The resting *posture* in which the neonate is found should be noted and its appropriateness for gestational age gauged. The normal term neonate lies with hips abducted and partially flexed and with knees flexed. The arms of the neonate are usually adducted and flexed at the elbow (Figures 11-1 and 11-2). The hand is normally loosely fisted, and the thumb may lie in the palm or adjacent to the fingers. At 28 weeks gestational age, the newborn's arms and legs are extended, with little tone. From 28 to 40 weeks gestational age, tone increases in a caudocephalic direction, with increased tone in flexion observed first in the legs (around 32–34 weeks) and later in the arms (around 34–36 weeks). In the premature neonate, the adductor muscles are hypotonic; although flexion is seen as gestational age increases, the limbs are often flat against the bed surface. In this posture, the legs are abducted, and the lateral thigh rests against the surface of the bed. This position, often referred to as the "frog leg" position, is abnormal in neonates greater than 36 weeks gestation. Neonates of 32 weeks gestation or greater who lie with their extremities completely extended are demonstrating abnormal postural tone. Depressed postural tone in the arms is suggested by flaccid extension of the arms or by some degree of flexion at the elbow but with open palmar surfaces facing up at 36 weeks or greater. In addition, cortical thumb—a persistent tightly fisted hand in which the thumb is firmly enclosed by the other fingers—may indicate neurologic abnormality. When inspection identifies any postural abnormality, it should be reconfirmed during the examination of tone and reflexes.

FIGURE 11-2 ▲ **Increase in active tone with maturity is illustrated. Note the ascending direction of tone.**

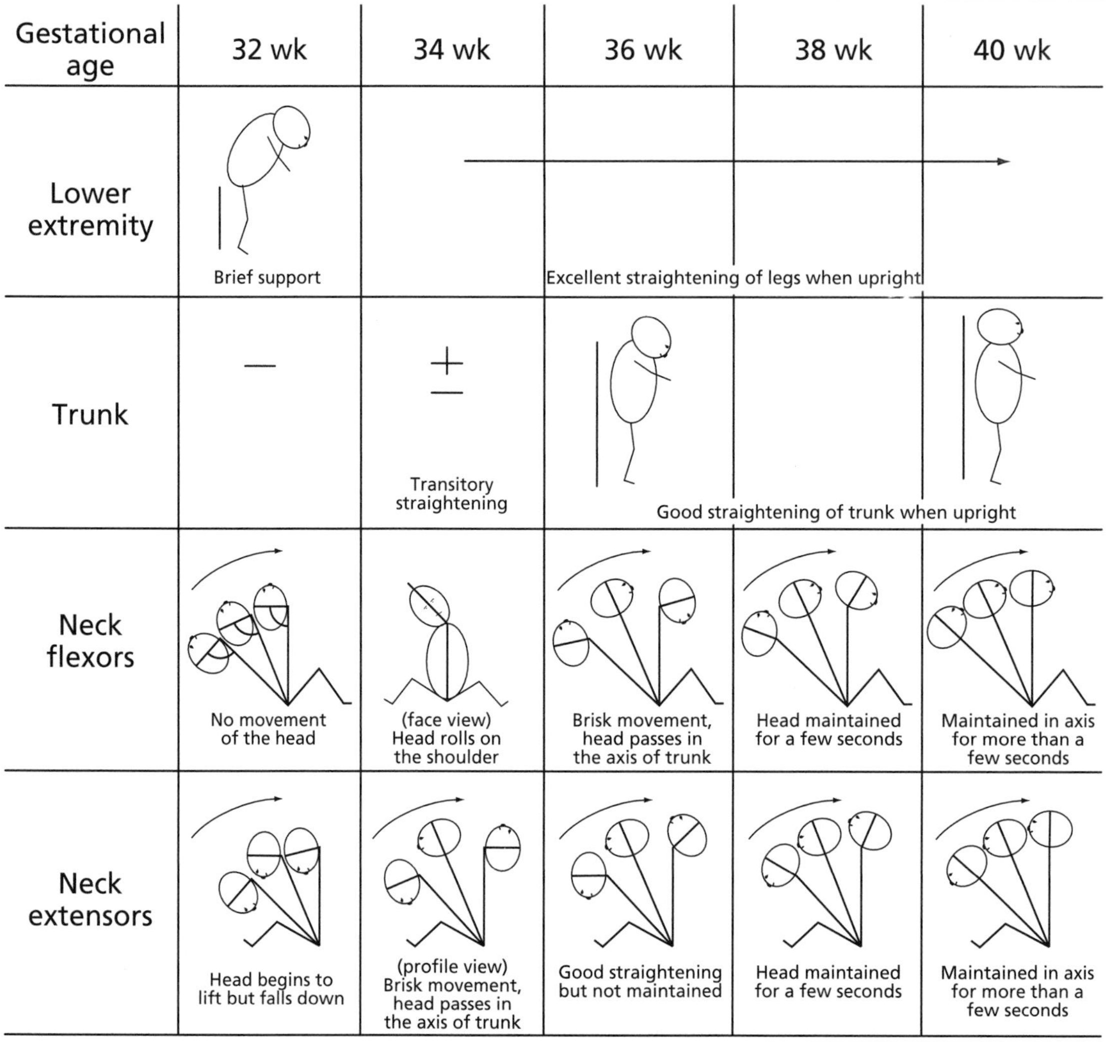

Gestational age	32 wk	34 wk	36 wk	38 wk	40 wk
Lower extremity	Brief support		Excellent straightening of legs when upright		
Trunk	—	± Transitory straightening	Good straightening of trunk when upright		
Neck flexors	No movement of the head	(face view) Head rolls on the shoulder	Brisk movement, head passes in the axis of trunk	Head maintained for a few seconds	Maintained in axis for more than a few seconds
Neck extensors	Head begins to lift but falls down	(profile view) Brisk movement, head passes in the axis of trunk	Good straightening but not maintained	Head maintained for a few seconds	Maintained in axis for more than a few seconds

From: Amiel-Tison C. 1991. Newborn neurologic examination. In *Rudolph's Pediatrics,* 19th ed., Rudolph AM, and Hoffman J, eds. Stamford, Connecticut: Appleton & Lange, 179. Reprinted by permission.

The *quality of movements* should also be evaluated in the active neonate. Term neonates move their limbs smoothly. In the preterm neonate, tremors and jitteriness may be present normally. Jitteriness can often be benign in term neonates and is sometimes seen with vigorous crying. It may also be a sign of disorders such as hypoglycemia, hypocalcemia, drug withdrawal, and hypoxic ischemic encephalopathy (Table 11-1). Jitteriness must be distinguished from seizure activity. Although the distinction can be subtle in the neonatal period, jitteriness is characterized by rapid alternating movements of equal amplitude in both directions. In contrast, the clonic movements seen during true seizures have a fast and slow component and are not as rapid. Noise, touch, or other environmental stimuli can elicit jitteriness, which can be stopped by flexing and holding the involved extremity. Seizures are generally not initiated by stimulation, nor can they be eliminated by flexing or holding. In addition, jitteriness is not associat-

TABLE 11-1 ▲ Distinguishing Seizure Activity from Jitteriness

Clinical finding	Seizure	Jitteriness
Abnormal gaze or eye movements	Yes	No
Stimulus sensitive	No	Yes
Cease with passive flexion	No	Yes
Autonomic changes	Yes	No
Predominant movement	Clonic jerking	Tremor

Adapted from: Volpe JJ. 1995. Neonatal seizures. In *Neurology of the Newborn*, 3rd ed. Philadelphia: WB Saunders, 182. Reprinted by permission.

ed with any subtle signs of seizure activity, such as abnormal eye movements.

The neonate's *state* should be noted both before and during the examination. Optimally, the examination is performed with the neonate in the quiet alert state. Timing the examination for 30 minutes to one hour before a feeding may increase the chances of the neonate being in this state. Prior to 28 weeks gestation, it is difficult to identify periods of wakefulness. Stimulation (such as a gentle shake) may result in eye opening and apparent alerting for short periods. At approximately 28 weeks gestation, there is an increase in the level of alertness, and both stimulated and spontaneous alerting can be seen. The more premature neonate has longer sleep cycles than the term neonate. Sleep-wake cycles are more apparent by 32 weeks gestation, and stimulation is usually not necessary to arouse and alert the neonate. By 37 weeks, increased alertness can be readily observed.

EXAMINATION OF THE HEAD

The status of the fontanels and sutures should be evaluated initially by gentle palpation in the noncrying neonate (Chapter 5). The examiner forms a general impression as to whether the fontanels are soft and flat or full or bulging. The size of the fontanels and sutures is next determined by palpation. A full or bulging fontanel with widened sutures may indicate increased intracranial pressure and hydrocephalus. Widening of the sutures alone, with a normal anterior fontanel, may be caused by abnormal ossification seen with intrauterine growth retardation. The head is palpated for other abnormalities, such as cephalhematoma and nondisplaceable sutures.

Head circumference is measured, plotted on a growth chart, and the percentile determined based on gestational age (Chapter 3). Neonates with head circumferences greater than the 90th percentile for gestational age and weight and height below the 90th percentile may have hydrocephaly, macrocephaly, or hydranencephaly. The skull configuration in hydrocephalus is frequently globular; and in neonates with Dandy-Walker syndrome, posterior ballooning of the skull may be evident. Abnormalities in skull configuration are also seen in some neonates with craniosynostosis. When a large head circumference and percentile for gestational age are identified, transillumination of the skull can be helpful. In a dark room and after the examiner's eyes have adapted to the reduced light, a rubber-cuffed flashlight or other transillumination device is applied firmly to the skull (Figure 5-1). A glow of more than 2 cm around the rubber cuff of the flashlight is abnormal. Neonates with small head circumferences (less than the 10th percentile for gestational age) may have microcephaly on the basis of chromosomal abnormality, intrauterine infection, or maternal drug and alcohol intake. Marked molding of the head following birth may give the erroneous impression of microcephaly, especially when the molding is conical.

Although not a routine part of the newborn physical examination, auscultation of the skull for bruits may be of value when arteriovenous malformation or aneurysm is suspected. Flow disturbances due to interference with the normal laminar flow through vessels may cause vessel wall vibrations heard as systolic murmurs and referred to as bruits. Bruits may be heard in Sturge-Weber syndrome, which is usually accompanied by facial hemangioma; it is therefore important to listen for bruits in neonates with this skin lesion. Arteriovenous malformations may lead to unexplained high-output cardiac failure in neonates, and an examination for bruits may assist in making the diagnosis. Auscultation is carried out with the bell of the stethoscope placed over the temporal, frontal, and occipital areas.

MOTOR EXAMINATION

Evaluation of muscle tone involves examination of resting posture (previously discussed), passive tone, and active tone of the major muscle groups. Tone can also be categorized as phasic, which correlates with passive tone and deep tendon reflexes, and postural, which correlates with active tone. Phasic tone is a brief, forceful contraction in response to a short-duration, high-amplitude stretch. Postural tone is a long-duration, low-amplitude stretch in response to gravity. The two tone types are tested separately and can vary independently.

PHASIC TONE

Phasic tone is evaluated by testing the resistance of the upper and lower extremities to movement and by the activity of the deep tendon reflexes. Resistance of the extremities to passive movements can be evaluated by the scarf sign (Chapter 3) and by arm and leg recoil. Minimal resistance is normal at 28 weeks; resistance increases with maturity. Tendon reflexes are elicited by sharp percussion with the examiner's finger or a small reflex hammer over the tendon, as discussed later. The biceps reflex and the patellar (or knee jerk) reflex are basic reflexes that can be tested in the neonate. These are most active in the first two days after birth and when the neonate is alert. Of all the tendon reflexes, the patellar is the most frequently demonstrated after birth. Innervation for the

knee jerk is at the second through fourth lumbar segments. It is tested by tapping the patellar tendon just below the patella while the examiner's hand supports the neonate's knee in a flexed position. The normal response is extension at the knee and visible contraction of the quadriceps. The biceps reflex is innervated at the fifth and sixth cervical nerve roots and is tested by holding the neonate's arm with the elbow in flexion and the examiner's thumb over the insertion of the biceps tendon. The examiner's thumb is tapped with a reflex hammer, and flexion of the biceps occurs.

Weak or absent reflexes may be seen in neonates less than 28 weeks gestational age, in those depressed from birth asphyxia or sepsis, and in those with dysfunction of the motor unit (i.e., the motor neuron, peripheral nerve, muscle and neuromuscular junction). Neonates with acute encephalopathy are frequently areflexic initially. As the neonate improves, reflexes return, but they may be depressed initially and later become increased or exaggerated. Exaggerated deep-tendon reflexes are also seen in neonates with drug withdrawal syndrome. Clonus is rapid movement of a particular joint brought about by sudden stretching of a tendon. Ankle clonus can be evaluated by holding the anterior portion of the neonate's foot with the hip and knee in flexion and dorsiflexing the forefoot. The response usually consists of several repetitive jerks (beats) of the foot or no movement at all. Sustained clonus (with more than eight to ten beats occurring) may indicate cerebral irritation.

POSTURAL TONE

Postural tone is best tested by the traction response (or pull-to-sit maneuver), which tests the ability to resist the pull of gravity. The traction response is tested by grasping the neonate's hands and pulling him slowly from the supine to a sitting position. The normal term neonate reinforces this maneuver by contracting the

FIGURE 11-3 ▲ Normal traction response seen in the full-term neonate.

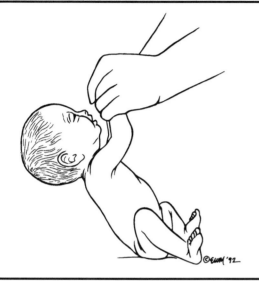

FIGURE 11-4 ▲ Traction response indicating hypotonia.

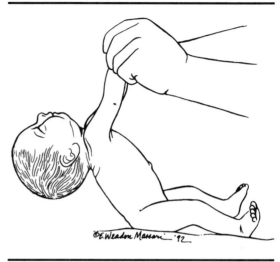

shoulder and arm muscles, followed by flexion of the neck. As the neonate is pulled to sit, his head leaves the bed almost immediately, lagging only minimally behind the body (Figure 11-3). When the infant reaches the sitting position, the head remains erect momentarily and then falls forward. During traction, flexion occurs in the elbows, knees, and ankles. In the term neonate, more than minimal head lag is abnormal and may indicate postural hypotonia (Figure 11-4). Neck flexion in response to traction is absent in premature neonates under 33 weeks. Because normal postural tone requires the integrated functions of the entire central nervous system, hypotonia (indicating depressed postural tone) may result from disturbances in the central nervous system, the peripheral nervous system, or the skeletal muscle. As with the other components of the neurologic examination, testing of postural tone should be done with the neonate in an awake alert state.

Testing muscle strength is imprecise in the neonate because differentiating between hypotonia and muscle weakness is difficult. The strength of the upper extremities is gauged by

using the grasp reflex and the pull-to-sit maneuver as described previously. The strength of the lower extremities is evaluated by observing the stepping reflex, readily elicited by 37 weeks gestation, and gauging the neonate's ability to support his weight when his feet are against a flat surface.

Movement should be evaluated and the presence of abnormal involuntary movements noted. At 28 to 32 weeks gestation, slow twisting movements of the trunk as well as rapid, wide-amplitude movements of the limbs are seen. By 32 weeks gestation, movements are more flexor and tend to occur in unison. At 36 weeks, active flexor movements of the lower extremities often occur in an alternating rather than bilateral symmetric pattern. The term neonate's upper and lower extremities move in an alternating pattern. Typical of the neonatal period are mass movements that occur in response to environmental stimuli and discomfort. During the first few weeks of life, coarse tremors or brief trembling of the chin may occur normally, as may occasional uncoordinated movements.

ABNORMALITIES OF TONE

The motor examination may detect hypotonia or hypertonia. *Hypotonia* is the most consistent abnormality observed in the neo-natal neurologic examination. A focal injury to the cerebrum can result in contralateral hemiparesis involving the face and upper extremities more than the lower extremities. Injury to the parasagittal cerebral region (which may be caused by cerebral perfusion abnormalities) results in weakness of the upper limbs more than the lower limbs. If spinal cord injury occurs, it is frequently in the cervical region and can result in flaccid weakness of the extremities; the face and cranial nerves are usually not affected. Neuromuscular junction diseases such as myasthenia gravis or infantile botulism cause generalized weakness and hypotonia. Disorders of the lower motor neurons (such as Werdnig-Hoffmann disease) cause flaccid weakness of the extremities with initial sparing of the face and cranial nerves. Fasciculation (spontaneous contraction of a group of fibers in a motor unit) can also be seen in Werdnig-Hoffmann disease and is best observed in the tongue. Inspection of the tongue reveals continuous and rapid twitching movements. Damage to nerve roots results in discrete patterns of focal weakness, the location of which depends upon the root involved. One example is the unilateral loss of movement seen in the arm of a neonate with brachial palsy.

Hypertonia is a less common finding in the neonatal period. If it is present, passive manipulation of the limbs often increases the tone. Opisthotonus (marked extensor hypertonia with arching of the back)

is sometimes seen with bacterial meningitis, severe hypoxic-ischemic brain damage, massive intraventricular hemorrhage, and tetanus. Table 11-2 lists patterns of abnormal muscle tone and their possible significance.

TABLE 11-2 ▲ Patterns of Abnormal Muscle Tone in the Neonate

Abnormality	Significance
Generalized increased or decreased tone	CNS insult or systemic illness
Increased arm flexor tone with increased leg extensor tone	Normal in crying neonate
	CNS irritability, hypoxic-ischemic encephalopathy, hemorrhage, increased intracranial pressure
Increased neck extensor tone more than neck flexor tone	Seen in crying neonates
	Hypoxic-ischemic injury
	Meningitis
	Increased intracranial pressure
Tight popliteal angle, increased as compared to leg tone	Intracranial hemorrhage
Asymmetric popliteal angles beyond 40 weeks	Hypertonia, hemiplegia

From: Hill A. 1992. Development of tone and reflexes in the fetus and newborn. In *Fetal and Neonatal Physiology,* Polin RA, and Fox WW, eds. Philadelphia: WB Saunders, 1581. Reprinted by permission.

ASSESSMENT OF DEVELOPMENTAL REFLEXES

Developmental reflexes are sometimes referred to as primary or primitive reflexes because they do not require functional brain above the diencephalon. Although there are

TABLE 11-3 ▲ Neonatal Reflexes

Reflex	Onset (Weeks)	Well-established (Weeks)	Disappearance (Months)
Suck	28	32–34	12
Rooting	28	32–34	3–4
Palmar grasp	28–32	32	2
Tonic neck	35	4	7
Moro	28–32	37	6
Stepping	35–36	37	3–4
Truncal incurvation	28	40	3–4
Babinski	34–36	38	12

Adapted from: Volpe JJ. 1995. *Neurology of the Newborn,* 3rd ed. Philadelphia: WB Saunders, 107; and Barness LA. 1991. *Manual of Pediatric Physical Diagnosis.* St. Louis: Mosby-Year Book, 17.

FIGURE 11-5 ▲ Development of reflexes with maturity from 28 to 40 weeks gestation.

Gestational age (wk)	28	30	32	34	36	38	40
Sucking reflex	Weak and not really synchronized with deglutition		Stronger and better synchronized with deglutition		Perfect		
Grasp reflex	Present but weak			Stronger		Excellent	
Response to traction	Absent		Begins to appear	Strong enough to lift part of the body weight		Strong enough to lift all of the body weight	
Moro reflex	Weak, obtained just once, incomplete		Complete reflex ⟶ ⟶ ➤ ⟶ ➤				
Crossed extension	Flexion and extension in a random pattern, purposeless reaction		Good extension but no tendency to adduction		Tendency to adduction but imperfect	Complete response with —Extension —Adduction —Fanning of the toes	
Automatic walking	—	—	Begins tiptoeing with good support on the sole and a righting reaction of the legs for a few seconds				
				Pretty good; very fast tiptoeing		• A premature who has reached 40 weeks. Walks in a toe-heel progression or tiptoes.	
						• A full term newborn of 40 weeks gestation. Walks in a heel-toe progression on the whole sole of the foot.	

Adapted from: Amiel-Tison C. 1991. In *Rudolph's Pediatrics,* 19th ed., Rudolph AM, and Hoffman J, eds. Stamford, Connecticut: Appleton & Lange, 178. Reprinted by permission.

many developmental reflexes, it is usual to test only those commonly present in most newborns. The normal timing of appearance and disappearance of the developmental reflexes is presented in Table 11-3. Development of reflexes with maturation from 28 to 40 weeks is shown in Figure 11-5.

SUCKING REFLEX

The sucking reflex is normally present at birth, even in the premature neonate, although it is weaker with decreasing gestational age. The stimulus consists of touching or gently stroking the lips. In response, the neonate's mouth opens and sucking movements are initiated. The examiner's gloved finger can be introduced into the mouth to evaluate strength and coordination of the suck.

ROOTING REFLEX

To evaluate the rooting reflex, stroke the cheek and corner of the neonate's mouth. The infant's head should turn toward the stimulus, and the mouth should open.

PALMAR GRASP

Stimulating the palmar surface of the neonate's hand with a finger should cause him to grasp the finger. Attempts to withdraw the finger lead to a tightened grasp. When the palmar grasp is tested with both hands, the term neonate can be lifted off the bed for a few seconds. If palmar grasp is weak or absent in a term neonate, cerebral, local nerve, or muscle injury may be present.

TONIC NECK REFLEX

To elicit the tonic neck reflex, place the neonate in a supine position and turn his head to one side. The neonate should extend the upper extremity on the side toward which the head is turned and flex the upper extremity on the opposite side (Figure 11-6). This is sometimes called the fencing position. If the response

FIGURE 11-6 ▲ The tonic neck reflex.

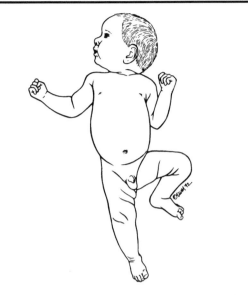

FIGURE 11-7 ▲ The Moro reflex.

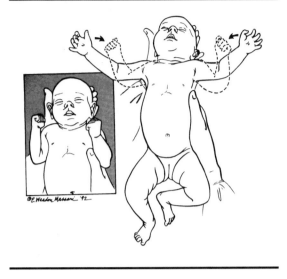

cannot be obtained or if even slight turning of the head consistently produces a marked tonic neck reflex, these can be important indicators of abnormality.

MORO REFLEX

The Moro reflex is a response to the sensation of loss of support. The most effective and reproducible method of stimulating it is to hold the neonate in a supine position with his head several centimeters off the bed. Then withdraw the hand supporting the head, and the infant's head falls back into the examiner's hand or against the surface of the bed. The infant's first response is a spreading movement in which the arms are extended and abducted and the hands are opened (Figure 11-7). That response is followed by inward movement and some flexion of the arms, with closing of the fists. An audible cry may accompany this reflex in neonates greater than 32 weeks gestational age. Premature neonates have incomplete responses, with abduction of the arms but without flexion, adduction, or cry. Complete absence of the reflex is abnormal and may occur in depressed neonates. Asymmetry of movements

may indicate a localized neurologic defect, such as brachial plexus injury.

A loud noise or bumping the side of the incubator or crib often produces a Moro-like response. This is usually a startle reflex—consisting of flexion of the extremities and palmar grasping—but not a complete Moro.

STEPPING REFLEX

When the neonate is held upright and the soles of the feet are allowed to touch a flat surface, alternating stepping movements can be observed. The stepping is more active 72 hours after birth.

TRUNCAL INCURVATION (GALANT) REFLEX

The truncal incurvation reflex is tested with the neonate in ventral suspension, with his anterior chest wall in the palm of the examiner's hand. Firm pressure with the thumb or a cotton swab is applied parallel to the spine in the thoracic area. A positive response is flexion of the pelvis toward the side of the stimulus.

BABINSKI REFLEX

The response to stimulation of the sole of the foot is usually plantar flexion. In the neo-

TABLE 11-4 ▲ Testing Cranial Nerve Function of Infants

Cranial Nerve	Function
I	Smell
II, III, IV, VI	Optical blink reflex—shine light in open eyes, note rapid closure.
	Regards face or close object.
	Eyes follow movement.
V	Rooting reflex, sucking reflex.
VII	Facial movements (e.g., wrinkling forehead and nasolabial folds) symmetric when crying or smiling.
VIII	Loud noise yields Moro reflex (until 4 months).
	Acoustic blink reflex—infant blinks in response to a loud hand clap 30 cm (12 in) from head. (Avoid making air current.)
	Eyes follow direction of sound.
IX, X	Swallowing, gag reflex.
XI	Head turns normally from side to side, shoulder height is equal.
XII	Coordinated sucking and swallowing. Pinch nose, infant's mouth will open and tongue rise in midline.

Adapted from: Jarvis C. 1992. *Physical Examination and Health Assessment*. Philadelphia: WB Saunders, 765. Reprinted by permission.

natal period, the Babinski reflex is positive if extension or flexion of the toes occurs. Consistent absence of any response is abnormal and may indicate central depression or abnormal spinal nerve innervation. In children older than 18 months, an abnormal response is extension or fanning of the toes; either response indicates upper motor neuron abnormalities.

ASSESSMENT OF SENSORY FUNCTION

The peripheral sensory system functions include touch and pain. The withdrawal reflex is stimulated to evaluate peripheral sensory function. Touching the sole of the foot with a pin provokes flexion of the stimulated limb and extension of the contralateral limb. Response is present in most neonates of 28 weeks gestation and above. In neonates, extension of the contralateral limb varies, and sometimes flexion of both limbs is seen. This assessment is rarely

performed as part of a routine neurologic examination but may be performed in cases of meningomyelocele or suspected spinal cord transection to delineate the level of abnormality.

EVALUATION OF THE CRANIAL NERVES (TABLE 11-4)

OLFACTORY-CRANIAL NERVE (I)

The neonate's sense of smell is rarely tested because disturbances in olfaction are rarely a feature of neurologic disease in the neonate. The sense of smell is present in neonates, and those of nursing mothers are able to discriminate between their mother's breast pad and that of another woman. Gross evaluation can be done using strong smelling substances such as anise, peppermint, or clove oil and evaluating for grimacing, sniffing, or startle responses.

OPTIC-CRANIAL NERVE (II)

Visual acuity, visual fields, and a funduscopic examination provide information on the function of the optic-cranial nerve. The ability of the neonate's eyes to fix on an object and follow it over a 60 degree arc is evaluated. The object may be the examiner's face, simple black-and-white pictures depicting facial features, or a ball held 10–12 inches from the neonate's eyes and moved from side to side. During the examination, occasional nystagmus (an involuntary rapid movement of the eyeball) may be seen in the neonate. Wandering or persistent nystagmus is abnormal and may indicate loss of vision. When a light is introduced into the periphery of the neonate's visual field, his head should turn toward it. Pupillary size and constriction in response to light are also evaluated. Funduscopic examination is performed, and the character of veins and arteries, the macula, and the optic disc are evaluated. A thorough examination of the optic disc requires pupillary dilation. Pupillary abnormalities and possible etiologies are shown in Table 11-5.

TABLE 11-5 ▲ Pupillary Abnormalities in the Neonatal Period

Etiology	Pupillary Reactivity
Bilateral increase in size	
Hypoxic-ischemic encephalopathy	Reactive early in course
	Unreactive later in course
Intraventricular hemorrhage	Unreactive
Local anesthetic intoxication	Unreactive
Bilateral decrease in size	
Hypoxic-ischemic encephalopathy	Reactive
Unilateral decrease in size	
Horner syndrome	Reactive
Unilateral increase in size	
Subdural hematoma	Unreactive
Unilateral mass	Unreactive
Third nerve palsy	± Unreactive
Hypoxic-ischemic encephalopathy	± Unreactive

Modified from: Volpe JJ. 1995. The neurologic examination: Normal and abnormal features. In *Neurology of the Newborn,* 3rd ed. Philadelphia: WB Saunders, 110. Reprinted by permission.

OCULOMOTOR (III), TROCHLEAR (IV), AND ABDUCENS-CRANIAL (VI) NERVES

These nerves supply the pupil and the extraocular muscles. Pupillary response to light is tested and should be present at 28 to 30 weeks gestation. Spontaneous movements of the eyes, their size, and symmetry are evaluated. The presence of ptosis, proptosis, sustained nystagmus, or strabismus is noted.

Movement of the eyes as the position of the head is turned is evaluated. The "doll's eye" maneuver consists of gently rotating the head from side to side and evaluating for deviation of the eyes away from the direction of rotation—for example, in a normal response, when the head is turned to the right, the eyes deviate to the left (Figure 11-8). If the eyes remain in a fixed position regardless of head rotation, brain stem dysfunction may be present. If the eyes move in the same direction as the head is rotated, brain stem or oculomotor nerve dysfunction may be present. When it is not possible to rotate the neonate's head, the semicircular canals can be stimulated by introducing cold water into the ear canal. In this maneuver, the eyes should deviate to the side of the cold water. This response is lost when the pontine centers are compromised.

TRIGEMINAL-CRANIAL NERVE (V)

The trigeminal-cranial nerve supplies the jaw muscles and is responsible for the sensory innervation of the face. The three divisions of this nerve are mandibular, maxillary, and ophthalmic. If unilateral facial paralysis is present, damage to the motor component of this nerve may cause the jaw to deviate to the paralyzed side when the mouth is open. Masseter strength is judged by placing a gloved finger in the neonate's mouth and evaluating the strength of the biting portion of the suck. The sensory component of this nerve can be estimated by response to touch (as in the rooting reflex) or by the response to gentle touching of the eyelashes with a piece of cotton. The corneal reflex can be tested by blowing air into the neonate's eye to elicit a blink or by gently touching the cornea with a small piece of cotton.

FACIAL-CRANIAL NERVE (VII)

The facial-cranial nerve controls facial expression. Facial symmetry is evaluated in the non-

FIGURE 11-8 ▲ The "doll's eye" maneuver.

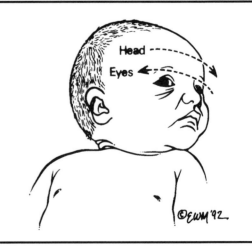

Cerebral
Hypoxic-ischemic encephalopathy
Cerebral contusion

Nerve
Traumatic nerve damage
Hematoma in posterior fossa

Neuromuscular junction
Myasthenia gravis

Nuclear injury
Möbius syndrome
Hypoxic-ischemic encephalopathy

Muscle
Myotonic dystrophy
Muscular dystrophy
Facioscapulohumeral dystrophy
Myopathy
Mitochondrial disorder
Muscle hypoplasia

Modified from: Volpe JJ. 1995. The neurological examination: Normal and abnormal features. In *Neurology of the Newborn,* 3rd ed. Philadelphia: WB Saunders, 112. Reprinted by permission.

crying, undisturbed neonate and in the crying neonate. Severe injury to the facial nerve may result in marked facial weakness. If the entire nerve is damaged, the neonate will be unable to wrinkle his brow or close his eyes well with crying, and the mouth will appear to draw to the normal side. Nasolabial creases will also be asymmetric. Causes of facial weakness are listed in Table 11-6.

AUDITORY-CRANIAL NERVE (VIII)

The auditory component of the auditory-cranial nerve can be grossly tested in the neonate by assessing response to a loud noise. The response may be a blink or a startle. Noting whether the neonate responds to your voice by turning his head toward you during the examination can also be used to estimate hearing. If the infant fails to respond to stimuli on repeat examinations, more accurate hearing tests (such

as auditory evoked potentials) should be performed. The vestibular component is tested by rotating the neonate from side to side and eliciting the "doll's eye" movement.

GLOSSOPHARYNGEAL-CRANIAL NERVE (IX)

Tongue movement is controlled by this nerve. It can be evaluated by inspecting tongue movement, eliciting a gag reflex, and noting the position of the uvula. If weakness of the palate is present, the uvula deviates toward the normal side.

VAGUS-CRANIAL NERVE (X)

The motor portion of the vagus-cranial nerve supplies the soft palate, pharynx, and larynx. Bilateral lesions of this nerve impair swallowing. Nerve function is evaluated by listening to the cry for abnormalities such as hoarseness, stridor, or aphonia and by the ability to swallow.

ACCESSORY-CRANIAL NERVE (XI)

Control of the sternocleidomastoid and the trapezius muscles is under the accessory-cranial nerve. Evaluation of the neonate's head position when the head is turned from one side to the other should be made. Paralysis of the sternocleidomastoid muscle is suggested by difficulty in turning the head to the affected side. Observations of shoulder height are made to evaluate the trapezius muscle function. When the upper fibers of the trapezius are paralyzed, the corresponding shoulder will be lower than the unaffected one.

HYPOGLOSSAL-CRANIAL NERVE (XII)

This nerve supplies the muscles of the tongue. Atrophy or abnormal movements of the tongue are assessed, as well as the gag, suck, and swallow reflexes. A weak suck and delayed swallowing are present with damage to the nerve. Other causes of impaired suck and swallow are listed in Table 11-7.

ASSESSMENT OF THE AUTONOMIC NERVOUS SYSTEM

The function of the segmental and peripheral centers of the autonomic nervous system is well established in the full-term neonate. This system has priority in maturation because it controls the activity of systems and organs essential for life. Vital signs, skin, and sphincters are areas that can be assessed. Observations of trends in temperature, blood flow, heart rate, blood pressure, respiratory rate, and pupillary response to light are made. The anal sphincter is observed to see if the opening is normal or patulous (distended). The anocutaneous reflex, or "anal wink," is tested by evaluating the response to cutaneous stimulation of the perianal skin. The normal response is contraction of the external sphincter. Bladder sphincter function is more difficult to assess. Constant dribbling of urine, or bladder distention and the need to credé the bladder, may indicate a neurogenic bladder. A normal variant demonstrating autonomic vasomotor instability in the neonate is the harlequin sign (Chapter 4). When the neonate is lying on his side, the dependent area becomes red, and the upper body appears pale in contrast.

ABNORMALITIES

PERINATAL ASPHYXIA

Neurologic examination plays a role in the assessment of the asphyxiated newborn. Perinatal asphyxia is an insult to the fetus and newborn resulting from lack of oxygen and perfusion. It is associated with tissue hypoxia and acidosis. The biochemical definition of asphyxia is acidosis, hypoxia, and hypercapnia. Hypoxic-ischemic encephalopathy—a result of asphyxia—is a syndrome characterized by recognizable clinical, biochemical, and pathologic features. The spectrum of hypoxic-ischemic encephalopathy can be divided into categories.

TABLE 11-7 ▲ Causes of Impaired Suck and Swallow in the Neonatal Period

Encephalopathy with bilateral cerebral involvement
Hypoxic-ischemic encephalopathy
Traumatic facial nerve damage
Bilateral laryngeal paralysis
Posterior fossa hematoma or mass
Arnold-Chiari malformation
Werdnig-Hoffmann disease
Möbius syndrome
Myasthenia gravis
Myotonic dystrophy
Muscular dystrophy
Myopathies
Facioscapulohumeral muscular dystrophy

Modified from: Volpe JJ. 1995. The neurological examination: Normal and abnormal features. In *Neurology of the Newborn*, 3rd ed. Philadelphia: WB Saunders, 115. Reprinted by permission.

Mild encephalopathy is associated with irritability, jitteriness, and hyperalertness. *Moderate encephalopathy* is characterized by lethargy, hypotonia, a decrease in spontaneous movements, and seizures. *Severe encephalopathy* is characterized by coma, flaccidity, disturbed brain stem function, and seizures.

The evolution of severe encephalopathy has been studied and is somewhat predictable. From birth to 12 hours, the neonate with severe encephalopathy usually demonstrates stupor or coma, periodic breathing, minimal movement, and seizures. Pupillary and oculomotor responses are intact. By 12 to 24 hours, the neonate's level of consciousness appears to improve, but this apparent improvement is accompanied by apneic spells, weakness, jitteriness, and severe seizures. Between 24 and 72 hours, the neonate's level of consciousness deteriorates, and stupor and coma may be associated with respiratory arrest. The pupils become fixed and dilated, and the doll's eye response is lost. Those neonates who survive 72 hours or longer usually demonstrate improvement, over days to weeks, in the level of consciousness, but hypotonia and weakness are common. Disturbances

TABLE 11-8 ▲ Maternal Drug Use and Fetal Central Nervous System Abnormality

Drug	Abnormality
Isotretinoin (Accutane)	Microcephaly, absence of the cerebellar vermis, hydrocephalus, Arnold-Chiari malformation, and Dandy-Walker syndrome
Antiepileptic drugs	Microencephaly, anencephaly, myelomeningocele, hydrocephalus
Primidone	Microcephaly, hydrocephalus, spina bifida, anencephaly
Cocaine	Microcephaly, cerebral infarction, encephalocele
Narcotics	Microcephaly, strabismus
Coumadin	Microcephaly, hydrocephalus, brain atrophy, Dandy-Walker syndrome
Ethanol	Microcephaly

Adapted from: Dodson WE. 1989. Deleterious effects of drugs on the developing nervous system. *Clinics in Perinatology* 16(2): 340–343, 348–353.

in suck, swallow, gag, and tongue movements may impair the ability to feed.

Specific patterns of limb weakness reflect the area of brain injury resulting from asphyxia. In term neonates, injury occurs predominantly to the parasagittal areas, zones between the cerebral arteries that are most affected by changes in blood flow and oxygenation. Weakness of the shoulder girdle and proximal upper extremities results from injury to this area of the brain. Focal ischemic injury in the area of the middle cerebral artery also presents frequently in the term neonate and is demonstrated by hemiparesis. In the premature neonate, decreased arterial blood flow affects the periventricular area and results in periventricular leukomalacia. Damage to the periventricular area results in weakness in the lower extremities.

MATERNAL DRUG USE

Drug use during pregnancy may affect the fetus and the newborn by producing malformations and withdrawal. Specific drugs and their relationship to central nervous system malformations and abnor-

mal neurologic signs are listed in Tables 11-8 and 11-9.

NEUROMUSCULAR DISORDERS

Components of the central and peripheral nervous systems are responsible for the control of movement and tone. Originating in the cerebral cortex and terminating in the muscle itself, these components compose what is known as the motor system. Generally, evidence of a central encephalopathy as the cause of abnormalities of the motor system is absent. Neonates may present with weakness and hypotonia but appear alert. Examination is directed toward evaluation of the muscle size, tone, tendon reflexes, muscle fasciculation, and fatiguing. Arthrogryposis, characterized by fixed position and limitation of limb movement, may be a major presenting feature of neuromuscular disease in the neonate. Atrophic muscles and decreased tendon reflexes are usually present.

SPINAL CORD INJURIES

Injuries to the spinal cord are usually seen following deliveries that overstretch the vertebral

TABLE 11-9 ▲ Maternal Drug Use and Neonatal Neurologic Abnormality

Drug	Abnormality
Isotretinoin (Accutane)	Hypotonicity, decreased reflexes, feeding problems, facial nerve paralysis, lack of visual responsiveness, seizures
Narcotics	Withdrawal symptoms; increased activity, tone, and arousal to stimulation
Phencyclidine	Hypertonicity, decreased reflexes, bursts of agitation, rapid changes in level of consciousness
Cocaine	Depressed interactive behavior, poor organizational responses to environmental stimuli

Adapted from: Dodson WE. 1989. Deleterious effects of drugs on the developing nervous system. *Clinics in Perinatology* 16(2): 340–343, 350–352.

axis or over-rotate the body in relation to the head. The majority of these injuries occur with breech presentations. Occasionally, a loud pop or snap is heard during the delivery. Clinical manifestations depend upon the level and severity of the injury. Transection injuries are irreversible; partial or complete recovery is possible with injuries caused by compression or ischemia. Following spinal cord injury, a state of shock and difficulty initiating respiration are common. Lesions above C3 or C4 paralyze the diaphragm. Lower cervical and upper thoracic cord lesions result in flaccidity of the legs and portions of the arms. Lack of perceptible response to pin prick can be demonstrated below the level of spinal injury.

DEFECTS IN CLOSURE OF THE ANTERIOR NEURAL TUBE

Anencephaly

Anencephaly is the result of defective closure of the anterior neural tube. The defect in the skull begins at the vertex and may extend to the foramen magnum. Dermal covering is absent; hemorrhagic and fibrotic cerebral tissue lies exposed to view. The cranium is underdeveloped, resulting in shallow orbits and protruding eyes. The most common variety of anencephaly involves the forebrain and variable amounts of the upper brain stem. Associated abnormalities (such as adrenal hypoplasia and lung defects) are frequently seen.

Encephalocele

Encephalocele is a restricted disorder of neural development involving closure of the anterior neural tube. There is a protrusion of meninges and sometimes cerebral tissue, which is covered by skin. The defect in the skull that allows protrusion is referred to as a bifid cranium.

Occasionally, cranium bifidum may be present without protrusion of meninges or fluid and instead appears as a small, tissue-covered opening on the skull. Noticeable tufts of normal hair may surround the defect. Encephaloceles most commonly occur in the midline of the occipital bone, but they may also occur in the parietal area, temporal area, or a frontal nasopharyngeal area. Occasionally, they appear to be protruding from the eye socket.

The severity of the clinical findings is related to the location, size, and contents of the sac. Encephaloceles may vary from tiny protrusions to massive protrusions the size of the skull. The sac may contain cerebral spinal fluid, meninges, and cerebral tissue. Severe deficits occur if brain tissue and part of the ventricular system are trapped in the defect. Microcephaly, spasticity, seizures, and cortical blindness are associated with structural defects of the occipital lobe. Skull x-rays are valuable in identifying the defect in the skull (the bifid cranium). Transillumination and ultrasound can be useful in identifying the extent of brain tissue in the sac.

DEFECTS IN CLOSURE OF THE POSTERIOR NEURAL TUBE

Spina bifida, meningocele, and myelomeningocele are defects arising from abnormal closure of the posterior neural tube (Figure 11-9).

Spina Bifida Occulta

A malformation arising from lack of closure or incomplete closure of the posterior portion of the vertebrae, spina bifida is the mildest form of all neural tube defects. It occurs most commonly in the lower lumbar and lumbosacral area and is covered with skin. The meninges and spinal cord are normal. The presence of tufts of hair, lipomas, or other abnormalities along the spine may indicate the presence of serious underlying defects. A dimple on the spine should be differentiated from a sinus. A dimple is a common finding and rarely indicates an underlying problem. It is usually located just superior to the anal opening. A *dermal*

FIGURE 11-9 ▲ Types of spina bifida and the commonly associated malformations of the nervous system.

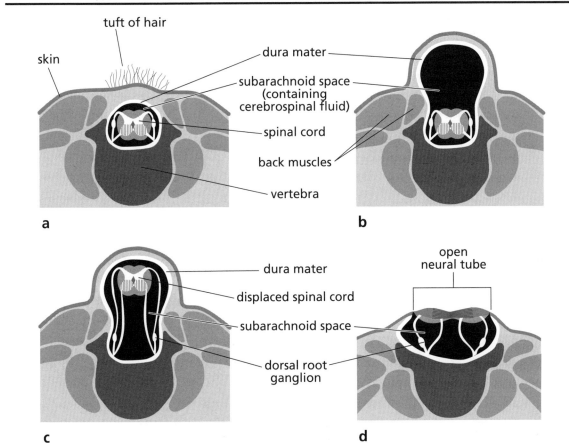

(a) Spina bifida occulta. About 10 percent of people have this vertebral defect in L5 and/or S1. It causes no back problems. (b) Spina bifida with meningocele. (c) Spina bifida with myelomeningocele. (d) Spina bifida with myeloschisis.

From: Moore KL. 1993. *The Developing Human*, 5th ed. Philadelphia: WB Saunders, 396. Reprinted by permission. (Modified from Patten BM. 1968. *Human Embryology*, 2nd ed. New York: McGraw-Hill. Used by permission of McGraw-Hill Book Company.)

sinus can occur anywhere along the midline of the back but is most frequently seen in the lumbar region. Although dimples generally have no clinical significance, sinuses may terminate in subcutaneous tissue, a cyst, or a fibrous band or may be associated with spina bifida and extend into an open spinal cord.

To inspect the dimple or sinus, try to visualize the skin covering the end of the site. This may be difficult with deep sinuses. Probing the site with instruments is contraindicated; in the case of an open spine, direct trauma to spinal elements as well as possible introduction

of bacteria into the defect could occur. With skin lesions other than dimples, evaluation is indicated. X-ray or ultrasound of the involved area is helpful in identifying the vertebral abnormalities and the relationship of the defect to the meninges and cord.

Meningocele

Lesions associated with spina bifida, meningoceles usually involve more than one vertebra. The meninges, covered by a thin atrophic skin, protrude through the bony defect. The spinal roots and nerves are normal, and neurologic deficits are unusual.

TABLE 11-10 ▲ Myelomeningocele and Sensory, Motor, Sphincter, and Reflex Function

Lesion	Innervation	Cutaneous Sensation	Motor Function	Working Muscles	Sphincter	Reflex
Cervical/thoracic	Variable	Variable	None	None	None	—
Thoracolumbar	T12	Lower abdomen	None	None	None	—
	L1	Groin	Weak hip flexion	Iliopsoas	None	—
	L2	Anterior upper thigh	Strong hip flexion	Iliopsoas and sartorius	None	—
Lumbar	L3	Anterior distal knee and thigh	Knee extension	Quadriceps	None	Patellar
	L4	Medial leg	Knee flexion, hip adduction	Medial hamstrings	None	Patellar
Lumbosacral	L5	Lateral leg, medial knee and foot	Foot dorsiflexion and eversion	Anterior tibial	None	Ankle jerk
	S1	Sole of foot	Foot plantar-flexion	Gastrocnemius, soleus, posterior tibial	None	Ankle jerk
Sacral	S2	Posterior leg and thigh	Toe flexion	Flexor hallucis	Bladder and rectum	Anal wink
	S3	Middle of buttock	Toe flexion	Flexor hallucis	Bladder and rectum	Anal wink
	S4	Medial buttock	Toe flexion	Flexor hallucis	Bladder and rectum	Anal wink

Note: To assess the degree of dysfunction and level of lesion, evaluate the neonate with myelomeningocele for the presence of cutaneous sensation, motor function, working muscles, sphincter control, and reflexes.

Adapted from: Volpe JJ. 1995. Neural tube formation and prosencephalic development. In *Neurology of the Newborn.* Philadelphia: WB Saunders, 10; and Noetzel M. 1989. Myelomeningocele: Current concepts of management. *Clinics in Perinatology* 16(2): 318. Reprinted by permission.

Myelomeningocele

Myelomeningoceles are lesions associated with spina bifida in which there is often bilateral broadening of the vertebrae or absence of the vertebral arches. In this type of lesion, the meninges, spinal roots, and nerves protrude. Remnants of the spinal cord are fused, and the neural tube is exposed on the dorsal portion of the mass. The majority of these lesions occur in the lumbar spine. Abnormalities in neurologic function depend upon the level of the lesion (Table 11-10). Attention should be paid to examination of the motor, sensory, and sphincter functions and the reflexes. Hydrocephalus is a frequent finding associated with myelomeningocele. The status of head size and percentile for gestational age, fontanel pressure, and width of sutures should be determined initially and periodically. Transillumination of the head following admission can be useful; serial brain ultrasounds are usually also done.

The hydrocephalus seen with myelomeningocele is frequently associated with the Arnold-Chiari malformation (inferior displacement of the medulla and fourth ventricle into the upper cervical canal and elongation and thinning of the upper medulla and lower pons). Inferior displacement of the lower cerebellum through the foramen magnum into the lower cervical canal is also a feature. Hydrocephalus is thought to result from aqueductal stenosis and blockage of the cerebrospinal fluid outflow from the fourth ventricle. Generally, the higher the defect is on the spine, the greater the degree of paralysis. Thoracic level defects may also be associated with marked abnormalities in spinal curvature and defects of the hips and lower extremities. Neurologic, neurosurgical, urologic, and orthopedic consultations are commonly required for these patients.

INTRACRANIAL HEMORRHAGE

PRIMARY SUBARACHNOID HEMORRHAGE

This common type of neonatal intracranial hemorrhage may occur in both the term and preterm neonate but is more common in the former. Bleeding occurs from vessels within the subarachnoid space, and the blood (hemorrhage) is usually most prominently located over the surface of the cerebral hemispheres (Figure 11-10). The etiology is thought to be trauma or hypoxia. Complications are rare.

Minor hemorrhages may go undetected because generally the neonate will be asymptomatic. Moderate degrees of hemorrhage may result in seizure activity in a neonate who otherwise appears well. One or more seizures can occur, but the neonate is stable between them.

Rarely, a massive subarachnoid hemorrhage may occur followed by rapid clinical deterioration and death. In those neonates surviving a major hemorrhage in the subarachnoid area, the development of hydrocephalus is possible. These neonates usually have histories of severe perinatal asphyxia and some degree of trauma. Hydrocephalus occurs with major hemorrhages as a result of decreased spinal fluid absorption by inflamed arachnoid villi, resulting in adhesions in the subarachnoid space. Adhesions may also occur around the outflow of the fourth ventricle, leading to obstruction and hydrocephalus.

SUBDURAL HEMORRHAGE

The least common type of intracranial hemorrhage, subdural hemorrhage is most often caused by trauma. It is more frequently seen in the term neonate. These hemorrhages are caused by (1) rupture of the tentorium; (2)

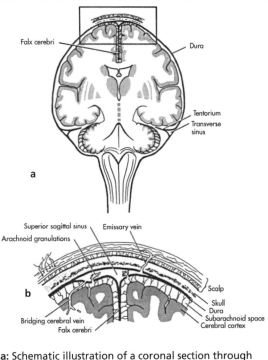

FIGURE 11-10 ▲ The brain and its coverings.

a: Schematic illustration of a coronal section through the brain and coverings. b: Enlargement of the area at the top of a.

From: deGroot J, and Chusid JG. 1988. Coverings of the brain. In *Correlative Neuroanatomy,* 12th ed. Stamford, Connecticut: Appleton & Lange, 211. Reprinted by permission.

occipital diastasis; (3) falx lacerations, and (4) rupture of superficial cerebral veins.[7]

The dura is a fibrous tissue with two layers: an outer periosteal layer and an inner meningeal layer. These layers separate in areas to form sinuses into which major veins drain. One of the layers of separation is called the falx. The falx divides the cerebral hemispheres. The superior and inferior sagittal sinus and the vein of Galen lie close to the falx. Another area of the dura called the tentorium separates the cerebral hemispheres from the cerebellum. The straight sinus, vein of Galen and transverse sinus lie in close proximity to the tentorium.[7]

Tentorial laceration may result in rupture of the vein of Galen, straight sinus, or transverse sinus (Figure 11-11). Clots extend into

FIGURE 11-11 ▲ Major cranial veins and dural sinuses.

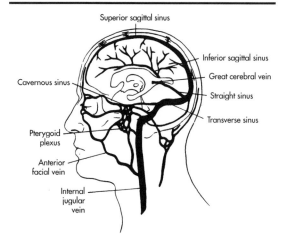

- Superior sagittal sinus
- Inferior sagittal sinus
- Great cerebral vein
- Straight sinus
- Transverse sinus
- Cavernous sinus
- Pterygoid plexus
- Anterior facial vein
- Internal jugular vein

From: Volpe JJ. 1995. Intracranial hemorrhage. In *Neurology of the Newborn*, 3rd ed. Philadelphia: WB Saunders, 376. Reprinted by permission.

the posterior fossa and, if large, cause compression of the brain. When the neonate has a large hemorrhage in this area, neurologic disturbances will be present from birth, with signs of midbrain–upper pons compression such as stupor, coma, lateral deviation of the eyes that does not change with the doll's eye maneuver, and unequal pupils with abnormal response to light. Opisthotonos may also be present. When bradycardia is seen, it generally indicates severe compression from a massive hemorrhage. As the size of the clot increases, stupor becomes coma, pupils become fixed and dilated, and the signs of lower brain stem compression such as abnormal eye movements and apnea occur.

Occipital diastasis is a traumatic injury that results in separation of the cartilaginous joint between the squamous and lateral portions of the occipital bone. This can lead to tearing of the dura and the occipital sinuses with massive bleeding below the tentorium. The same clinical features as described for tentorial laceration occur. Smaller degrees of hemorrhage and hematoma formation in the posterior fossa lead to a different clinical evolution of signs. Initially, the neonate may have no abnormal neu-

rologic signs. They begin to develop over hours or days as continued seepage of blood and gradual enlargement of the hematoma occur. Clinical signs of increased intracranial pressure ensue, followed by signs of disturbance of the brain stem, including respiratory depression, apnea, oculomotor abnormalities, and facial paresis. Seizures are also commonly seen.

When *falx laceration* has occurred with bleeding from the superior sagittal sinus, hematoma development in the cerebral fissure occurs. Marked neurologic signs develop only when the clot has extended infratentorially, and then the clinical signs are those described for tentorial laceration.

Rupture of the superficial cerebral veins results in blood collecting over the cerebral convexities. Three neurologic syndromes have been associated with hemorrhage in this area. The first and most common that occurs with minor hemorrhages is either hyperirritability and a hyperalert appearance or no clinical signs at all.

The second presentation includes signs of focal cerebral disturbances. Seizures are common; hemiparesis with eye deviation to the side opposite the hemiparesis can occur. The doll's eye maneuver remains normal because this is a cerebral lesion, not a brain stem lesion. Dysfunction of the third cranial nerve, the oculomotor, on the side of the hematoma, results in a poorly reactive or nonreactive pupil on the side of the lesion.

The third presentation is secondary to chronic subdural effusion. The neonate has few or no clinical signs in the neonatal period but presents months later with an enlarging head.

PERIVENTRICULAR-INTRAVENTRICULAR HEMORRHAGE

Periventricular-intraventricular hemorrhage (PV-IVH) is the most common cause of intracranial hemorrhage seen in the premature neonate. The incidence of intraventricular hemorrhage increases with decreasing gestational age. The correlation with gestational age is related to the site of bleeding, the subependymal germinal matrix. In this area of the brain, there is a matrix of poorly supported, thin-walled capillaries. It is located near the caudate nucleus at or slightly posterior to the foramen of Monro. At 28 weeks gestational age, the vessels in this area begin to involute, and involution continues so that the subependymal germinal matrix is no longer present by term.

Hemorrhage that starts in the periventricular germinal matrix can be localized in this area, or it may rupture into the ventricular system and, if large enough, cause distention of the lateral ventricles. Adjacent cerebral tissue can also be damaged as a result of hemorrhage in the germinal matrix, resulting in a parenchymal clot or infarction.

Large intraventricular hemorrhages have a high incidence of associated hydrocephalus. Most commonly, hydrocephalus occurs as a result of inflammation of the arachnoid villi, which absorb cerebrospinal fluid. With hemorrhage, they become inflamed or scarred from blood and particulate matter in the cerebrospinal fluid. Obstruction to absorption of cerebrospinal fluid then occurs. Obstruction less commonly occurs at the outlet of the third ventricle, the aqueduct of Sylvius, when debris or tissue reaction combine to lead to a blockage.

As stated previously, the germinal matrix is a poorly supported structure with thin-walled vessels that are adjacent to the lateral ventricles. Autoregulation of cerebral blood flow is lost in sick premature neonates. This renders the vessels of the subependymal germinal matrix vulnerable to blood flow alterations. Hemorrhage can result after a period of increased blood flow, decreased blood flow, increased central venous pressure, or with coagulation abnormalities. The majority of periventricular-intraventricular hemorrhages occur in the first day of life,

and 90 percent are identified using ultrasound by 72 hours of age.

Three clinical syndromes have been described and are thought to be related to the severity of the hemorrhage. A catastrophic course is the least common but most dramatic presentation. Stupor progresses to coma, shallow respirations progress to apnea, generalized seizures occur, pupils become fixed and nonreactive to light, the doll's eye maneuver is abnormal, the eyes are fixed to vestibular stimulation, and marked hypotonia is present. A falling hematocrit, hypotension, bradycardia, metabolic acidosis, and a bulging fontanel are also accompanying findings.

A less dramatic course has been described in which the neonate presents with signs of a progressively decreasing level of consciousness, hypotonia, lethargy, subtle eye movement abnormalities, and partial response to the doll's eye maneuver. The deterioration occurs over many hours, with periods of apparent stabilization followed by recurrence of abnormal signs. This progression of neurologic symptoms with periods of apparent stabilization may be seen over a period of several days.

The third type of syndrome is a clinically silent course in which a screening ultrasound detects the hemorrhage.

Rarely, intraventricular hemorrhage is seen in the term neonate. In these neonates, the site of hemorrhage is most commonly the choroid plexus within the ventricle. Trauma and hypoxic events are thought to be the pathogenic mechanisms.

SUMMARY

A careful neurologic assessment of the newborn is mandatory for optimal management. A normal exam is reassuring to the parents and the examiner. An abnormal exam serves as a guide for attempting to clarify the etiology of abnormal responses, documenting changes over time, and providing optimal care for the neonate.

REFERENCES

1. Amiel-Tison C. 1986. *A Neurologic Assessment During the First Year of Life.* Oxford: Oxford University Press, 7.

2. Prechtl H. 1977. *The Neurological Examination of the Full-Term Newborn Infant.* London: Heinemann, 1.

3. Dubowitz L, and Dubowitz V. 1981. *The Neurological Assessment of the Preterm and Full-Term Newborn Infant.* London: Heinemann, 9.

4. Jones KL. 1988. P. hamartoses. In *Smith's Recognizable Patterns of Human Malformation,* 4th ed. Philadelphia: WB Saunders, 452.

5. Tallman B, et al. 1991. Location of port-wine stains and the likelihood of ophthalmic and or central nervous system complications. *Pediatrics* 87(3): 323–327.

6. Volpe JJ. 1995. Injuries of extracranial, cranial, intracranial, spinal cord, and peripheral nervous system structures. In *Neurology of the Newborn,* 3rd ed. Philadelphia: WB Saunders, 782–785.

7. Volpe JJ. 1995. Intracranial hemmorhage. In *Neurology of the Newborn,* 3rd ed. Philadelphia: WB Saunders, 376–383.

BIBLIOGRAPHY

- Barness LA. 1991. *Manual of Pediatric Physical Diagnosis.* St. Louis: Mosby-Year Book.

- Brazelton TB. 1984. Neonatal Behavioral Assessment Scale. In *Clinics in Developmental Medicine,* No. 88. London: Spastics International Medical Publication; Philadelphia: JB Lippincott.

- Capute A, et al. 1978. *Primitive Reflex Profile.* Baltimore: University Park Press.

- Coen RW, and Koffler H. 1987. *Primary Care of the Newborn.* Boston: Little, Brown.

- Dekaban A. 1965. *Neurology of Infancy.* Baltimore: Williams & Wilkins.

- Dodson WE. 1989. Deleterious effects of drugs on the developing nervous system. *Clinics in Perinatology* 16(2): 342–353.

- Fenichel GM. 1980. *Neonatal Neurology.* New York: Churchill Livingstone.

- Fenichel GM. 1990. *Neonatal Neurology,* 2nd ed. New York: Churchill Livingstone.

- Goldbloom RB. 1992. *Pediatric Clinical Skills.* New York: Churchill Livingstone.

- Hill A, and Volpe J. 1989. Perinatal asphyxia: Clinical aspects. *Clinics in Perinatology* 16(2): 435–457.

- Hogan GR, and Ryan NJ. 1977. Neurological evaluation of the newborn. *Clinics in Perinatology* 4(1): 31–42.

- Noetzel M. 1989. Myelomeningocele: Current concepts of management. *Clinics in Perinatology* 16(2): 318.

- Painter MJ, and Bergman L. 1982. Obstetrical trauma to the neonatal central and peripheral nervous system. *Seminars in Perinatology* 6(1): 89–104.

- Roland E. 1989. Neuromuscular disorders in the newborn. *Clinics in Perinatology* 16(2): 519–547.

- Scanlon JW, Nelson T, and Grylack LJ. 1979. *A System of Newborn Physical Examination.* Baltimore: University Park Press.

- Stevenson DK, and Sunshine P. 1989. *Fetal and Neonatal Brain Injury.* Philadelphia: BC Decker.

- Taeuscher H, and Yogman M. 1987. *Follow-Up Management of the High-Risk Infant.* Boston: Little, Brown.

NOTES

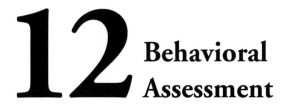

12 Behavioral Assessment

Catherine Witt, RNC, MS, NNP
Connie Rusk, RNC, MS, NNP

In the past 20 years, awareness of the newborn's capabilities of interacting with the environment has increased. Assessing the neonate's neurologic status and cognitive abilities requires evaluating how the infant responds to and interacts with his environment. In order to respond appropriately to an infant as caregivers or parents, we must first understand the infant's capabilities and behavioral cues.

In addition to providing clues about the infant's neurologic well-being, behavioral assessment allows caregivers to design individualized, developmental care for hospitalized infants. Studies by Als and associates and by Becker and colleagues show that appropriate, individualized developmental care of preterm infants decreases the length of hospitalization.[1,2] Other studies indicate an enhancement of developmental outcomes when the infant's behavioral and physiologic cues are supported in the nursery.[3,4]

Parents and infants benefit from the parent's awareness of the infant's behavioral capabilities and temperament. Parental ability to interpret their infant's behavior has been shown to strengthen parent-infant interaction during the first year of life.[5-8] When parents can interpret their infant's cues and respond appropriately, the infant is able to control his environment as well as respond to it.

APPROACH TO BEHAVIORAL ASSESSMENT

Behavioral assessment relies primarily on the examiner's observational skills. The practitioner must observe the infant's ability to organize himself and recognize how the infant changes states and reacts to environmental stimuli.

It is important to follow the basic principles of physical examination when assessing the infant's behavior. Perinatal history will provide important information on factors that will affect the infant's ability to interact with the environment. Matters such as time elapsed since birth, type of labor and delivery, and drugs administered to the mother must be considered. Gestational age will have a significant impact on the behavioral findings as well as the infant's ability to tolerate the exam. The infant's overall health is also important; an infant with respiratory distress will exhibit different behaviors than one who is not in distress.

The environment is an important consideration that may affect the outcome of the exam. A warm, quiet, softly lit room provides the best environment in which to observe the infant's response to stimuli and ability to control his state. Performing the exam in the presence of the infant's parents or caregivers provides a valuable opportunity for them to get to know their infant.

The infant's state of consciousness, or "state," is another important consideration.[9] His response to stimuli and behavioral cues will vary according to his state. State depends on a variety of factors, such as time of last feeding, recent events (e.g., blood tests or circumcision), and the infant's individual sleep-wake cycle. Preterm infants exhibit different state behaviors than full-term infants.

ASSESSMENT TOOLS

Perhaps the best-known tool for behavioral assessment of the term infant is the Neonatal Behavioral Assessment Scale (NBAS) developed by Brazelton.[9] The NBAS assesses the newborn's response to 28 behavioral items, each scored on a 9-point scale, and 18 elicited responses, each scored on a 4-point continuum. Such items as reflexes, state regulation, orientation to visual and auditory stimuli, habituation, motor performance, and interaction with caregivers are assessed. The infant's best performance on each item is scored. These items provide information about the newborn's ability to respond and adapt to his environment. The exam was designed for healthy newborns from about 36 to 44 weeks gestation. A complete behavioral assessment using the NBAS takes about 30 minutes and is best administered by a trained examiner. However, even limited aspects of the exam by an untrained examiner can be used to provide helpful information about the infant's neurobehavioral status.[9,10]

Als and associates developed an instrument for assessing the preterm infant. Their assessment of preterm infant behavior (APIB) examines five behavioral parameters: *autonomic*, which

refers to physiologic changes such as pulse, respiration, and skin color; *state,* or state of consciousness; *motor,* which assesses tone, posture, and movements; *attention/interaction,* or the ability to attend to and react with the environment; and *self-regulatory,* the infant's ability to maintain state and self-console.[11] These parameters can be used to assess the preterm infant's ability to cope with the NICU environment. Once an infant's coping ability and organization are assessed, a plan of care that individualizes interactions for that infant can be developed.[4,11,12] As with the NBAS, training is required to become proficient at administering the complete exam. However, an awareness of various behavior dynamics will increase the examiner's assessment of the infant's well-being.

IDENTIFYING STATE OF CONSCIOUSNESS

State refers to the level of consciousness exhibited by the infant. This is determined by his level of arousal and ability to respond to stimuli. The infant's behavior, function, and reaction to his environment will depend upon which state he is in, ranging from deep sleep to vigorous crying. Healthy infants can use state to exert control over environmental input, but this ability is limited in the preterm or sick infant. Behavioral assessment begins with evaluating the infant's ability to control his state, move smoothly from one state to another, and maintain alertness.[9,13,14]

State is determined by observing an infant's level of arousal and accompanying behaviors or cues. A number of scoring systems have been developed for identifying infant states. Brazelton's scoring system is probably the most widely used and easiest to follow, particularly in the term infant.[9] In the preterm infant, more definitive state definitions may be useful, such as those developed by Als.[11,15]

SLEEP STATES

Deep sleep is characterized by closed eyes with no eye movements, regular breathing, and no spontaneous activity. There is a delayed response to external stimuli, and then only a brief arousal followed by a return to deep sleep. Isolated sucking movements or startles may be noted. Preterm infants may demonstrate a difference between very deep, still sleep and deep sleep with startles or muscle twitching.

Light sleep consists of low levels of activity with greater response to external stimuli (Figure 12-1). Rapid eye movement (REM) may be observed. Preterm infants may exhibit irregular respirations. Infants in light sleep may startle or make brief fussing or crying noises. Parents may need support in delaying response to these brief episodes during the light sleep phase. Active sleep is greater in preterm infants than in term infants, who spend more time in deep sleep and alert states.[15]

TRANSITIONAL STATE

Drowsiness is characterized by a variable activity level, with smooth movements and occasional mild startles. The eyes open and close and appear dull and heavy lidded. The infant will react to stimuli, but the response is delayed. From the drowsy state, the infant may either return to a sleep state or move to a more alert status. Caregivers may arouse an infant to a quiet alert state by providing an auditory or visual stimulus (Figure 12-2).

AWAKE STATES

Quiet alert refers to the state in which the infant interacts most with the environment. The infant exhibits a brightening and widening of the eyes and an alert appearance. Attention is focused on available stimuli, whether visual or auditory. A minimal amount of motor activity is noted and respirations are regular. This state provides the greatest opportunity for infant interaction with caregivers. Term newborns commonly experience a period of a quiet alertness in the first few hours after birth, providing an opportune time for parents to interact with their infant (Figures 12-3 and 12-4).

Preterm infants may have difficulty maintaining a quiet alert stage for long. They may become "hyperalert," with an inability to decrease or end fixation on a stimulus (Figure 12-5). Preterm infants may also appear awake and alert but be unable to involve themselves in interaction.[11,15]

The *active alert* state is characterized by increased motor activity with heightened sensitivity to stimuli. The infant may have periods of fussiness but can be consoled. The eyes are open but are less bright and attentive than in the quiet alert state. Respirations are irregular. The term infant may be able to use self-consoling techniques to return himself to a quiet alert state. The preterm infant will usually become distressed and unable to organize himself. Intervention by caregivers may help him return to a quiet alert state (Figure 12-3).

Crying is accompanied by increased motor activity and color changes. The infant is very responsive to unpleasant stimuli, both internal and external. Some infants are able to console themselves from time to time and return to a lower state, while others need help from caregivers. Preterm infants may exhibit a very weak cry or may be unable to cry. They do demonstrate color changes, alterations in motor activity, and other signs of stress, such as apnea, vomiting, or decrease in oxygen saturation.

MAINTENANCE OF STATE

Although the states can be distinguished from one another, the infant makes frequent transitions between them. He may change from one state to another several times in the course of the exam. The full-term infant should display smooth transitions between states. Excessive lethargy or irritability is

FIGURES 12-1 through 12-9 ▲ Progression of infant through states of light sleep to crying, demonstrating time out signals with visual stimuli.

FIGURE 12-1 ▲ Light sleep.

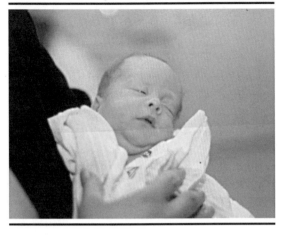

FIGURE 12-2 ▲ Drowsy.

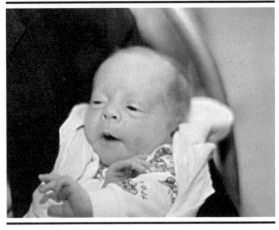

FIGURE 12-3 ▲ Quiet alert.

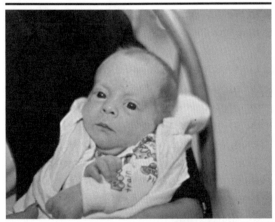

FIGURE 12-4 ▲ Signs of attentiveness.

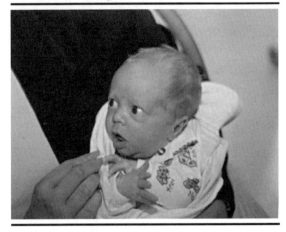

FIGURE 12-5 ▲ Hyperalert response to stimulus.

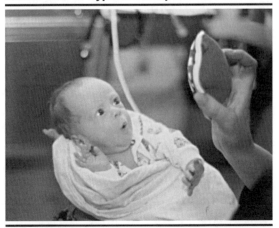

FIGURE 12-6 ▲ **Self-consoling behavior; hand to mouth.**

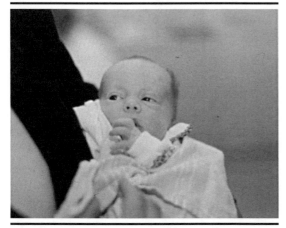

FIGURE 12-7 ▲ **Sign of overstimulation in response to stimulus.**

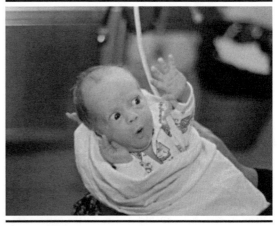

FIGURE 12-8 ▲ **Sign of overstimulation in response to stimulus.**

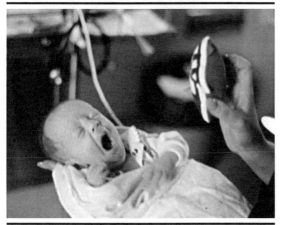

FIGURE 12-9 ▲ **Crying as a response to continued stimulus.**

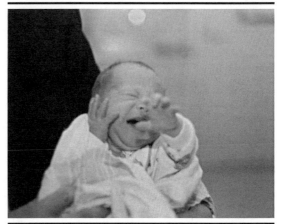

abnormal. The preterm or neurologically impaired infant may exhibit sudden changes between sleep and awake states, but abrupt changes in the full-term healthy infant are a cause for concern.

The ability to maintain an alert state varies among infants. Some have difficulty becoming alert initially and then are unable to maintain this state for any length of time. Others have trouble filtering out noxious stimuli and progress rapidly to active alert or crying. Swaddling or a quiet, darkened environment may help these infants remain alert and focus on a single stimulus.

The examiner should note the amount of time the infant spends in the quiet alert state or focusing on a stimulus. Infants who have difficulty remaining alert can be frustrating for caregivers, especially parents. The examiner may spend time teaching parents ways to help the infant maintain a quiet alert state.

Preterm infants have brief periods of alertness but have difficulty maintaining this state. Brazelton describes the "cost of attention" as the amount of energy the infant must expend to maintain an alert state.[9] This cost of attention varies, depending on the health and maturity of the infant. Premature or sick infants show fatigue or stress sooner than full-term healthy infants.

Signs of stress or fatigue include color changes, irregular respirations, apnea, changes in tone, irritability or lethargy, and vomiting. The infant may change states rapidly from crying to sleep or become hyperalert. The examiner must be able to recognize these signs of stress and fatigue and discontinue the exam when appropriate. After the infant has had a period of rest, the examiner may be able to begin again. The amount of energy required—the cost to the infant—should be noted.

ORGANIZATION

Organization reflects the infant's ability to integrate physiologic and behavioral systems in response to the environment without disruption in state or physiologic functions.[3,16] Physiologic systems include such parameters as heart rate, respiratory rate, oxygen consumption, and digestion. The behavioral system includes state and motor activity.

The organized infant maintains stable vital signs, smooth state transitions, and smooth movements when interacting with the environment. He is able to self-console or be consoled easily and can habituate to or block out overwhelming stimuli. The disorganized infant will react to the environment with sudden state changes and will exhibit frantic, jittery movements; color changes; and irregular respirations. Some infants will respond with hypotonia. The ability to maintain organization depends on the infant's maturity level and overall well-being. Individual temperament may also play a role in organizational ability.

In evaluating organization of motor behavior the practitioner assesses the infant's ability to control his motor activity and the kind of movements he makes, both random and purposeful. Hand to mouth maneuvers in an attempt to self-console are purposeful movements achieved by the mature, well-organized infant (Figure 12-6). When a cloth is placed over the face of a full-term neonate, he will attempt to remove it by arching, rooting, and swiping at it. As during most assessments of behavioral maturity, the preterm infant will have a limited ability to respond to stimuli with purposeful movements of muscle groups.

Infants who are easily overwhelmed will benefit from care designed to enhance their organizational ability. Clustering care to allow for uninterrupted sleep, arousing the infant slowly, and introducing one stimulus at a time supports the disorganized infant. Containing

TABLE 12-1 ▲ Signs of Overstimulation (Time-Out)

Gaze aversion
Frowning
Sneezing
Yawning
Hiccuping
Vomiting
Mottled skin
Irregular respirations
Apnea
Increased oxygen requirement
Heart rate changes
Finger splaying
Arching
Stiffening
Fussing, crying

TABLE 12-2 ▲ Signs of Attention (Approach)

Quiet alert state
Focused gaze
Dilated pupils
Regular respirations
Regular heart rate
Rhythmic sucking
Reaching or grasping
Hand to mouth movements

extremities, decreasing noise and lights, and handling gently are also helpful.

RECOGNIZING THE SENSORY THRESHOLD

Sensory threshold refers to the level of tolerance for stimuli within which the infant can respond appropriately. When he reaches or exceeds his threshold, the infant has become overstimulated and exhibits signs of stress and fatigue (Table 12-1). Preterm and neurologically impaired infants may have low thresholds, as may some healthy term newborns. What would normally be considered routine care (e.g., talking to the infant during feeding) may be overstimulating to an infant with a low sensory threshold. These infants may do better when presented with a single (rather than multiple) stimulus.

EVALUATING BEHAVIORAL RESPONSES

The mature newborn has a unique ability to regulate physiologic and emotional response to a variety of stimuli. It is his way of learning to control the effects of the surrounding environment. Evaluating these reactions to the environment allows the practitioner to design a plan

of care that is unique to that infant. This also facilitates parental teaching and involvement.

OBSERVING BEHAVIORAL CUES

An infant's behavior includes a variety of cues that indicate his physical, psychological, and social needs. Caregivers who respond appropriately to these cues develop a reciprocal relationship with the infant. Responding to an infant's behavioral cues also reinforces his behavioral organization.[3,14]

Signs of approach (or attention) indicate that the infant is ready to interact with the caregiver or the environment. Approach behaviors include an alert, focused gaze; regular breathing; and dilated pupils. The infant may also exhibit grasping, sucking, or hand to mouth movements (Table 12-2 and Figure 12-6).[17]

Avoidance behaviors (time-out signals) indicate that the infant is becoming tired, overstimulated, or stressed, and needs a break from the stimulus or interaction. Avoidance behaviors include averting the gaze, frowning, sneezing, yawning, vomiting, and hiccuping. The infant may also display finger splaying, arching, stiffening, or crying (Table 12-1 and Figures 12-7 through 12-9). Color changes, apnea, irregular breathing, and decreased oxygen saturation also indicate the infant's need for time-out.[14,17] State changes may be an avoidance behavior, as demonstrated by the infant who shuts down entirely by falling asleep during repeated or prolonged painful procedures.

HABITUATION

The infant's ability to alter his response to a repeated stimulus is referred to as *habituation*. When a stimulus is repeated, the infant's initial response to it will gradually disappear. Habituation provides a defense mechanism for shutting out overwhelming or disturbing stimuli.

Habituation should be assessed with the infant in a light sleep or a quiet alert state.[9,16] The stimulus can involve the visual, auditory, or tactile senses. Visual habituation can be assessed by shining a light briefly into the infant's eyes from 10 to 12 inches away. Repeat the stimulus every five seconds to a maximum of ten times or until the infant ceases to respond (whichever comes first). Note the presence of startles, facial grimaces, blinking, and respiratory changes. If habituation occurs, responses will become delayed and eventually disappear. Infants who are able to habituate successfully usually do so within five to nine flashes.

The infant's ability to habituate to an auditory stimulus can be tested in the same manner, but using an object that makes a noise (e.g., a bell or rattle). Holding the object 10 to 15 inches from the baby, shake it for about one second. Reactions may include startles, facial grimaces, and respiratory changes. Note the infant's ability to decrease his reactions as the stimulus is repeated. As they do with visual habituation, most term infants decrease their reaction after five to nine repetitions.

Habituation to tactile stimulation can be determined by pressing the sole of the foot with a smooth object. Repeat the stimulus every five seconds. The infant may begin with a generalized body response, pulling both feet away. The response will gradually decrease to only the involved foot or will disappear altogether.

The ability to habituate varies among infants. Some (including those who are preterm) have difficulty tuning out noxious stimuli.[18] They are easily distracted and then become irritable and disorganized, displaying signs of stress and fatigue. Their inability to ignore other environmental sights and sounds may make feeding difficult. These infants may need to be fed in a quiet, darkened room or presented with one stimulus at a time during their quiet alert state. Teaching parents how to read their infant's cues regarding care and adaptability can make parenting a more satisfying experience.

RESPONSE TO STIMULI

VISUAL STIMULI

The newborn has the ability to focus on and react to a variety of stimuli in the environment. The examiner should observe and record the infant's response to visual and auditory stimuli. For optimal evaluation, responses should be assessed with the infant in the quiet alert state.

Two tests for visual response can be performed on the newborn. The first is a response to light. When a light is directed toward the infant's eyes, he should grimace and close his eyelids. The second test evaluates the infant's ability to fixate on an object and track it. Term infants are able to fixate briefly on an object (a face or a mobile, for example). The newborn's visual field is fairly narrow, with the ability to focus on objects at a distance of about 10 to 12 inches. Objects closer or farther away will be ignored. The newborn should be able to follow or track an object horizontally about 60 degrees and vertically about 30 degrees, often with some head movement.[9,17]

Preterm infants demonstrate both response to light and ability to fixate on simple patterns by about 30 weeks gestation.[17] They may take longer to fixate on an object, and they have less visual acuity than a full-term newborn.

AUDITORY STIMULI

When in the alert state, newborns will respond to an auditory stimulus with brightening of the eyes and face and turning of the head in search of the sound. A rattle, bell, or music box will work well as an auditory stimulus. Keep in mind that a newborn may tune out a noxious auditory stimulus. With the baby's head in midline, initiate the stimulus 6–12 inches away from the baby's ear, out of his visual range. He should alert and turn toward the sound. Alternate on each side with sounds of varying rhythm and intensity.

EVALUATING CONSOLABILITY

Infants' abilities to quiet when in a crying state vary. The well-organized infant demonstrates observable activities to self-console during the course of the exam. These include bringing the hands to the mouth, sucking on the fist or tongue, and/or using environmental stimuli (visual or auditory) to self-console (Figure 12-6).[9] Infants who make limited attempts or who show decreased ability to self-console may be more irritable or sensitive to stimuli.[9,19]

An infant should respond to consoling attempts by caregivers. Irritable infants may be easily disturbed by stimuli from the environment and may be slower to respond (or may not respond at all) to attempts to console them. The examiner should try holding, rocking, speaking quietly to the infant, swaddling or flexing his extremities near the trunk to prevent startle activity, or offering nonnutritive sucking. Decreasing such environmental stimuli as light, noise, or sudden movement may be helpful. A common mistake is trying several interventions at the same time (e.g., rocking, talking softly, *and* offering a pacifier). A combination of activities may overstimulate some infants. Therefore, limit the interventions. If one intervention fails, try a different one.

IDENTIFYING TEMPERAMENT

Temperament refers to the way an individual interacts with his environment. Even as infants, individuals react to stimuli in different ways. Chess and Thomas describe nine different behaviors which define differences in temperament.[20,21] A description of each behavior follows:

Activity level refers to motor activity such as playing, dressing, eating, crawling, and walking. Sleep-wake cycles and their durations are also used in scoring activity level. Some infants are very active, with short sleep cycles; others are more quiet.

Rhythmicity refers to the regularity of functions such as hunger, sleep-wake patterns, and elimination.

Approach or withdrawal describes the individual's reaction to a new stimulus such as food, a new toy, or a new person. Approach responses are positive; withdrawal responses are negative reactions to the new situation.

Adaptability is the individual's response to new situations once the initial response has passed. Adaptability examines the ability to adjust to the new situation or environment.

Threshold of responsiveness refers to the amount of stimulation required to generate a response, either positive or negative.

Quality of mood describes the overall mood of the individual or the amount of pleasant, friendly, happy behavior versus unpleasant, unfriendly, or fussy behavior.

Intensity of reaction is the level of energy in a response, whether positive or negative.

Distractibility is the ability of extraneous stimuli to interfere with the individual's current behavior.

Attention span or persistence refers to the length of time an individual will pursue a specific activity, especially when obstacles interfere with it.

Based on these behaviors, three categories of temperament can be defined and frequently identified in the newborn:

1. The "easy" baby demonstrates regularity, positive approaches to new situations, adaptability to change, and an overall positive mood.

2. The "difficult" baby has an irregular schedule, trouble adapting to new situations, a low threshold for stimulus, and intense, often negative moods.

3. The "slow-to-warm" infant is characterized by mild intensity, positive or negative moods, and slow adaptation to new situations and people. These infants need repeated, slow exposure to a situation before responding positively.

Understanding and accepting a child's temperament can help parents create an environment that will maximize their child's positive characteristics and minimize frustrations. Parents of a slow-to-warm child can allow extra time for him to adapt to new situations. The infant with a low sensory threshold may be easier to care for if activity is limited to one or two stimuli at a time.

SUMMARY

An infant's behavior may be difficult to elicit and interpret, but it is an integral part of the complete examination. It allows the examiner and the caregiver an opportunity to evaluate some aspects of the infant's neurologic status and help establish guidelines for developmental care of both the term and preterm infant. Behavioral assessments can also help teach parents how to read and respond to their newborn's cues and signals. Behavioral assessment encourages a view of the infant as a whole individual. Care and support of infants and families are therefore enhanced.

REFERENCES

1. Als H, et al. 1986. Individualized behavioral and environmental care for the very low birth weight preterm infant at high risk for bronchopulmonary dysplasia: Neonatal intensive care unit and developmental outcome. *Pediatrics* 78(6): 1123–1132.

2. Becker PT, et al. 1991. Outcomes of developmentally supportive nursing care for very low birth weight infants. *Nursing Research* 40(3): 150–155.

3. D'Apolito K. 1991. What is an organized infant? *Neonatal Network* 10(1): 23–29.

4. Burns K, et al. 1994. Infant stimulation: Modification of an intervention based on physiologic and behavioral cues. *Journal of Obstetric, Gynecologic, and Neonatal Nursing* 3(7): 581–589.

5. Anderson CJ. 1981. Enhancing reciprocity between mother and neonate. *Nursing Research* 30(2): 89–93.

6. Liptack GS, et al. 1983. Enhancing infant development and parent-practitioner interaction with the Brazelton Neonatal Assessment Scale. *Pediatrics* 72(1): 71–78.

7. Myers BJ. 1982. Early intervention using Brazelton training with middle class mothers and fathers of newborns. *Child Development* 53(2): 462–471.

8. Beal JA. 1986. The Brazelton Neonatal Behavioral Assessment Scale: A tool to enhance parental attachment. *Journal of Pediatric Nursing* 1(3): 170–177.

9. Brazelton TB. 1995. *Clinics in Developmental Medicine*, 3rd ed. London: MacKeith Press, 85–100.

10. Gorski P, Lewkowicz D, and Huntington L. 1987. Advances in neonatal and infant behavioral assessment: Toward a comprehensive evaluation of early patterns of development. *Journal of Developmental and Behavioral Pediatrics* 8(1): 39–50.

11. Als H, et al. 1982. Manual for the assessment of preterm infant's behavior. In *Theory and Research in Behavioral Pediatrics*, Fitzgerald HE, Lester BM, and Yogman MW, eds. New York: Plenum Press, 65–132.

12. Cole JG, et al. 1990. Changing the NICU environment: The Boston City Hospital model. *Neonatal Network* 9(2): 15–23.

13. Zuckerman BS, and Frank DA. 1992. Infancy and toddler years. In *Developmental and Behavioral Pediatrics*, Levine MD, Carey WB, and Crocker AC, eds. Philadelphia: WB Saunders, 27–38.

14. Creger P. 1992. Developmental support in the NICU. In *Core Curriculum for Neonatal Intensive Care Nursing*, Beachy P, and Deacon J, eds. Philadelphia: WB Saunders, 426–442.

15. Holditch-Davis D. 1993. Neonatal sleep-wake states. In *Comprehensive Neonatal Nursing: A Physiologic Approach*, Kenner C, Brueggemeyer A, and Gunderson LP, eds. Philadelphia: WB Saunders, 1075–1093.

16. Gorski PA, Davison MF, and Brazelton TB. 1979. Stages of behavioral organization in the high risk neonate: Theoretical and clinical considerations. *Seminars in Perinatology* 3(1): 61–72.

17. Blackburn S, and VandenBerg K. 1993. Assessment and management of neonatal neurobehavioral development. In *Comprehensive Neonatal Nursing: A Physiologic Approach*, Kenner C, Brueggemeyer A, and Gunderson LP, eds. Philadelphia: WB Saunders, 1094–1130.

18. Long LG, Lucey JF, and Phillip AG. 1980. Noise and hypoxemia in the ICN. *Pediatrics* 65(1): 61–72.

19. Budreau G, and Kleiber C. 1991. Clinical indicators of infant irritability. *Neonatal Network* 9(5): 23–30.

20. Chess S, and Thomas A. 1992. Dynamics of individual behavioral development. In *Developmental and Behavioral Pediatrics*, 2nd ed., Levine MD, Carey WB, and Croker AC, eds. Philadelphia: WB Saunders, 84–94.

21. Brazelton TB. 1992. *Touchpoints: Your Child's Emotional and Behavioral Development*. Reading, Massachusetts: Addison-Wesley, 76–78, 106–107.

NOTES

NOTES

13 Assessment of the Dysmorphic Infant

Elizabeth Kirby, RNC, MS, NNP

The majority of physical examinations of newborn infants reveal no abnormality, but 4 to 5 infants in every 100 will have some dysmorphogenesis, although it is usually minor.[1] The initial examination in the delivery room is generally brief but necessary to exclude the possibility of major anomalies or significant distress. Early identification of problems helps the health care provider alert the nursery about special preparations and personnel needed to stabilize the infant. Early identification also ensures early and appropriate support and guidance for the parents. The examination on admission to the nursery during the transition period should be one of careful scrutiny, to detect any irregularity.

The most important tool used in assessing the dysmorphic infant is that of critical inspection. When watching a dysmorphologist or geneticist perform an assessment, it is easy to see the attention to detail, down to the loops, whorls, and arches on the fingertips. The examiner must be able to see each individual feature and body part in isolation and also in its relationship to the whole. The practitioner must also know what is normal to ensure that even subtle variations are evaluated.

MATERNAL AND FAMILY HISTORIES

As with any complete physical assessment, it is important to begin with the family and previous obstetrical histories. Many abnormalities may have a familial or genetic link. Multiple previous early fetal losses may indicate lethal abnormalities. Complications in the maternal history and during the obstetrical course should be noted as indicators of possible consequences to fetal development. The majority of serious problems occur during the embryonic period (the third to eighth week), which is when many women are just becoming aware of their pregnancy. These problems may include structural malformations such as anencephaly (before 26 days), diaphragmatic hernia (before six weeks), and transposition of the great vessels of the heart (before 34 days).[2] This is the time of biochemical and morphologic differentiation and major organ system development. An insult in the first two weeks results either in survival of the embryo or in loss of the pregnancy because, from zygote to embryo, the cell mass is so fragile that any significant insult results in abortion. If the insult is not significant enough to destroy the embryo, only a few cells may be damaged, and the

FIGURE 13-1 ▲ Embryonic and fetal development.

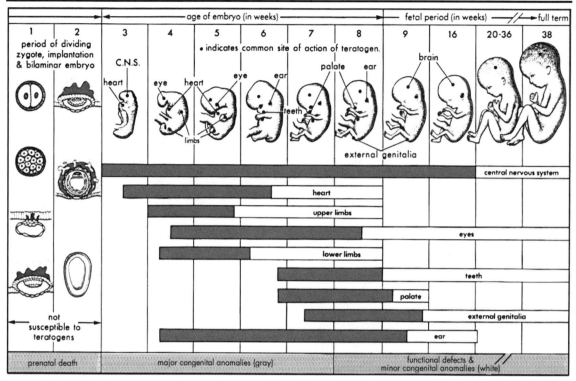

Schematic illustration of the critical periods in human development. During the first two weeks of development, the embryo is usually not susceptible to teratogens. During these pre-embryonic stages, a teratogen either damages all or most of the cells, resulting in its death, or damages only a few cells, allowing the conceptus to recover and the embryo to develop without birth defects. *Gray denotes highly sensitive periods* when major defects may be produced (e.g., amelia, absence of limbs). White indicates stages that are less sensitive to teratogens when minor defects may be induced (e.g., hypoplastic thumbs).

From: Moore KL, and Persaud TVN. 1993. *The Developing Human*, 5th ed. Philadelphia: WB Saunders, 156. Reprinted by permission.

embryo will recover. During the final stage of pregnancy, the fetal period (ninth week through term), the primary activity of the fetus is growth. The occurrence of true malformations is rare because most organ systems have completed differentiation and now must grow and mature.[1] Figure 13-1 illustrates embryonic and fetal development.

NORMAL/UNUSUAL/ABNORMAL CONTINUUM

Physical assessment findings may be described as *normal, unusual,* or *abnormal.*

These findings may be imagined along a continuum, with increasing severity of problems in form and function pushing the evaluation of the infant to the right on that continuum (Figure 13-2). Within each category, there is a range of findings that are accepted and degrees of variation that are expected. The difference between any two points on the continuum may be very subtle.

NORMAL TO UNUSUAL FINDINGS

Normal findings are expected on a newborn examination. There is no single standard, but

FIGURE 13-2 ▲ The continuum of findings.

Normal ──────────────▶	Unusual ──────────────▶	Abnormal ──────────
Normal variants Familial traits	Minor anomalies	Major anomalies

TABLE 13-1 ▲ Anomalies Found on Physical Examination

General	Lack of symmetry, problems of relationship, inappropriate size and structure
Head	Anencephaly—failure of the neural tube to close at its cephalic end, resulting in malformation of the cranial vault
	Encephalocele—failure of neural tube closure with a resultant outpouching of the encephalon, which may or may not include brain tissue; usually found at the glabella or nape of the neck **(Figure 13-3a)**
Head shape	Craniosynostosis—premature closure of any or all suture lines, resulting in cessation of cranial growth perpendicular to that suture
Head size	Microcephaly—related to brain growth and the pressure the brain exerts on the skull to enlarge and accommodate it
	Macrocephaly—associated with increases in interior volume; hydrocephaly, hydranencephaly **(Figure 13-3b)**
Scalp	Cutis aplasia—punched-out scalp lesion or area of ulceration that is bald; associated with trisomy 13 **(Figures 4-19 and 5-9)**
Hair	Texture—steely or wooly hair may be associated with some syndromes
	Hair line—low or unusual hair line may be associated with genetic aberration
	Whorls—the hair stream has a specific developmental pattern that is associated with brain growth; three or more whorls suggest brain malformation
Eyes	Lid: ptosis—drooping eyelid associated with nerve paralysis or trauma; coloboma—notch in lid
	Iris: coloboma—notch or keyhole defect
	Lens: cataract—opacity of the lens most commonly associated with intrauterine infection, especially the TORCH viruses **(Figure 13-3c)**
	Position: telecanthus—appearance that the eyes are too widely set because the palpebral fissures are at too great a distance from each other; orbs at an appropriate distance
	Hypertelorism—eyes too widely spaced; distance from inner to outer canthi should equal distance between inner canthi
	Mongolian slant—outer canthus higher than inner canthus (trisomy 21) **(Figure 13-8)**
	Antimongolian slant—outer canthus below inner canthus
	Epicanthal folds—crease at inner canthus due to lack of "tenting" by nasal bridge (trisomy 21)
Nose	Flat nasal bridge—failure of formation, gives the appearance of a flat facies
	Choanal atresia (bilateral)—membranous or bony obstruction of the nares; baby is blue when sleeping and pink when crying
Mouth	Cleft lip/palate—unilateral or bilateral failure of closure of the frontal ridge **(Figure 13-9)**
	Smooth philtrum—associated with fetal alcohol syndrome/effect
	High arched palate—caused by *in utero* position of tongue and sucking activity
	Macroglossia—large tongue; associated with trisomy 21 and Beckwith-Wiedemann syndrome
Chin	Micrognathia—small chin; associated with Robin sequence **(Figure 5-19)**
Ears	Low set—failure of the primitive ear to migrate toward the crown; common in many syndromes **(Figure 5-13)**
	Rotated—failure to migrate to the vertical axis
Neck	Cystic hygroma—most common fluctuant mass on the neck **(Figure 5-20)**
	Webbing—redundant skin at the posteriolateral portion of the neck **(Figure 5-21)**
Chest	Accessory nipples—generally in the same line as normal nipples
Abdomen	Two-vessel cord—cord begins with four vessels, only one is normally obliterated; may be associated with renal or cardiovascular anomalies
	Omphalocele—failure of abdominal contents to reenter abdominal cavity, with resultant herniation into the umbilical cord **(Figure 13-3d)**
	Gastroschisis—vascular accident that results in an abdominal wall defect; generally found on the right side of the cord **(Figure 13-3e)**
	Prune belly—congenital absence of abdominal musculature **(Figure 8-1)**
GU (male)	Hypospadius—4 degrees of severity, dependent on the placement of the meatus **(Figures 9-14 to 9-16)**
	Chordee—curvature of the penile shaft
	Ambiguous genitalia—failure of differentiation of the newborn genitalia
Anus	Imperforate—may occur at several levels; more common in males **(Figure 8-7)**
Spine	Scoliosis—lateral curvature of the spine **(Figures 10-11a and b)**
	Lordosis—AP curvature of the thoracic spine
	Kyphosis—AP curvature of the lumbar spine
	Spina bifida—failure of the bony spine to close
	Occulta—indicated by a dimple or patch of hair over the spinal column **(Figure 10-18)**
	Myelomeningocele—open spinal column exposing the spinal cord and its coverings
Extremities	Length—should be appropriate to trunk length
	Shape—some bowing noted in lower extremities of the normal newborn; extreme bowing seen with some forms of dwarfism
	Absent bones—radius and ulna most common **(Figure 10-21)**
	Syndactyly—failure of digits to separate, resulting in soft tissue or bony fusion of digits **(Figure 10-29)**
	Polydactyly—duplication of digits **(Figures 10-30 and 10-31)**
	Clinodactyly—curvature of digits, most commonly the fifth
	Simian crease—single flexion crease due to hand closure without the thumb and fingers in opposition **(Figure 13-14)**
	Clubfoot—may be positional, with stretching/shortening of soft tissues, or may be "true," with bony malformations **(Figure 10-24)**

FIGURE 13-3 ▲ Anomalies found on physical examination.

Encephalocele at the glabella.

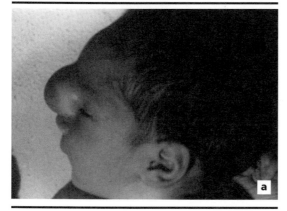

Macrocephaly, secondary to hydrocephaly.

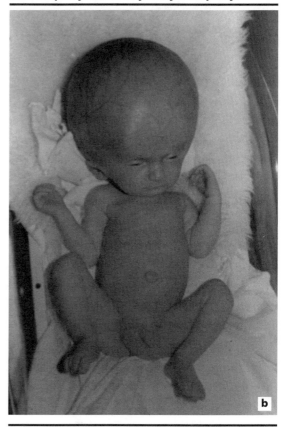

Congenital cataract.

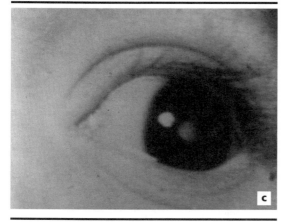

Omphalocele.

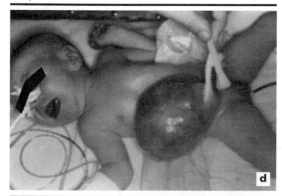

Gastroschisis.

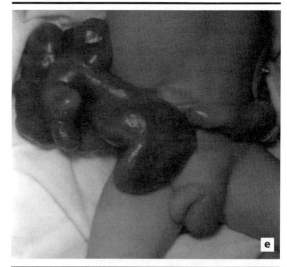

All photos courtesy of J. Hernandez, MD, The Children's Hospital, Denver, Colorado.

an accepted range of morphology. Most discussions of "normal" relate to Caucasian features. There can be significant ethnic and racial variation that remains within the range of normal for that group. For example, while examining white infants from Wales and black infants from Nigeria, Omotade found similar inner canthal distances between the two groups, but the outer canthal distance and palpebral fissure length were greater in the African group.[3]

Normal findings include what are called normal variants and familial traits. *Normal* (or minor) *variants* are those features that differ from race to race or among ethnic groups. *Family traits* are unusual features that may be significant or very subtle but are identified by the family as a feature that persists in its phenotype. This may be viewed as an indicator of parentage. Often these features are so subtle as to be difficult to identify specifically, but simply cause the child to have an unusual appearance—hence the inappropriate term "funny-looking kid." Slight hypotelorism or a saddle nose doesn't instantly alert the examiner to a grossly dysmorphic appearance, but may be labeled as unusual. Family traits may also be of consequence, as in the case of polydactyly that may persist generation to generation. The ability to isolate each feature as the assessment proceeds and then to view the features in relation to each other allows the examiner to detect not only gross abnormalities but also these subtle variations.

Gestational age (Chapter 3) also accounts for extensive variation in the normal newborn. From the extremely premature to the postmature baby, the variety of features changes dramatically. Lanugo, for example, may be expected at 28 weeks but is described as hirsutism at term.

Unusual to Abnormal Findings

Dysmorphic features are termed *anomalies* (Table 13-1 and Figure 13-3a–e). Anomalies are further categorized as *minor* or *major*. Minor

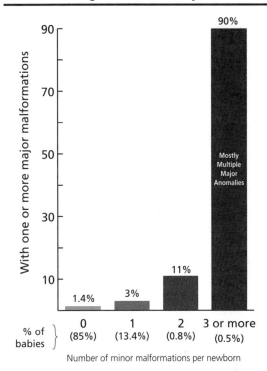

FIGURE 13-4 ▲ Frequency of major malformations in relation to the number of minor anomalies detected in a given newborn baby.

From: Marden PM, Smith DW, and McDonald MJ. 1964. Congenital anomalies in the newborn infant, including minor variations. *Journal of Pediatrics* 64: 357. Reprinted by permission.

anomalies are those of little cosmetic or functional consequence and require little or no intervention. Major anomalies do cause serious cosmetic or functional consequences and require medical intervention.

Dysmorphic features—anomalies—are segregated, by cause, into three major categories: malformations, deformations, and disruptions. Malformations and disruptions are usually major anomalies. Major anomalies are more likely to occur to areas of complex morphogenesis, like the face, hands, or major organ systems. Many of the deformations qualify as minor anomalies because their effect is self-limiting. Torticollis, for example, can usually be

TABLE 13-2 ▲ Minor Anomalies

Head	Neck
Aberrant scalp hair patterning	Mild webbed neck
Flat occiput	Branchial cleft fistula
Bony occipital spur	**Hands**
Third fontanel	Rudimentary polydactyly
Eyes	Duplication of thumbnail
Epicanthal folds	Single palmar crease
Epicanthus inversus	Unusual dermatoglyphics
Upward-slanting palpebral fissures	Clinodactyly
Downward-slanting palpebral fissures	Short fingers
Short palpebral fissures	**Feet**
Dystopia canthorum	Syndactyly
Minor hypertelorism	Gap between toes
Minor hypotelorism	Short great toe
Minor ptosis	Recessed toes
Coloboma	Thickened nails
Ears	Prominent calcaneus
Primitive shape	**Skin**
Lack of helical fold	Hemangioma (other than face and neck)
Asymmetric size	Pigmented nevi
Posterior angulation	Mongolian spot (Caucasians)
Small size	Depigmented spot
Protuberant ears	Unusual placement of nipples
Absent tragus	Café au lait spots
Double lobule	**Body**
Auricular tag	Diastasis recti
Auricular pit	Umbilical hernia
Narrow external auditory meatus	Minor hypospadias
Nose	Deep sacral dimple
Small nares	**Skeletal**
Notched ala nasi	Cubitus valgas
Oral Regions	Prominent sternum
Borderline small mandible	Depressed sternum
Incomplete form of cleft lip	Shieldlike chest
Bifid uvula	Genu valgum
Aberrant frenulum	Genu varum
	Genu recurvatum

Adapted from: Cohen MM. 1990. Syndromology: An updated conceptual overview. *International Journal of Oral Maxillofacial Surgery* 19(2): 81–88 (adapted from: Marden PM, Smith DW, and MacDonald MJ. 1964. Congenital anomalies in the newborn infant, including minor variations. *Journal of Pediatrics* 64: 357).

reversed by breastfeeding the infant so that the muscles on the affected side are stretched.

On the continuum, minor anomalies fall to the abnormal side of unusual. Major anomalies are considered abnormalities.

There is an interesting relationship between major and minor anomalies, which was first investigated in 1964 by Marden, Smith, and MacDonald. In patients with no minor anomaly, they found that the probability of occurrence of a major anomaly was only 1.4 percent. Patients with one minor anomaly have a 3 percent probability of occurrence of a major anomaly. The probability of occurrence of a major anomaly increases to 11 percent when two minor anomalies are found (Figure 13-4). Individuals with three minor anomalies have a 90 percent probability of occurrence of a major anomaly; in most cases, multiple major anomalies, usually involving organ systems, are seen.[4] Table 13-2 categorizes common minor anomalies by body area.

ANOMALIES

As mentioned earlier, anomalies—dysmorphic features—are categorized by cause into three main groups: malformations, deformations, and disruptions.

MALFORMATIONS

Malformations are birth defects that arise from abnormal tissue. Their basis may be viewed as intrinsic (due to genetic error) or extrinsic (due to exposure to teratogens, maternal infection, or maternal metabolic imbalances).

Genetic, or intrinsic, causes of malformation fall into three categories: single-gene defects, polygenic defects, and chromosomal aneuploidy.

Intrinsic: Single-Gene Defect

Single-gene defects may be expressed when one gene from one parent has the aberration; this is the dominant form of inheritance. The recessive form requires the aberrant genetic material to be found in both genes, one donated by each parent. Because expressivity may vary, the parents' phenotype may not be stunningly abnormal. In many forms of dominant inheritance, both parents are normal; the genetic aberration is a new mutation. The other single-gene method of inheritance is when the abnormal gene is on the X chromosome. With X-linked inheritance, the errant genetic information is transmitted on the parental X (sex) chromosome. Once it is transmitted, the most common expression is that daughters are carriers and sons are affected; daughters may also be affected, but to a lesser degree.

Intrinsic: Polygenic Defects

Polygenic transmission is thought to be the cause of many of the major anomalies. Proving polygenic causes is difficult because, theoretically, multiple genes each have some influence on the outcome. Polygenic transmission includes common malformations such as cleft lip and neural tube defects (Figure 13-5).[2]

Intrinsic: Chromosomal Aneuploidy

The third major genetic cause of malformations is chromosomal aneuploidy. Each individual normally has 22 pairs of chromosomes called autosomes and 2 sex chromosomes. Aneuploidy is either too many or too few chromosomes.

An embryo with *monosomy*, or 45 chromosomes, usually is aborted early in pregnancy. Turner syndrome, more appropriately called ovarian dysgenesis, is seen with 44 autosomes and a single X sex chromosome. These concepti rarely survive. When they do, the result is a

FIGURE 13-5 ▲ Chromosomal aberrations.

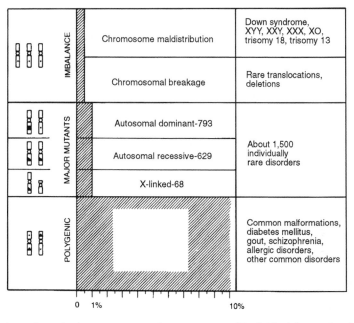

The scale at the base represents the percentage of individuals born who do have, or will have, a problem in life secondary to a genetic difference. The three categories of genetic aberrations are depicted to the left. The dots within the chromosomes represent "normal" genes, the bar represents a dominant mutant gene, the hash-bar represents a recessive mutant gene, and the triangles denote minor gene variants.

From: Jones KL. 1988. *Smith's Recognizable Patterns of Human Malformation,* 4th ed. Philadelphia: WB Saunders, 642. Reprinted by permission.

female child with small stature, lymphedema, ovarian dysgenesis, narrow palate and jaw, anomalous external ears with associated hearing loss, blue sclera, cataracts, webbed neck, and low posterior hairline (Figure 13-6). There can be other skeletal, cardiac, and renal findings. Mental retardation may occur but is felt to be the result of a chromosomal abnormality of other than the sex chromosome.

The other common form of aneuploidy is *trisomy,* the result of 47 chromosomes. The most frequent cause of trisomy formation is nondisjunction—the failure of the egg or sperm to divide the genetic material equally between germ cells. Advanced maternal age is thought to be a major cause of nondisjunction, due to "sticky" genetic material. The result is a division that produces germ cells with 24 chro-

FIGURE 13-6 ▲ Turner syndrome.

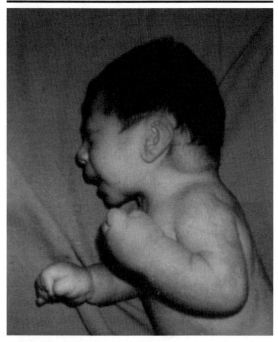

Lymphedema (hands), webbed neck, low posterior hair line, low-set ears

Courtesy of J. Hernandez, MD, The Children's Hospital, Denver, Colorado.

FIGURE 13-7 ▲ Diagram showing the first meiotic nondisjunction in a female resulting in an abnormal oocyte with 24 chromosomes and how subsequent fertilization by a normal sperm produced a zygote with 47 chromosomes.

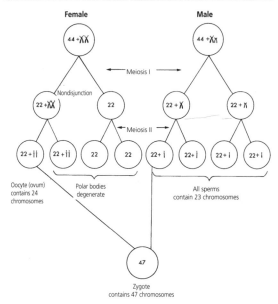

From: Moore KL. 1993. *The Developing Human*, 5th ed. Philadelphia: WB Saunders, 145. Reprinted by permission.

mosomes and with 22 chromosomes rather than the normal 23 (Figure 13-7). When a 24-chromosome germ cell combines with a normal germ cell containing 23 chromosomes, the total number of chromosomes is 47. The most common autosomal trisomies are of chromosome 21 (Down syndrome), chromosome 18, and chromosome 13. Table 13-3 provides

additional information about these three trisomies, and Figures 13-8 through 13-10 illustrate them.

The other method of trisomy formation occurs when a parent has a balanced translocation. A portion of a chromosome may be broken off and attached to another chromo-

TABLE 13-3 ▲ Trisomies of the Autosomes

Disorder	Incidence	Characteristics
Trisomy 21 (Down syndrome)	1:800	Mental deficiency; brachycephaly, flat nasal bridge; upward slant of the palpebral fissures; protruding tongue; simian crease, clinodactyly of the fifth finger; congenital heart defects; gastrointestinal malformation
Trisomy 18	1:8,000	Mental deficiency; growth retardation; prominent occiput; short sternum; ventricular septal defect; micrognathia; low-set, malformed ears; flexed, overlapping fingers, hypoplastic nails; rocker-bottom feet
Trisomy 13	1:25,000	Mental deficiency; cardiac defects; sloping forehead; malformed ears, scalp defects; microphthalmia; bilateral cleft lip and/or palate; polydactyly; posterior prominence of the heel

From: Moore KL. 1993. *The Developing Human*, 5th ed. Philadelphia: WB Saunders, 147. Reprinted by permission.

FIGURE 13-8 ▲ Trisomy 21 (Down syndrome).

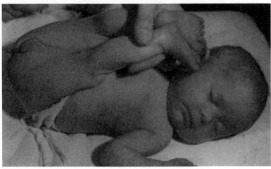

Typical facies and significant decrease in tone.

Courtesy of J. Hernandez, MD, The Children's Hospital, Denver, Colorado.

FIGURE 13-9 ▲ Trisomy 13.

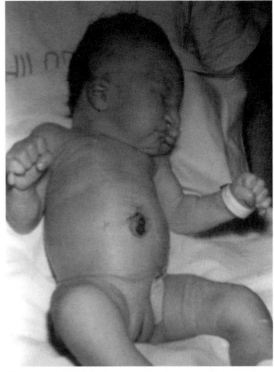

Bilateral cleft lip and palate, low-set ears, beak nose, and polydactyly.

Courtesy of J. Hernandez, MD, The Children's Hospital, Denver, Colorado.

some. The individual with this karyotype is normal because the appropriate amount of genetic material is present. If the gene with the attached piece of chromosome is donated to the gene pool of the embryo, the embryo will have excessive amounts of that material. The expression of this type of aneuploidy varies.

There are also trisomies of the sex chromosomes. Generally not obvious until adolescence, these are not within the scope of this text.

Extrinsic Causes

The term *teratogen* comes from the Greek "to make monsters." Teratogenic agents are the extrinsic factors—environmental or maternal—that affect fetal development. Table 13-4 lists known teratogenic agents in humans. Environmental factors include exposure to heavy metals (mercury and lead) and to many household, industrial, and agricultural chem-

FIGURE 13-10 ▲ Trisomy 18.

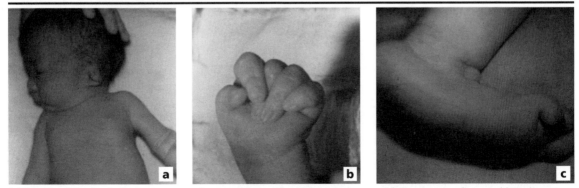

(a) Prominent occiput; short sternum; micrognathia; malformed, low-set ears. (b) Overlapping fingers. (c) Rocker-bottom feet.

Courtesy of J. Hernandez, MD, The Children's Hospital, Denver, Colorado.

TABLE 13-4 ▲ Teratogenic Agents

Drug	FDA Risk Category*	Risk
Alcohol (ethanol)	X	Fetal alcohol syndrome •Intrauterine growth retardation •Facial malformation •Major organ defects, especially cardiac •Microcephaly •Mental retardation
Aloe (oral) (laxative)	D	Can cross the placenta, may cause meconium passage
Alprazolam (sedative/antianxiety)	D	Cleft lip Cleft palate Lethargy, respiratory depression, and withdrawal
Amitriptyline (antidepressant)	D	Malformation of the extremities
Amphetamines (appetite suppressants)	C	Drug withdrawal Agitation Poor feeding
Anabolic steroids (increase RBC production)	X	Birth defects Masculinization of females Fetal death
Barbiturates (sedative/anticonvulsant)	D	Cleft lip Congenital heart disease Microcephaly Withdrawal Increased bleeding
Carbamazepine (anticonvulsant)	C	Cleft lip Cleft palate
Chlordiazepoxide (antianxiety/sedative)	D	Cleft lip Cleft palate Lethargy, respiratory depression, and withdrawal
Chlorpropamide (oral) (diabetes)	C	Birth defects Severe prolonged hypoglycemia
Clomiphene	X	No indication during pregnancy ? Birth defects
Clonazepam (antianxiety/sedative)	D	Birth defects Cleft lip Cleft palate Lethargy, respiratory depression, and withdrawal
Cocaine	X	Prematurity, small for gestational age Abruption, neurologic damage Respiratory difficulty Withdrawal
Coumadin (Warfarin) (anticoagulant)	X	Birth defects, including abnormal bone growth, hydro- cephalus, eye abnormalities, growth retardation Increased risk of hemorrhage during birth
Cyclophosphamide	D	Malformations, abnormal growth
Danazol (hormone)	X	Malformation of female genitalia
Diazepam (antianxiety/sedative)	D	Birth defects, including cleft lip and palate Lethargy, respiratory depression, and withdrawal
Diethylstilbestrol (hormone)	X	Birth defects Female: increased risk of vaginal cancer Male: increased risk of testicular cancer
Disulfiram (prevention of alcohol abuse)	X	Birth defects
Doxepin (antidepressant)	C	Birth defects

* C: Animal studies have shown an adverse effect on the fetus, but there are no adequate studies in humans. Benefits from use in pregnant women may be accepteble despite potential risks.
  D: May cause risk to the human fetus, but the potential benefits of use in pregnant women may be acceptable despite the risks.
  X: Animal or human studies show fetal abnormalities, or adverse reaction reports indicate evidence of fetal risk. The risks involved clearly outweigh potential benefits.

TABLE 13-4 ▲ Teratogenic Agents (continued)

Drug	FDA Risk Category*	Risk
Doxycycline (antibiotic)	D	Staining of teeth Abnormal bone growth Birth defects
Ergotamine (antimigraine)	X	Miscarriage Abnormal bone growth
Estrogens (female hormones)	X	Female: malformations of the genitalia, increased risk of vaginal cancer
Etretinate (vitamin)	X	Major birth defects
Flurazepam	D	Birth defects, including cleft lip and palate Lethargy, respiratory depression, and withdrawal
Glipizide (oral hypoglycemic agent)	C	Birth defects Severe hypoglycemia
Halazepam (antianxiety/sedative)	D	Birth defects, including cleft lip and palate Lethargy, respiratory depression, and withdrawal
Heroin (narcotic)	X	Small for gestational age Stillbirth Withdrawal
Hydroxychloroquine (antiarthritis, antimalaria)	C	Damage to eye tissue
Imipramine (antidepressant)	D	Birth defects
Iodide (expectorant)	X	Fetal goiter
Isotretinoin (Accutane) (antiacne)	X	Birth defects
Lovastatin (cholesterol reduction)	X	Birth defects
Lysergic acid diethylamide (LSD) (hallucinogen)	X	Chromosomal damage Birth defects
Marijuana	X	Birth defects Intrauterine growth retardation Central nervous system depression
Measles (rubeola) vaccine (live-attenuated virus vaccine)	C	Unknown
Menotropins (ovulation stimulant)	X	Birth defects
Meprobamate (sedative/tranquilizer)	D	Malformations Congenital heart defects Sedation
Methimazole (antithyroid)	D	Goiter Cutis aplasia
Methotrexate (anticancer)	X	Birth defects, fetal growth deficiency
Methysergide (antimigraine)	X	Miscarriage Premature labor
Midazolam (antianxiety/sedative)	D	Birth defects, including cleft lip and palate Lethargy, respiratory depression, and withdrawal
Minocycline (antibiotic)	D	Staining of teeth Abnormal bone growth Fetal malformations
Misoprostol (antiulcer)	X	Miscarriage
Mumps vaccine (live-virus vaccine)	C	Unknown
Nicotine polacrilex (smoking cessation aid)	C	Birth defects
Oxazepam (antianxiety/sedative)	C	Birth defects, including cleft lip and palate Lethargy, respiratory depression, and withdrawal
Phencyclidine (PCP) (hallucinogen)	X	Facial malformations Feeding and behavior problems
Phenobarbital (anticonvulsant/sedative)	D	Fetal malformations

continued on the next page.

TABLE 13-4 ▲ **Teratogenic Agents** (continued)

Drug	FDA Risk Category*	Risk
Phenytoin (anticonvulsant)	D	Facial anomalies Limb defects Mental retardation
Potassium iodide (expectorant)	D	Goiter
Prazepam (antianxiety/sedative)	C	Birth defects, including cleft lip and palate Lethargy, respiratory depression, and withdrawal
Primidone (anticonvulsant)	D	Fetal malformation
Propylthiouracil (antithyroid)	D	Goiter
Quinine (antimalaria, muscle relaxant)	X	Malformations
Rubella vaccine (live-virus vaccine)	C	Birth defects
Spironolactone (diuretic)	X	Male: malformation of genitalia
Temazepam (sedative)	D	Birth defects, including cleft lip and palate Lethargy, respiratory depression, and withdrawal
Testosterone (male hormone)	X	Genital malformation
Thalidomide	X	Amelia (absence of limbs), phocomelia (short limbs)
Tolbutamide (oral hypoglycemic agent)	C	Birth defects Severe hypoglycemia
Triamcinolone (corticosteroid inhaler)	C	Cleft palate (animals)
Triazolam (sedative)	X	Birth defects, including cleft lip and palate Lethargy, respiratory depression, and withdrawal
Trimethadione (anticonvulsant)	D	Birth defects Mental retardation Cleft lip and palate Congenital heart malformation Growth retardation

Known Environmental Teratogens

Heavy metals (lead, mercury)		Mental retardation, miscarriage, brain damage, low birth weight, blindness
Pesticides		Suggested: birth defects, miscarriage, stillbirth, growth retardation
Radiation		Birth defects
Solvents and cleaners, gasoline, glue, paint thinner, nail polish remover, lighter fluid		Birth defects, miscarriages, growth retardation

Known Maternal Metabolic Diseases with Teratogenic Effects

Alcoholism		Fetal alcohol effect/syndrome
Diabetes		Related to class (severity): macrosomia, birth defects, birth trauma, hypoglycemia
Hyperthyroidism		Goiter
Hypothyroidism		Hypothyroidism
Phenylketonuria		Phenylketonuria, mental retardation, microcephaly, congenital heart defects

Known Maternal Infections with a Teratogenic Effect

Cytomegalovirus		Congenital defects, hearing loss, mental retardation
Herpes simplex		Miscarriage, malformation
Human parvovirus B19		Fifth disease, nonimmune hydrops fetalis, fetal death
Rubella		Congenital heart disease, deafness, cataracts, mental retardation
Systemic lupus erythematosus		Complete heart block
Varicella zoster		Prematurity, neonatal death

Adapted from: Abrams RS. 1990. *Will It Hurt the Baby? The Safe Use of Medications During Pregnancy and Breast Feeding.* New York: Addison Wesley; and *Nursing 96 Drug Handbook.* 1996. Springhouse, Pennsylvania: Springhouse Corporation.

TABLE 13-5 ▲ Common Deformations

Location	Deformation	Cause
Cranium	Craniosynostosis	Premature fusion of one or more sutures stops bone growth perpendicular to the suture but permits it parallel to the suture.
	Molding	The cranial bones move to accommodate travel through the birth canal.
	Craniotabes	Prolonged pressure on the cranium interferes with bone mineralization.
	Occipital shelf	Breech presentation presses the head against the uterine fundus.
	Nasal deviation	This may be true dislocation of the cartilage from the vomerine ring or an optical illusion caused by asymmetry of soft tissue.
	Folded helix	The ear is held in a folded position against the uterus or a fetal body part.
	Micrognathia	There is pressure from a chin-to-chest position.
	Mandibular asymmetry	There is pressure from a chin-to-shoulder position.
	Torticollis	The sternocleidomastoid muscle is shortened from compression of the head to one side.
Thorax	Pulmonary hypoplasia	There is constraint by the thoracic cage due to a relatively small uterus or oligohydramnios.
	Pectus	There is carinatum or excavatum due to lateral compression of the chest.
	Scoliosis	There is significant constraint, frequently from a transverse lie *in utero*.
Nerves	Palsies	There is pressure on a peripheral nerve, which may lead to ischemia.
Extremities	Contracture	A joint is immobilized in a fixed position.
	Calcaneovalgus	A foot is held in a dorsiflexed position *in utero*.
	Metatarsus adductus	The forefoot is compressed with the legs crossed.
	Equinovarus ("clubfoot")	A foot is inverted from pressure on the folded legs.
	Genu recurvatum	There is hyperextension of the knee secondary to breech position *in utero*.

Adapted from: Graham JM. 1988. *Smith's Recognizable Patterns of Human Deformation,* 2nd ed. Philadelphia: WB Saunders.

icals. Radiation in varying doses (from the atomic bomb to 5 rads from x-ray exposure) has been shown to cause skeletal malformations, growth retardation, microcephaly, anencephaly, and fetal demise. The maternal influences on malformations are primarily from infection, metabolic disorders, and drug and alcohol use. The effect on the fetus is related to the dose and route of the exposure as well as to the time during development when exposure takes place.

Deformations

Deformations are those abnormalities caused by pressure exerted by mechanical forces on the fetus. These usually occur late in gestation, after the major organ systems are formed. A common source of the mechanical force is intrauterine constraint. The cause of inadequate uterine space may be maternal or fetal. Maternal causes include abnormal uterine structure (such as bifid uterus), fibroid tumors, small maternal size, or a primigravida status. Fetal contribution to *in utero* constraint may include macrosomia, multiple gestation, unusual presentation, and oligohydramnios. Most deformations affect the musculoskeletal system and diminish over time (Table 13-5).

FIGURE 13-11 ▲ Constriction defect from amniotic band.

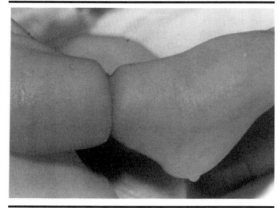

Courtesy of J. Hernandez, MD, The Children's Hospital, Denver, Colorado.

Disruptions

Disruptions occur when normal tissue, appropriately developed, is broken down. Classic examples of disruption are congenital amputation of an extremity or a facial cleft caused by amniotic bands. If the amnion tears, strips may develop and become wrapped around a digit or an extremity (Figure 13-11). Amputation occurs due to ischemic insult (Figure 13-12). Disruption of the face occurs when a strip of the amnion is caught in the mouth (probably during fetal swallowing) and causes an ischemic insult to the facial structures it transects (Fig-

FIGURE 13-12 ▲ Amputation of digits.

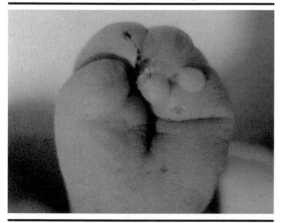

Courtesy of David A. Clark, MD, Louisiana State University.

FIGURE 13-13 ▲ Amniotic bands.

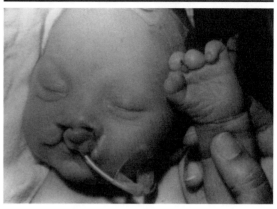

Facial cleft and digit amputation

Courtesy of J. Hernandez, MD, The Children's Hospital, Denver, Colorado.

ure 13-13). Another mechanism for amniotic disruption is when a window is created by a perforation in the amniotic envelope. The embryo may then come into contact with the inner surface of the chorion. The delicate tissue of the embryo may adhere to this surface, with resultant breakdown of the tissue.

FIGURE 13-14 ▲ Simian crease.

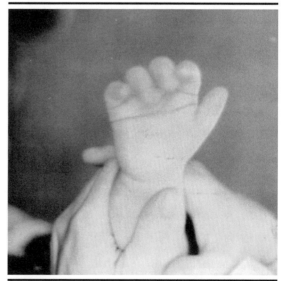

Courtesy of Eva Sujansky, MD, Associate Professor of Pediatrics, University of Colorado Health Sciences Center.

FIGURE 13-15 ▲ **Malformation sequence.**

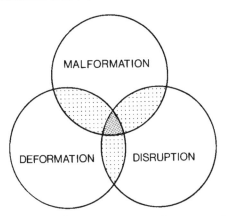

An initiating malformation may give rise to secondary deformation or disruption, and vice versa. The terminology, such as *malformation sequence*, refers to the *initiating* defect and its consequences. When the nature of the initiating defect is unresolved between the three types, the term *malformation* is generally utilized.

From: Jones K. 1988. *Smith's Recognizable Patterns of Human Malformation*, 4th ed. Philadelphia: WB Saunders, 2. Reprinted by permission.

SYNDROMES, SEQUENCES, AND ASSOCIATIONS

A *syndrome* is a pattern of recognizable anomalies that can result in multisystem abnormalities. When seen in combination, these anomalies lead to a diagnosis. Many syndromes are not identifiable with routine laboratory tests (chromosome analysis, amino acid, organic acid, or lysosome evaluation). The diagnosis is founded on repeated case descriptions of similarly affected individuals over medical history. As with the expressivity of any individual phenotype, not all anomalies need be present for diagnosis. For example, only 45 percent of individuals with trisomy 21 syndrome have a simian crease (Figure 13-14).[2]

A *sequence* occurs when a single defect can be identified as the causal factor for other anomalies (Figure 13-15). This snowball effect is seen in Potter syndrome, or renal agenesis. The absence of kidneys and subsequent lack of urine production causes oligohydramnios. Lack of appropriate amniotic fluid volume causes

FIGURE 13-16 ▲ **Constraint deformities.**

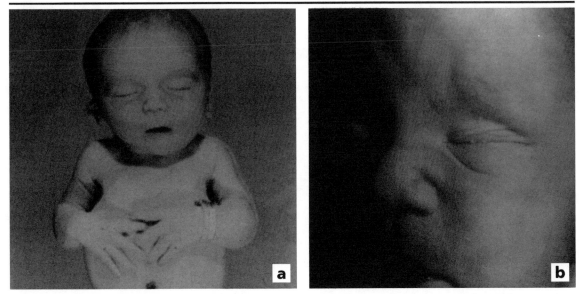

(a) Secondary to Potter syndrome: narrow, flaired thorax, folded ear. (b) Typical Potter facies: flattened nose, ear anomalies, furrowed brow.

Courtesy of J. Hernandez, MD, The Children's Hospital, Denver, Colorado.

intrauterine compression and impairment of fetal breathing. The outcome is pulmonary hypoplasia and constraint deformities, including the classic Potter facies (Figure 13-16).

An *association* is a combination of defects that occur together, but in a less fixed group than a syndrome. Associations are frequently named by an acronym, with each letter standing for a defect commonly found in the association. For example, the VATER or VATERS association is an acronym for the following:

V **v**ertebral anomalies (70 percent occurrence)

ventricular septal defect and other cardiac defects (53 percent occurrence)

A **a**nal anomalies (80 percent occurrence)

TE **t**rach**e**oesophageal fistula with esophageal atresia (70 percent occurrence)

R **r**adial dysplasia (65 percent occurrence)

renal anomaly (53 percent occurrence)

S **s**ingle umbilical artery (35 percent occurrence)[2]

SUMMARY

The ability to master the physical examination of the dysmorphic infant comes with practice. That practice, in most settings, is enhanced by the experience of performing thorough well-baby examinations that follow a consistent, logical approach so that nothing is overlooked. With practice over time, the examiner learns to appreciate the variety within the continuum of normal and unusual, as well as dysmorphic findings.

REFERENCES

1. Aase JM. 1992. *Diagnostic Dysmorphology.* New York: Plenum, vii, 10.

2. Jones K. 1988. *Smith's Recognizable Patterns of Human Malformation,* 4th ed. Philadelphia: WB Saunders, 639, 642, 11, 602.

3. Omotade OO. 1990. Facial measurements in the newborn (towards syndrome delineation). *Journal of Medical Genetics* 27(6): 358–362.

4. Marden PM, Smith DW, and MacDonald MJ. 1964. Congenital anomalies in the newborn infant, including minor variations. *Journal of Pediatrics* 64: 357.

BIBLIOGRAPHY

- Abrams RS. 1990. *Will It Hurt the Baby? The Safe Use of Medications During Pregnancy and Breast Feeding.* New York: Addison Wesley.

- Avery G. 1987. *Neonatology, Pathophysiology, and Management of the Newborn,* 3rd ed. Philadelphia: JB Lippincott.

- Avery M. 1988. *Schaffer's Diseases of the Newborn,* 6th ed. Philadelphia: WB Saunders.

- Bankier A. 1990. Annotation: Approach to the dysmorphic child. *Journal of Pediatric Child Health* 26(2): 69–70.

- Benson RC. 1983. *Handbook of Obstetrics and Gynecology,* 8th ed. Los Altos, California: Lange Medical Publications.

- Cohen MM. 1990. Syndromology: An updated conceptual overview. *International Journal of Oral Maxillofacial Surgery* 19(2): 81–88.

- Cunningham F, MacDonald P, and Grant N. 1989. *Williams Obstetrics,* 18th ed. Norwalk, Connecticut: Appleton & Lange.

- Graham JM. 1988. *Smith's Recognizable Patterns of Human Deformation,* 2nd ed. Philadelphia: WB Saunders.

- Miller ME. 1984. Approach to the dysmorphic newborn. In *Assessment of the Newborn,* Zia M, Clarke TA, and Merritt TA, eds. Boston: Little, Brown, 129–139.

- Moore KL. 1993. *The Developing Human,* 5th ed. Philadelphia: WB Saunders.

- Scanlon JW, et al. 1979. *A System of Newborn Physical Examination.* Baltimore: University Park Press.

- Shepard TH. 1984. Teratogens: An update. *Hospital Practice* 19(1): 196–200.

NOTES

Antepartum Tests and Intrapartum Monitoring

Barbara E. Carey, RNC, MN, NNP, CPNP

COMMON ANTEPARTUM TESTS

Assessment of fetal activity, or movement counts by the mother, is a noninvasive technique for monitoring fetal well-being. This is thought to be an effective, noninvasive method of reducing fetal stillbirth.[1] Usually, monitoring begins at 28 weeks gestation.[2,3] The mother rests for one hour daily in a quiet room at the same time each day. During that rest period, she records the fetal movements on an activity chart. Most practitioners consider a baseline of four fetal movements per hour acceptable.[2] If fewer than four fetal movements are detected further testing is indicated.

Amniocentesis is indicated for mothers over 35 years of age to screen for chromosomal abnormalities and for those with known hereditary disorders to identify if the disorder is present in the fetus. Pregnancies affected by Rh disease are monitored by examining the amniotic fluid for optical density. A low α-fetoprotein level in the mother may indicate that trisomy 21 is present in the fetus and may indicate the need for amniocentesis for chromosomal analysis. Known consanguinity in the parents or a previous child with a chromosomal or hereditary disease are other indications

for amniocentesis for chromosomal analysis. Amniocentesis has traditionally been performed at 18 to 20 weeks gestation, but earlier amniocentesis is offered by some practitioners at 13 to 14 weeks gestation.[1,2] There is an increased risk of rupture of membranes if the test is performed before 13 weeks gestation.[2] For chromosomal analysis, the cells taken from the amniotic fluid can take from 10 to 14 days for karyotyping. At later gestational ages, amniocentesis can be done to evaluate fetal lung maturity.

Chorionic villus sampling is indicated for suspected chromosomal or biochemical defects in the fetus. Chorionic tissue has the same genotype as the fetus, and testing can be performed at 10 to 12 weeks. Results are available within 24 hours because living tissue is analyzed. Sampling can be by the transabdominal or transcervical approach.[1,2]

Ultrasound examination is useful in helping to determine gestational age, for detecting altered or abnormal growth, and for identifying the presence of malformations. In the first trimester, it can be used to locate the gestational sac and the embryo or embryos and to determine crown to rump length. Pregnancy can be detected by

TABLE A-1 ▲ Biophysical Profile Scoring: Variables and Scoring Criteria

Biophysical Variable	Normal (score = 2)	Abnormal (score = 0)
Fetal breathing movements (FBM)	At least one episode of FBM of at least 30 seconds duration in 30 minutes of observation	Absent FBM or no episodes of more than 30 seconds in 30 minutes
Gross body movements	At least three discrete body/limb movements in 30 minutes (episodes of active continuous movement are considered to be a single movement)	Two or fewer episodes of body/limb movements in 30 minutes
Fetal tone	At least one episode of active extension with return to flexion of fetal limb(s) or trunk; opening and closing of hand considered normal tone	Either slow extension with return to partial flexion or movement of limb in full extension or absent fetal movement
Qualitative pockets of amniotic fluid (AF) volume	At least one pocket of AF that measures at least 1 cm in two perpendicular planes	Either no AF or a pocket of less than 1 cm in two perpendicular planes
Reactive fetal heart rate (FHR) episodes	At least two episodes of FHR accelerations of more than 15 beats per minute and of at least 15 seconds duration associated with fetal movement in 30 minutes	Less than two accelerations of FHR or accelerations of less than 15 beats per minute in 30 minutes

From: Manning FA. 1993. The fetal biophysical profile: Current status. *Obstetrics and Gynecology Clinics of North America* 17(1): 153. Reprinted by permission.

ultrasound as early as five weeks from the last menstrual period. In the second and third trimesters, ultrasound can be used to evaluate for fetal loss, fetal age, or a four-chamber heart and to detect abnormalities of the bladder, kidneys, brain, spine, and extremities. Placental maturity can be determined by grading the placenta from Grade 0 to Grade III. Changes in the chorionic plate, placental surface, and basal layers of the placenta can be evaluated to provide supporting information to help date the pregnancy. The status of amniotic fluid volume can be evaluated, and the umbilical cord can be inspected.[1] Hydrops fetalis can also be detected and monitored.

Doppler velocimetry evaluates blood flow in the umbilical arteries during diastole. A decrease in diastolic flow indicates an increase in downstream placental resistance. Absent or reversed flow is an ominous sign and may indicate uteroplacental insufficiency.[4,5] This test is used to detect a compromised fetus in diabetic, chronic hypertensive, or preeclamptic pregnancies. It has been used to detect twin-to-twin transfusion *in utero*.

The **nonstress test** (NST) is an indirect test of placental function that assesses fetal heart

rate acceleration and variability. External fetal monitoring is done, and uterine activity is monitored. Observations of the baseline fetal heart rate, accelerations, and decelerations are made. Fetal movements and changes in fetal heart rate with movement are assessed. Generally, patients are monitored for 20 to 60 minutes.[2,6] Fetal movements can be spontaneous, or they can be induced by manipulation of or by vibroacoustic stimulation to the mother's abdomen.[2] Accelerations in the fetal heart rate of at least 15 beats per minute correlate positively with fetal well-being. The results are classified as reactive, which indicates that two accelerations in fetal heart rate of at least 15 beats per minute occurred with fetal movement in a 20-minute period, or nonreactive, which indicates that none or fewer than two periods of fetal heart rate acceleration occurred. If test results are nonreactive, testing time may be increased, or the test may be repeated later the same day.[2] In some cases, a contraction stress test or a biophysical profile will be the next step.

A **contraction stress test** is a method of determining fetal well-being by evaluating the response of fetal heart rate to uterine contrac-

TABLE A-2 ▲ Interpretation of Fetal Biophysical Profile Score Results and Recommended Clinical Management

Score	Interpretation	Perinatal Mortality Within One Week Without Intervention	Management
10 of 10 8 of 10 (normal fluid) 8 of 8 (non-stress test not done)	Risk of fetal asphyxia extremely rare	Less than 1/1,000	Intervene only for obstetrical and maternal factors. No indication for intervention because of fetal disease.
8 of 10 (abnormal fluid)	Probable chronic fetal compromise	89/1,000	Determine that renal tissue is functioning and membranes are intact. If so, deliver for fetal indications.
6 of 10 (normal fluid)	Equivocal test; possible fetal asphyxia	Variable	Deliver if the fetus is mature. If the fetus is immature, repeat the test within 24 hours and deliver if the score is less than 6 of 10.
6 of 10 (abnormal fluid)	Probable fetal asphyxia	89/1,000	Deliver
4 of 10	High probability of asphyxia	91/1,000	Deliver
2 of 10	Fetal asphyxia almost certain	125/1,000	Deliver
0 of 10	Fetal asphyxia certain	600/1,000	Deliver

From: Manning FA. 1993. The fetal biophysical profile: Current status. *Obstetrics and Gynecology Clinics of North America* 17(1): 154. Reprinted by permission.

tions. It is a nonspecific test of placental reserve. Uterine contractions normally increase fetal heart rate variability and may result in increased fetal movement. Uterine contractions are induced by pitocin or by nipple stimulation. Three contractions in a ten-minute period are evaluated. A negative test indicates the absence of late deceleration of the fetal heart rate with contractions. A positive test shows late deceleration in fetal heart rate with contractions. In cases of positive stress tests and suspicious or technically poor tests, a biophysical profile may be ordered.[2,6,7]

The **biophysical profile** is a more extensive evaluation of the fetus using ultrasound in addition to nonstress testing. Scoring and recommended management approaches are explained in Tables A-1 and A-2. In addition to nonstress testing, ultrasound evaluations of fetal breathing, movement, tone, and amniotic fluid are obtained.[8]

Alpha-**fetoprotein** is evaluated at 15–18 weeks of pregnancy to screen for neural tube defects, which are associated with elevated levels of this protein. Maternal serum or amniotic fluid can be used to determine levels. High levels are also associated with multiple gestation, congenital nephritis, exstrophy of the bladder, omphalocele, intrauterine growth retardation, and fetal death. A lower than normal level is associated with trisomies 21, 18, and 13. The addition of two other tests to the α-fetoprotein level can be helpful in determining the presence of trisomy 21.[9] These are **unconjugated estriol** and **human chorionic gonadotropin**. A lower than normal unconjugated estriol level with an elevated human chorionic gonadotropin level in the second trimester correlates with trisomy 21 in the fetus. These three tests are sometimes referred to as triple markers for trisomy 21. Use of the triple-marker tests along with the indicator of maternal age

TABLE A-3 ▲ Fetal Scalp Blood Values

Value	Normal	Metabolic Acidosis	Respiratory Acidosis
pH	≥ 7.25	< 7.25	< 7.25
PO$_2$ (mmHg)	≥ 20	Variable	< 20
PCO$_2$ (mmHg)	≤ 50	> 50	> 50
HCO$_3$ (mmol/liter)	≥ 20	< 20	< 20
BE (mmol/liter)	< –6	> –6	< –6

From: Manning FA. 1989. Fetal biophysical assessment by ultrasound. In *Maternal-Fetal Medicine: Principles and Practice,* Creasy RK, and Resnik R, eds. Philadelphia: WB Saunders, 366. Reprinted by permission.

has led to a prediction rate accuracy of 60 percent for trisomy 21.[1,9]

Maternal serum estriol levels increase as pregnancy advances; a sharp or progressive decrease in levels may indicate fetal compromise. Estriol is a steroid produced by the placenta. Serial sampling is necessary to compare values. The normal range of estriol plasma concentrations is 9 to 22 µg/dl. Falsely low levels are seen with maternal corticosteroid use and with impaired maternal renal and hepatic function.[6,9]

Human placental lactogen is a hormone released by cytotrophoblasts into the maternal circulation. Production increases until about 37 weeks gestation and then may stabilize or decrease slightly. Low levels may indicate uteroplacental insufficiency and are seen with maternal hypertension. Serial levels are recommended. Because high placental lactogen levels are seen in multiple gestation, erythroblastosis, and poorly controlled diabetes, however, levels are not helpful indicators in women with these conditions. The normal range of levels near term is 5.4 to 7 µg/ml.[6,9]

Hemoglobin A$_{1c}$ peptide levels (HgbA$_{1c}$) are used in diabetic pregnancies and reflect net hyperglycemia over previous weeks. Higher first-trimester levels are associated with a higher incidence of congenital anomalies and cardiac defects and reflect poor metabolic control.[1] Tight control of blood sugar before pregnancy and in the first trimester is recommended to avoid hyperglycemic exposure of the fetus.

HgbA$_{1c}$ levels should be less than 8 percent and blood glucose levels, below 150 mg/dl.[1]

The **lecithin-sphingomyelin ratio** (L/S ratio) is used to determine fetal lung maturity and is done on amniotic fluid. Levels of 2 or higher indicate fetal lung maturity. Falsely high levels are seen if the amniotic fluid is contaminated by blood, meconium, or vaginal secretions. Mature L/S ratios are not always accurate in the diabetic pregnancy and in those affected by erythroblastosis fetalis. Use of a lung profile with a phosphatidylglycerol (PG) level (see below) is more accurate in determining fetal lung maturity in these pregnancies.[1,6,7]

The **shake test,** done on amniotic fluid, is a rapid and inexpensive bedside screening test for lung maturity. Lung maturity is indicated by a complete ring of bubbles in a dilution of amniotic fluid and ethanol. Persistence of an intact ring of bubbles at the air-liquid interface after 15 minutes is considered positive, indicating pulmonary maturity. Contamination of the fluid with blood or meconium results in false positives.[1]

The **lung profile** evaluates amniotic fluid for the L/S ratio and for PG and phosphatidylinositol levels. PG appears in the amniotic fluid as phosphatidylinositol begins to fall. The presence of PG indicates mature lungs and is not affected by a diabetic or erythroblastotic pregnancy. Contamination of the amniotic fluid does not alter test accuracy. Some institutions use the lung profile for the L/S ratio and PG measurement only.[1,9]

TABLE A-4 ▲ Normal Cord Blood Gas Values

Value	Vein	Artery
pH	≥ 7.25	≥ 7.20
PO$_2$ (mmHg)	≥ 30	≥ 15
PCO$_2$ (mmHg)	< 40	< 50
HCO$_3$ (mMol/liter)	> 19	> 18
BE (mMol/liter)	< –6	< –8

From: Manning FA. 1989. Fetal biophysical assessment by ultrasound. In *Maternal-Fetal Medicine: Principles and Practice,* Creasy RK, and Resnik R, eds. Philadelphia: WB Saunders, 366. Reprinted by permission.

A commercial test, the Amniostat FLM (Irvine Scientific Products, Irvine, California), is available and detects PG in a sample of amniotic fluid. The test takes approximately 15 minutes. A positive test indicates pulmonary maturity.

The recently introduced TDx FLM assay (Abbott Laboratories, Abbott Park, Illinois) is an automated fetal lung maturity test that also can be performed in less than an hour. This test determines the relative concentrations of surfactant and albumin in a sample of amniotic fluid. The manufacturer's recommended interpretation of the surfactant/albunin values is as follows:[10,11]

- a value <30 mg/gram is considered definitely immature.
- a value between 30 and 50 mg/gram is considered transitionally immature and risky.
- a value in the range of 50–70 mg/gram is considered transitionally mature and should be treated with caution.
- a value >70 mg/gram indicates lung maturity.

INTRAPARTAL MONITORING

Fetal heart rate monitoring is commonly used during labor to identify fetal distress. Beat-to-beat fetal heart rate is recorded, with simultaneous recording of uterine activity. The normal baseline fetal heart rate is 120 to 160 beats per minute and should be accompanied by good baseline fetal heart rate variability. The following fetal heart rate abnormalities may occur.

Decreased or lost beat-to-beat variability can be due to fetal hypoxia. It is also seen when narcotics, sedatives, or analgesic drugs have been administered to the mother. A decrease in variability can be seen with fetal sleep. Other factors that can lead to decreased or lost variability are administration of magnesium sulfate to the mother, fetal immaturity, and fetal tachycardia.[1,9]

Fetal tachycardia, indicated by a fetal heart rate greater than 160 beats per minute, can be associated with maternal fever, chorioamnionitis, and certain medications such as atropine, terbutaline, and others that may cause a decrease in uterine blood flow. A small percentage of fetuses whose mothers are hyperthyroid demonstrate tachycardia. Rates of 200 to 300 beats per minute are seen with fetal supraventricular tachycardia. Tachycardia is frequently seen in the recovery phase following fetal bradycardia related to a hypoxic episode but can also been seen with the gradual onset of fetal hypoxemia.

Fetal bradycardia is indicated by a heart rate less than 120 beats per minute. It is often referred to as physiologic, not related to hypoxemia, if accompanied by good baseline variability. Some practitioners think that a baseline fetal heart rate of 90 to 120 with good variability represents a normal heart rate.[1,2] Sustained low heart rates with normal variability can also be seen with fetal heart block, fetal central nervous system anomalies, and administration to the mother of β-adrenergic receptor blocking drugs such as propranolol. Loss of variability with bradycardia can be associated with fetal hypoxia.

Early fetal heart rate decelerations are a benign response to uterine pressure on the fetal head. Baseline fetal heart rate and variability are normal.

Variable decelerations of fetal heart rate are caused by umbilical cord compression as uterine contraction activity peaks. Transient fetal hypoxemia and acidosis occur with compression of the arteries.

Late decelerations reflect fetal hypoxemia. Initially, the late deceleration pattern may be mediated by the vagus nerve, but with continued, prolonged, hypoxia the heart rate is low because of myocardial depression. Other factors leading to this pattern are maternal hypotension; hypercontractility of the uterus due to oxytocin;

regional anesthesia; and major maternal emergencies such as hemorrhage, seizures, or respiratory arrest.[9]

Sinusoidal patterns of fetal heart rate appear as baseline oscillations of fetal heart rate similar to a sine wave, with fixed periodicity and loss of variability. They are associated with severe fetal anemia and are seen with Rh-sensitized fetuses and with large fetofetal transfusion, fetomaternal transfusion, and fetal hemorrhage as into a cavernous hemangioma.[1,9]

Fetal blood sampling is indicated in the case of confusing fetal heart rate patterns. Blood can be obtained from the scalp or presenting part for use in determining the fetal acid-base balance. A pH greater than 7.25 is normal. A pH less than 7.25 is considered abnormal and may indicate fetal hypoxemia.[1] When the result is between 7.20 and 7.25, the test is often repeated. Fetal blood gas status can also be determined using percutaneous umbilical vessel sampling, also called cordocentesis. Table A-3 lists normal values for fetal blood gases.

Cord blood gases are often obtained following delivery in depressed neonates and those with abnormal monitoring results during the intrapartum period. Information from the cord blood gases often aids understanding of the events surrounding the birth of a neonate with low Apgar scores. Routine cord blood gases are obtained in many institutions.[1] Normal values are listed in Table A-4.

REFERENCES

1. Creasy RK, and Resnik R. 1989. Fetal breathing and body movement. In *Maternal-Fetal Medicine: Principles and Practice,* 2nd ed. Philadelphia: WB Saunders, 277–284.
2. Tabsh K, and Theroux N. 1993. A primer of biophysical evaluation of the fetus. In *Neonatology for the Clinician,* Pomerance JJ, and Richardson CJ, eds. Norwalk, Connecticut: Appleton & Lange.
3. Baskett TF, and Liston RM. 1989. Fetal movement monitoring: Clinical application. *Clinics in Perinatology* 16(3): 613–622.
4. Farmakides G, et al. 1994. Doppler velocimetry. *Clinics in Perinatology* 21(4): 849–856.
5. Morrow R, and Ritchie K. 1989. Doppler ultrasound fetal velocimetry and its role in obstetrics. *Clinics in Perinatology* 16(4): 771–779.
6. Klaus M, and Fanaroff A. 1993. Antenatal and intrapartum care of the high risk neonate. In *Care of the High-Risk Neonate,* 4th ed. Philadelphia: WB Saunders, 7–8.
7. Knuppel RA, and Druckker JE. 1986. Diabetes mellitus in pregnancy. In *High-Risk Pregnancy: A Team Approach.* Philadelphia: WB Saunders, 404–406.
8. Manning FA. 1993. The fetal biophysical profile: Current status. *Obstetrics and Gynecology Clinics of North America* 17(2): 147–162.
9. Huddleston JF, Freeman RK, and Browne PC. 1992. Estimation of fetal well-being. In *Neonatal-Perinatal Medicine: Diseases of the Fetus and Infant,* 5th ed, Fanaroff AA, and Martin RJ, eds. St. Louis: Mosby-Year Book, 103–104, 117–118.
10. Herbert WNP, et al. 1993. Role of the TDx FLM assay in fetal lung maturity. *American Journal of Obstetrics and Gynecology* 168(3): 808–812.
11. Russell JC, et al. 1989. Multicenter evaluation of TDx test for assessing fetal lung maturity. *Clinical Chemistry* 35(6): 1005–1010.

NOTES

Glossary of Terms

Abduction: Drawing a limb or limbs away from the midline of the body or the digits away from the axial line of the limb. The lower the neonate's gestational age, the greater the amount of hip abduction seen.

Acetabulum: The cup-shaped cavity in which the femoral head articulates.

Achondroplasia: Congenitally shortened lower extremities, seen when the ratio of upper body length to lower body length exceeds 1.7:1.

Acrocyanosis: Bluish discoloration of the palms of the hands and the soles of the feet. This condition is normal in otherwise normal neonates immediately after birth, but should not persist longer than 48 hours.

Active alert state: A wakeful state of infant consciousness characterized by increased motor activity and sensitivity to stimuli. The eyes are less attentive than in the quiet alert state, and periods of fussiness may be seen. In this state, preterm infants may become distressed and unable to focus.

Active sleep: A sleeping state of infant consciousness characterized by low activity but with some response to external stimuli (startle, brief crying noises). Rapid eye movements may be seen.

Adduction: Drawing a limb or limbs toward the midline of the body or the digits toward the axial line of the limb. In the neonate, hip adduction increases with gestational age.

Adventitious sounds: Abnormal breath sounds or sounds not normally found within the lungs.

Agenesis: Absence or failure of development of any organ or part.

Allis's sign: A procedure for observing femoral length. With the infant's feet flat on the bed and the big toes and femurs aligned, flex the infant's knees. Face the feet and observe the height of the knees. A positive Allis sign is present if one knee is higher than the other.

Anal wink: Reflexive contraction of the anal sphincter in response to gentle stroking of the anal area. This reflex aids inspection of sphincter placement and tone in the newborn. Also called *anocutaneous reflex.*

Anencephaly: A defect in the newborn's skull (beginning at the vertex and extending, in some cases, to the foramen magnum) resulting from defective closure of the anterior neural tube. Hemorrhagic and fibrotic cerebral tissue protrudes, uncovered, through the defect. Generally, anencephaly involves the forebrain and some amount of the upper brainstem. The infant displays an underdeveloped cranial vault, shallow orbits, and protruding eyes. Abnormalities of other systems are also seen.

Anomaly: A deviation from the norm, especially a defect of congenital or hereditary origin. A **minor anomaly** is one that is of little cosmetic significance and requires minimal or no intervention. Many deformations fall into this category. A **major anomaly** is cosmetically significant and requires medical intervention. Most malformations and disruptions are categorized as major anomalies. The greater the number of minor anomalies seen in an infant, the higher the risk of a major anomaly also being present.

Anterior axillary line: A reference line (used to describe the location of physical findings) that passes vertically through the anterior axillary fold.

Anterior vascular capsule of the lens: Within the first 24 to 48 hours of life, transient embryologic vascular systems that nourish the eye during active intrauterine growth can be seen on the anterior vascular capsule of the infant's lens using an ophthalmoscope. Because these systems appear at week 27 and disappear by the end of week 34 of gestation, the degree of their presence in the neonate's lens can be used to determine gestational age.

Antimongolian slant: Description of an eye in which the outer canthus is lower than the inner canthus.

Aphonia: Loss of the voice.

Apical impulse: The forward thrust of the left ventricle during systole, usually seen in the newborn in the fourth intercostal space at or left of the midclavicular line. An apical impulse downward and to the left suggests left ventricular dilatation. A very sharp apical impulse indicates high cardiac output or left ventricular hypertrophy.

Aplasia cutis congenita: (Also called cutis aplasia.) A congenital abnormality of unknown cause, aplasia cutis congenita most often appears on the scalp (over the parietal bones or near the sagittal suture) and is characterized by the absence of some or all layers of the skin. It may be an isolated defect or may be associated with chromosomal disorders such as trisomy 13.

Apnea: A lapse of 20 seconds or more between respiratory cycles, with bradycardia or color changes. Apnea is commonly seen in premature neonates, and is outgrown as the infant approaches term. It is abnormal in near-term or term infants.

Appropriate for gestational age (AGA): An infant whose weight, length, and/or occipital-frontal circumference falls between the tenth and the ninetieth percentiles for gestational age when plotted on a standard growth chart.

Areola: The darkened area surrounding the nipple. In a full-term infant, it is raised and stippled, with 0.75–1 cm of palpable breast tissue. The distance between the outside of the two areolae should be less than 25 percent of the chest circumference.

Arnold-Chiari malformation: A congenital anomaly marked by inferior displacement of the medulla and fourth ventricle into the upper cervical canal and elongation and thinning of the upper medulla and lower pons, along with interior displacement of the lower cerebellum through the foramen magnum into the lower cervical canal. It is generally associated with hydrocephalus and myelomeningocele.

Arrhythmia: An irregularity in the heart rhythm. Arrhythmias are common—and usually benign—in the newborn. **Sinus arrhythmia** is characterized by irregularity of the R-R interval with an otherwise normal cardiac cycle. **Premature atrial beat**, seen in perhaps a third of healthy term and premature infants, is an early beat arising from a supraventricular focus, with normal ventricular conduction. **Premature ventricular beat** is an early beat arising from an irritable ventricular focus, with abnormal ventricular conduction producing a wide QRS complex.

Arthrogryposis: Congenital limitation of movement of limbs due to nonprogressive contracture of the joint.

Ascites: Accumulation of serous fluid in the peritoneal cavity.

Asphyxia, perinatal: Acidosis, hypoxia, and hypercapnia caused by lack of oxygen and carbon dioxide exchange and decreased perfusion in the fetus or the newborn. It may result in hypoxic-ischemic encephalopathy.

Association: A combination of defects that occur together more frequently than would be normal by chance, but that is less fixed than the pattern seen in a syndrome. Associations are generally named by acronyms formed from the initial letter of each defect in them.

Asymmetrically growth retarded: An infant who has not grown at the expected rate—that is, who ranks at less than the tenth percentile for gestational age on standard growth charts—for one of the three growth parameters: weight, length, and occipital-frontal head circumference.

Atelectasis: Incomplete expansion of all or part of a lung.

Atresia, anal: Congenital absence of the anal canal and/or orifice, indicated by lack of stool passage, progressive abdominal distention, and finally vomiting. Also called *imperforate anus.*

Atresia, bilateral choanal: Obstruction of the posterior nasal passages. Infants affected are cyanotic at rest and pink when crying because they are breathing through an open mouth.

Atresia, esophageal: Congenital lack of continuity of the esophagus, characterized by excessive salivation.

Auscultation: A physical assessment technique involving listening for body sounds—chiefly those of the heart and lungs, but also those of the pleura and abdomen. *Direct* auscultation is performed without the aid of a stethoscope; *indirect (mediate)* auscultation involves use of the stethoscope.

Avulsion: A tearing away.

Barrel chest: An abnormality of the bony structure of the chest in which the anterior-posterior diameter of the chest is greater than normal. It is seen with TTN, meconium aspiration, and hyperinflation.

Behavioral assessment: Evaluation of the infant's ability to interact with the environment; includes assessment of organization, changes in state of consciousness, and response to stimuli. Behavioral assessment also includes evaluation of motor maturity and muscle tone, strength, and coordination.

Behavioral cues: Signs infants give to indicate their physical, psychological, and social needs. **Signs of attention** (also called *signs of approach*) indicate a readiness to interact. These cues include an alert, focused gaze; and regular breathing; they may also include grasping, sucking, or hand-to-mouth movements. **Time-out signals** (also called *avoidance behaviors*) indicate the need for a respite from interaction. These cues include an averted gaze, frowning, sneezing, yawning, vomiting, and hiccups, sometimes accompanied by finger splaying, arching, and stiffening. Color changes, apnea, irregular breathing, and decreased oxygen saturation may also be seen.

Bell's palsy: Paralysis of the facial nerve with a resultant characteristic distortion of the face—unilateral.

Bones, cranial: There are four cranial bones: the *frontal, occipital, parietal,* and *temporal.* See Figure 5-3 for locations.

Bowel sounds: Metallic, tinkling sounds heard every 15–20 seconds when the four abdominal quadrants are auscultated beginning within 15 minutes after birth. Hyperactive sounds immediately after feeding, with the intensity of the sounds diminishing as the next feeding approaches, are normal. Auscultation of *friction rubs* (resembling the sound of rubbing a finger over a cupped hand held near the ear) may indicate peritoneal irritation. When heard in the newborn over the lung fields, bowel sounds are likely referred sounds from the abdomen. If they persist, however, they could indicate diaphragmatic hernia.

Brachial palsy: A functional paralysis of part or all of the arm, resulting from birth trauma and more common in large babies. Its cause is stretching injuries to the components of the brachial plexus during delivery. The upper arm is more commonly affected than the lower or the entire arm. The Moro reflex is absent on the affected side, but the grasp reflex remains. Neurologic function returns within several days of birth as hemorrhage and edema resolve, if the nerve roots are not injured.

Brachycephaly: Broad skull shape caused by craniosynostosis (premature fusion) of the coronal suture, limiting forward growth of the skull.

Bradycardia, sinus: A heart rate less than 80 beats per minute in a newborn. Transient bradycardia, with origin in the sinus node, is commonly seen in both full-term and premature newborns, generally in response to vagal stimulation.

Bradypnea: Excessively slow respirations. In the neonate, persistent respirations of less than 40 per minute are associated with central nervous system depression from such factors as maternal drug ingestion, asphyxia, or birth injury.

Branchial sinus: An abnormal opening seen anywhere along the sternocleidomastoid muscle. It may communicate with deeper structures, with potential for infection.

Bronchial breath sounds: Seldom heard in the neonate, bronchial sounds are the loudest of the normal breath sounds. They are found over the trachea and are marked by a short inspiration and a longer expiration.

Bronchopulmonary dysplasia (BPD): Chronic neonatal lung disease characterized by bronchiolar metaplasia and interstitial fibrosis.

Bronchovesicular breath sounds: Normally found over the manubrium and the intrascapular regions, bronchovesicular sounds are intermediate in intensity between bronchial and vesicular breath sounds. In these sounds, inspiration and expiration are equal in quality, intensity, pitch, and duration.

Bruit: (1) A murmur-like sound auscultated over the fontanels or the lateral skull. It may signify intracranial arteriovenous malformation in an infant with congestive heart failure. (2) A sound, resembling a systolic murmur, heard with dilated, tortuous, or constricted vessels during auscultation of the skull. It is produced by the vibration of vessel walls within the skull, caused by flow disturbances that interfere with the normal laminar flow through the vessels. Bruits may be heard with Sturge-Weber syndrome. (3) If heard over the newborn's abdomen and not eliminated by changing the infant's position, bruits may indicate umbilical vein or hepatic vascular system abnormalities, renal artery stenosis, or hepatic hemangiomas.

Brushfield spots: White specks scattered linearly around the circumference of the iris. These spots are associated with Down syndrome, but may also be seen as a normal variant.

Bulla: An elevation of the skin filled with serous fluid (a vesicle) greater than 1 cm in diameter.

Café au lait patch: A tan or light brown macule or patch with well-defined borders. One patch is found in up to 19 percent of normal children, and these patches are of no pathologic significance when they are less than 3 cm in length and less than six in number. A greater number of patches or patches larger than 3 cm may indicate a cutaneous neurofibromatosis, an autosomal dominant genetic disorder.

Candida diaper dermatitis: A moist, erythematous rash caused by or associated with *Candida albicans* and consisting of small white or yellow pustules over the buttocks and perianal region (and occasionally the thighs).

Canthus: The angle at either end of the opening between the eyelids. The eye has two canthi, the inner (adjacent to the nose) and the outer.

Capillary filling time: A measurement used to assess cardiac perfusion in the newborn. Press the infant's skin with a finger until it blanches; then count the seconds required for the color to return. This should take no more than 3-4 seconds in a normal infant. Check filling time in both a central and a peripheral area.

Caput succedaneum: Edema occurring in and under the presenting part of the fetal scalp during delivery, generally due to pressure restricting venous and lymph flow. The edema has poorly defined edges, pits on pressure, and usually crosses suture lines. It resolves within a few days. *Caput succedaneum* is the most common form of birth trauma to the head.

Caput: The head.

Caudocephalad: From the lower extremities toward the head.

Cephalhematoma: Collection of blood (hemorrhage) between the periosteum and the skull, generally resulting from birth trauma. The edges are clearly demarcated and bounded by suture lines. Cephalhematomas are most commonly seen over the parietal and occipital bones. Over time, a cephalhematoma may liquefy and become fluctuant on palpation; resolution can take weeks to months.

Chordee: Ventral bowing of the penis, which produces a downward curvature on erection. It is often seen with hypospadias.

Chromosomal aneuploidy: Too many or too few chromosomes, resulting in a genetic malformation. Normal infants have 46 chromosomes (22 pairs of autosomes and 2 sex chromosomes). Forms of aneuploidy include monosomy and trisomy.

Clavicle: One of the pair of bones linking the sternum with a scapula. Commonly called the *collarbone.*

Cleft lip: A congenital defect in the upper lip.

Cleidocranial dysostosis: Syndrome characterized by congenital complete or partial absence of the clavicles. Defective cranial ossification, large fontanels, and delayed suture closure are often seen with complete absence. This anomaly is characterized by excessive scapulothoracic motion.

Clonus: Involuntary repetitive muscle contraction and relaxation.

Clubfoot *(talipes equinovarus):* One of the common congenital deformities of the foot, seen more often in male infants than in female, and varying in severity. The forefoot is adducted and points medially, there is pronounced varus of the heel, and the foot and toes point downward. In unilateral presentation, the affected foot is smaller, with thickened joints.

Coloboma: A malformation characterized by absence of or a defect in the tissue of the eye. It is sometimes seen as a keyhole-shaped pupil and associated with other anomalies.

Congenital absence of the radius: A bilateral anomaly in half the infants who exhibit it, radial absence presents with a deviated hand and wrist, a shortened forearm with a bowed ulna, an absent or hypoplastic thumb, and limited elbow movement. The condition may require surgery.

Congenital absence of the tibia or fibula: This unusual anomaly more frequently affects the fibula than the tibia and is more often unilateral than bilateral. There may be partial or complete absence of the bone. Foot deformity and leg length discrepancies are generally seen in the absence of either long bone.

Congenital constricting bands (Streeter dysplasia): Bands of tissue (thought to be amniotic in origin) encircling one or more extremities of the newborn. These bands can produce shallow indentations of the soft tissue or constrictions severe enough to cause partial or complete amputation of the extremity. Treatment depends on the severity; a surgical consultation may be required.

Congenital heart disease (CHD): A spectrum of cardiac anomalies present at birth. There is increased risk of CHD in infants of mothers with CHD, in infants with an older sibling who has CHD, and in low birth weight infants. An increased incidence of CHD is also associated with extracardiac anomalies, including those of the gastrointestinal, renal, and urogenital systems; tracheoesophageal fistulas; and diaphragmatic hernias.

Congenital hip dysplasia: An abnormality in which the hip joint develops abnormally, causing instability of the hip ranging from minimal to dislocation. The causes of congenital hip dysplasia may include lack of acetabular depth, laxity of the ligaments, and/or intrauterine breech position. Congenital hip dysplasia is more often seen in Caucasian than in African-American or Oriental infants; it is more common in females than in males, and the left hip is affected more often than the right. In multiple births, it is more common in the first born. A positive Allis' sign may indicate congenital hip dysplasia. It is associated with other orthopedic anomalies and deformities.

Consolability: An infant's ability to quiet himself when in the crying state or to respond to attempts by a caregiver to quiet him. An infant with well-developed organization generally exhibits self-consoling behaviors, including bringing the hands to the mouth, sucking on the fist or tongue, or using environmental stimuli as a distraction.

Consolidation: An area of increased lung tissue density.

Cost of attention: A term used by T.B. Brazelton to describe the amount of energy an infant must expend to maintain an alert state of consciousness. The cost of attention depends on both the health and maturity of the infant.

Crackles: Adventitious breath sounds involving a series of brief crackling or bubbling sounds. (Crackles were previously termed rales.) **Fine crackles**, usually heard at the end of inspiration, resemble the sound made by rubbing a lock of hair. They may be associated with RDS or BPD. **Medium crackles** sound like a carbonated fizz. They are believed to reflect the passage of air past sticky surfaces, as found with pneumonia or TTN. **Coarse crackles** (also called *rhonchi*) are loud, bubbly sounds associated with mucus or fluid accumulation in the large airways.

Craniosynostosis: Premature fusion of one or more sutures, stopping bone growth perpendicular to the suture but permitting it parallel to the suture.

Craniotabes: Areas of soft (demineralized) bone in the skull, usually in the occipital and parietal bones along the lambdoidal suture. Craniotabes is sometimes seen with hydrocephalus.

Cremasteric reflex: Contraction of the cremaster muscle resulting in a drawing up of the ipsilateral testis when the inner thigh is stroked or stretched longitudinally.

Cri du chat syndrome: A chromosomal disorder in which the short arm of the fifth chromosome is missing. It presents with a catlike cry in the newborn and other associated anomalies.

Crust: Dried serous exudate, blood, or pus.

Crying: A wakeful state of infant consciousness characterized by crying (in term infants), increased motor activity, color changes, and exaggerated response to unpleasant stimuli. Some term infants console themselves by returning to a lower state of consciousness. Preterm infants may have a very weak (or even absent) cry, but exhibit the other signs of stress indicative of this state.

Cryptorchidism: Failure of one or both testes to descend into the scrotum. It can be unilateral (most often occurring on the right side) or bilateral. In full-term infants who present with undescended testes at birth, about half show descent by six weeks of age; in 75 percent of preterm infants, the testes descend by three months of age. Testes do not usually descend spontaneously after nine months of age. Inguinal hernia is commonly seen with cryptorchidism.

Cutis marmorata: Bluish mottling or marbling of the skin in response to chilling, stress, or overstimulation, usually disappearing when the infant is warmed.

Cyanosis, central: Bluish discoloration of the skin and mucous membranes due to significant arterial oxygen desaturation. It presents when at least 5 gm of unbound (to oxygen) hemoglobin are present per 100 ml of blood. An important indicator of congenital heart disease, cyanosis due to cardiac causes does not improve on administration of 100 percent oxygen and also increases with crying. In cyanotic infants without increased respiratory effort, the cause of the cyanosis is most likely congenital heart disease. Central cyanosis may also occur in the presence of persistent pulmonary hypertension, lung disease, sepsis, or neurologic disease. Central cyanosis must be differentiated from acrocyanosis (peripheral cyanosis) and circumoral cyanosis, both of which are normally seen in the first few days after birth.

Cyanosis, circumoral: Bluish discoloration of the lips and area surrounding the mouth.

Darwinian tubercle: A normal variant appearing as a small nodule on the upper helix of the ear.

Deep sleep state: A sleeping state of infant consciousness characterized by closed eyes, regular breathing, and lack of spontaneous activity. Response to external stimuli is delayed.

Defect, polygenic: A malformation resulting from the effects of multiple genes.

Defect, single-gene: A genetically caused malformation. The form of inheritance may be dominant (carried by one gene from one parent), recessive (requiring one gene from each parent), or X-linked (carried on the X chromosome and expressed in male offspring, with female offspring being carriers).

Deformation: A congenital abnormality caused by pressure exerted by mechanical forces on the fetus generally late in gestation after the major organ systems are formed. The source of the pressure is generally uterine constraint (maternal or fetal). Most deformations occur to the musculoskeletal system.

Depigmentation lesion: A white, macular lesion with an irregular, leaf-like border. These lesions may be early indicators of tuberous sclerosis, a progressive degenerative neurologic disease.

Dermis: Inner, vascular layer of the skin containing fibrous and elastic tissues, sweat and sebaceous glands and ducts, hair follicles and shafts, blood vessels, and nerves. Also called *corium.*

Diaphragmatic hernia: Protrusion of abdominal contents through an opening in the diaphragm.

Diastasis recti: A palpable midline gap between the rectus muscles of the abdominal wall.

Bulging may be seen when the infant cries. Diastasis recti is often seen in otherwise normal infants and is benign unless a hernia is present.

Diastole: Dilatation of the heart (particularly of the ventricles), coincident with the interval between the second (S2) and the first (S1) heart sounds.

Disruption: A congenital abnormality caused by the breakdown of normal tissue *in utero.* Most disruptions result from amniotic bands wrapping around fetal extremities or entering the fetus' mouth.

Doll's eye maneuver: Used to evaluate movement of the eyes as the head is turned. The infant's head is gently rotated from side to side, the eyes should deviate away from the direction of rotation, i.e., turning the head to the right, the eyes should deviate to the left.

Dorsiflexion: Flexion toward the back, as in flexion of the foot so that the forefoot is higher than the ankle.

Drowsiness: The transitional state of infant consciousness between sleep and wakefulness. The infant exhibits a variable activity level, with dull, heavy-lidded eyes that open and close periodically. Movements are smooth, and there is response to stimuli, but not immediately.

Dysmorphogenesis: Abnormal development of form or structure, as seen in congenital malformations. Dysmorphic features are also called *anomalies.*

Ecchymosis (plural: ecchymoses): A non-blanching area of subepidermal hemorrhage, initially bluish black in color, then changing to greenish brown or yellow. Ecchymoses may be seen on the labia of female infants and the scrotal area of male infants after breech deliveries.

Edema: Abnormally large amounts of fluid in the intercellular tissue spaces of the body,

usually the subcutaneous tissues. Most newborns have some edema around the face and eyes due to excess fluid volume after delivery. After difficult deliveries, edema of the scalp or in dependent areas is often seen. In *pitting edema,* indentations produced by pressure remain for prolonged periods. In *nonpitting edema,* the tissues cannot be pitted with pressure.

Ejection click: A snappy, high-frequency heart sound normal during the first 24 hours of life; after that, it is considered abnormal. If present, it is best heard just after the first heart sound and resembles in timing, but not in quality, a widely split S1 heart sound.

Embryonic period: The third to the eighth week of pregnancy, the period during which differentiation and major organ system development take place. Insults to the embryo during this period can result in major anomalies in the newborn.

Encephalocele: A restricted disorder of anterior neural tube closure producing a defect in the skull called *cranium bifidum.* In some cases, a skin-covered protrusion (sac) containing meninges and cerebral spinal fluid (and sometimes cerebral tissue) is present. In other cases, the defect appears as a small tissue-covered opening (often surrounded by tufts of abnormal hair) on the skull, with no protrusion of skull contents. The most common location for encephaloceles is the midline of the occipital bone, but they are also seen in the parietal, temporal, or frontal nasopharyngeal areas. Size varies from tiny to massive; severity depends on location, size, and the contents of the protrusion. Skull x-rays can identify the cranium bifidum, and transillumination and ultrasound help identify the contents of the protrusion.

Encephalopathy, hypoxic-ischemic: A syndrome resulting from perinatal asphyxia. It can be categorized as **mild** (associated with irritability, jitteriness, and hyperalertness), **moderate** (characterized by lethargy, hypotonia, decreased spontaneous movement, and seizures), or **severe** (characterized by coma, flaccidity, disturbed brainstem function, and seizures). The pattern of limb weakness displayed by an affected infant reflects the area of the brain injured by the asphyxia. In term neonates, injury to the parasagittal areas (resulting in weakness of the shoulder girdle and proximal upper extremities) or the middle cerebral artery (presenting as hemiparesis) predominates. In the premature newborn, injury is often to the periventricular area, resulting in weakness in the lower extremities.

Epicanthal fold: A vertical fold of skin on either side of the nose that covers the lacrimal caruncle. These folds are normal in Oriental infants but suggestive of Down syndrome in neonates of other races.

Epidermis: Outermost layer of the skin, itself composed of five layers. The top layer is the *stratum corneum* (dead cells that are constantly being sloughed off and replaced); lower layers contain keratin-forming cells and melanocytes.

Epispadias: Location of the urethral meatus on the *dorsal* surface of the penis. It is a less common abnormality than hypospadias. In **balanic epispadias**, the meatus is found at the base of the balanus (glans); in **penile epispadias**, it is on the penile shaft; and in **penopubic epispadias**, it is found, not on the penis at all, but directly below the symphysis.

Epstein's pearls: Epidermal inclusion cysts seen in the newborn at the junction of the hard and soft palates of the mouth and on the gums. They usually disappear by a few weeks of age.

Erb's palsy: Damage (generally due to birth trauma) to the upper spinal roots C5 and C6, resulting in paralysis of an arm (but usually without involvement of the hand). See also **Brachial palsy.**

Erythema toxicum neonatorum: A benign rash consisting of small white or yellow papules or vesicles with an erythematous base. Seen in up to 70 percent of term infants between 24 and 48 hours of age, the rash occurs most often on the face, trunk, or extremities.

Everted: Turned out and away from the midline of the body.

Exophthalmos: Abnormal protrusion of the eyeball. It may be associated with hyperthyroidism.

Expected date of confinement (EDC): Delivery due date. Generally 280 days (40 weeks) from the onset of the mother's last menstrual period.

Expressivity: The extent to which an inheritable trait is manifest in the individual carrying the gene.

Exstrophy of the bladder: A visible fissure between the anterior abdominal wall and the urinary bladder. In male infants, it is commonly accompanied by epispadias.

Extension: The straightening of a limb at a joint.

Family traits: Unusual features (subtle or significant) identified by a family as characteristic of its phenotype.

Fasciculation: The spontaneous localized contraction of a group of fibers in a motor unit, visible through the skin. In Werdnig-Hoffmann disease, these continuous and rapid twitching movements can be seen in the tongue.

Fetal period: The ninth week of pregnancy through birth. The fetus becomes more and more resistant to teratogens as this period progresses.

Fibrils: Tiny fibers or filaments connecting the dermis and the epidermis.

Fistula, rectourethral: An abnormal connection between the rectum and the urethra, indicated by the presence of meconium in the urethral orifice.

Fistula, rectovaginal: An abnormal connection between the rectum and the vagina, indicated by the presence of meconium in the vaginal orifice.

Flexion: The act of bending or the condition of being bent. The bending of a limb at a joint. In the neonate, the degree of arm, knee, and hip flexion is indicative of gestational age.

Flexion contracture: Resistance of a muscle to passive flexion. The newborn's hips generally have a flexion contracture; when the right hip is flexed to stabilize the pelvis and flatten the lumbar spine, a flexion contracture of the left hip may be seen. The infant's elbow also shows a flexion contracture for the first few weeks of life, making it difficult to examine.

Fontanel: A membrane-covered space (soft spot) in the infant's skull reflecting incomplete ossification of the skull. Fontanels occur where two sutures meet. The **anterior fontanel** occurs at the intersection of the metopic, coronal, and saggital sutures. The **posterior fontanel** occurs where the sagittal and lambdoidal sutures meet. The **sphenoid fontanel** is at the juncture of the coronal and squamosal sutures. The **mastoid fontanel** occurs at the intersection of the squamosal and lambdoidal sutures. A defect of the parietal bone along the sagittal suture may appear to be—but is not—a true fontanel (third fontanel). It may be a normal variant or may be associated with Down syndrome or congenital hypothyroidism.

Forcep marks: Red, bruised, or abraded areas on the cheeks, scalp, and face of infants born after application of forceps. Observation of forcep marks calls for examination for facial palsy, fractured clavicles, skull fractures, or other complications of birth trauma.

Frog leg position: A resting posture, normal in premature neonates of 36 or fewer weeks gestation, in which the legs are abducted and the lateral thigh rests against the bed surface. This position is abnormal if seen in newborns older than 36 weeks gestation.

Funnel chest *(pectus excavatum)*: An abnormality of the bony structure of the chest in which the sternum is indented. It is seen in infants with Marfan syndrome and rickets.

Gastroschisis: Protrusion of abdominal contents and other organs through an abdominal wall defect lateral to the midline; the protrusion is not covered by a membrane. A gastroschisis is associated with fewer congenital malformations than is an omphalocele.

Gestational age: The length of time between fertilization of the egg and birth of the infant.

Glabella: The area above the nose and between the eyebrows (bridge of the nose).

Growth parameters: Measurements used to determine whether an infant is small, appropriate, or large for gestational age. The three parameters are weight, length, and occipital-frontal head circumference.

Habituation: A newborn's ability to alter his response to a repeated stimulus, decreasing and finally eliminating the response on repetition of the stimulus. Habituation is a defense mechanism.

Harlequin sign: A sharply demarcated red color in the dependent half of the body, with the superior half of the body appearing pale, when the infant is placed on his side. Rotating the infant to the other side reverses the coloring. Harlequin color change occurs in both healthy and sick infants but is more common in low birth weight infants. It has no pathologic significance.

Heart rate: The normal heart rate for a full-term neonate is 80-160 beats per minute.

Heart sounds: **S1**, the first heart sound, is best heard at the mitral or tricuspid area. It is usually loud at birth, but decreases in intensity by two days of life. **S2**, the second heart sound, is best heard at the aortic or pulmonic area. It is usually single at birth but is split in two-thirds of infants by 16 hours of age and in 80 percent by 48 hours of age. Wide splitting of S2 is abnormal. **S3**, commonly heard in premature infants with PDA, is best heard at the apex of the heart during early diastole. **S4**, a pathologic sound, is heard at the apex of the heart in infants with conditions characterized by decreased compliance.

Heave: A point of maximum impulse that is slow rising and diffuse, generally associated with ventricular dilatation or volume overload. Also called a *lift*.

Helix: The upper and outer margin of the pinna of the ear.

Hemangioma, cavernous: A raised, lobulated, soft and compressible bluish-red tumor, with poorly defined margins. The cavernous hemangioma consists of large, mature vascular elements lined with endothelial cells and involves the dermis and subcutaneous tissues of the skin. It increases in size during the first 6–12 months of life, and then involutes spontaneously. Two syndromes—Kasabach-Merritt and Klippel-Trenaunay-Weber—may be associated with cavernous hemangiomas.

Hemangioma, strawberry: A raised, lobulated, soft and compressible bright red tumor, with sharply demarcated margins, on the head, neck, trunk, or extremities. (Tumors occurring in the throat can obstruct the airway.) Caused by dilated capillaries, with associated endothelial proliferation in the dermal and subdermal layers of the skin, the strawberry hemangioma occurs in up to 10 percent of newborns. It gradually increases in size for about six months and then spontaneously regresses over a period of up to several years.

Hematocele: A circumscribed collection of blood in a cavity of the scrotum, generally due to trauma to the scrotum during delivery.

Hematocolpos: Retention of blood in the internal genitalia due to an imperforate hymen. It may be palpated as a suprapubic mass, accompanied by a bluish, bulging hymen.

Hemiparesis: Muscle weakness or partial paralysis affecting one half of the body.

Hepatomegaly: Enlargement of the liver.

Hermaphroditism: Anomalous differentiation of the gonads, with presence of both ovarian and testicular tissue and ambiguous morphologic sex criteria. Hermaphroditism is suspected when only one testis is confirmed in a male-appearing infant. See also **Pseudohermaphroditism.**

Hernia, epigastric: Protrusion of fat through a defect on the midline above the umbilicus and below the sternum, presenting as a firm palpable mass. Palpation may elicit a pain response. Surgical intervention is necessary.

Hernia, femoral: A small bulge adjacent and medial to the femoral artery. It is more common in females than in males.

Hernia, inguinal: Muscle wall defect in the inguinal area through which bowel loops or gonads enter the scrotal sac (in males) or the soft tissues (in females). The hernia usually presents as bulging in the groin area and is more common in male than in female infants.

Hernia, umbilical: Skin- and subcutaneous-tissue-covered protrusion of part of the intestine at the umbilicus. It is seen with some frequency in low birth weight and African-American male infants and in infants of other races with hypothyroidism. The hernia usually reduces by two years of age, but intervention is required with strangulation of abdominal contents or large size.

Holosystolic: Occurring throughout systole. Also called *pansystolic*.

Hydranencephaly: Partial or complete absence of the cerebral hemispheres, with the space being filled with cerebrospinal fluid.

Hydrocele: A circumscribed collection of clear fluid in the scrotum, which may resolve spontaneously by six months of age. A hydrocele may communicate with the inguinal canal, however, and may be associated with a hernia. **Hydrocele of the cord** presents as a palpable sausage-shaped, smooth bulge above the testes.

Hydrocephalus: Accumulation of cerebrospinal fluid (often under increased pressure) within the skull, due to obstruction of the cerebrospinal fluid pathways causing dilatation of the cerebral ventricles. It may be congenital or may develop after birth and is characterized by head enlargement, forehead prominence, brain atrophy, mental deterioration, and convulsions. The skull is often globular in shape.

Hydrometrocolpos: Collection of secretions in the vagina and uterus due to an imperforate hymen. It may be palpated as a small midline lower abdominal mass or a cystic movable mass as the quantity of secretions increases.

Hygroma, cystic: The most commonly seen neck mass in newborns, a cystic hygroma is soft, fluctuant, and can range from only a few centimeters in size to massive. It is usually seen laterally or over the clavicle and transilluminates well.

Hymenal tag: A small appendage or flap on the hymen, normal in female infants. It disappears in several weeks.

Hyperplasia, sebaceous gland: Numerous white or yellow papules (less than 0.5 mm in size) on the nose and upper lips. These enlarged sebaceous glands spontaneously decrease in size with age and require no treatment.

Hypertelorism: Widely spaced eyes—those with greater than a palpebral fissure length between them.

Hypertonia: Increased resistance of the skeletal muscles to passive stretching. In the presence of hypertonia, passive manipulation of the limbs often increases the tone.

Hypertrophy: Enlargement or overgrowth of an organ or part.

Hypertrophy of the clitoris: The most common genitourinary abnormality in female infants, suggesting pseudohermaphroditism.

Hypoplastic nails: Nails that are incompletely developed. Edema of the hands can give the appearance of hypoplastic nails.

Hypospadias: Location of the urethral meatus on the **ventral** surface of the penis. In **balanic (glanular) hypospadias,** the meatus is located at the base of the balanus (glans). In **penile hypospadias,** the meatus is found between the glans and the scrotum. It is often accompanied by chordee, flattening of the glans, and an absent ventral foreskin. In **penoscrotal (perineal) hypospadias,** the meatus is found at the penoscrotal junction. Gender ambiguity is associated with penoscrotal hypospadias, as is bifid scrotum, small penis with a large meatus, and undescended testes.

Hypotelorism: Closely spaced eyes—those with less than a palpebral fissure length between them.

Hypotonia: Depressed postural muscle tone.

Inner canthal distance: The measurement between the inner canthi of the two eyes. If the eyes are normally spaced, this distance should be equal to the length of the palpebral fissure.

Inspection: A physical assessment technique involving careful visual attention to, measurement of, and notation of the status of external body parts and systems, for the purpose of forming a judgment.

Intrauterine growth retarded (IUGR) neonate: A newborn who did not grow *in utero* at the expected rate for weight, length, or occipital-frontal head circumference. Although the term is often used synonymously with small for gestational age (SGA), the two terms do not necessarily mean the same thing. A neonate may be growth retarded but may not fall below the tenth percentile for gestational age.

Intussusception: Prolapse of one part of the intestine into the channel of the adjoining part. May present as a sausage-like mass in the right or left upper abdominal quadrant during palpation.

Inverted: Turned inward toward the midline of the body.

Jaundice: Yellow coloring of the skin and whites of the eyes, generally appearing first on the head and face and then progressing toward the feet. Jaundice is due to excess bilirubin in the blood (hyperbilirubinemia).

Jitteriness: A series of movements seen at times in normal preterm neonates and in normal term neonates with vigorous crying. (Persistent jitteriness may indicate a disorder.) Jitteriness is characterized by rapid movements of equal amplitude in alternating directions, generally occurs in response to a stimulus, can be stopped by flexing and holding the involved extremity, and is not associated with abnormal eye movements or other signs of seizure. Jitteriness must be distinguished from seizure activity. See also **Seizure.**

Karyotype: Representation by diagram of the chromosomal characteristics of an individual or species.

Karyotyping: Chromosomal evaluation.

Keratin: An insoluble, fibrous protein that is the main component of certain protective and/or supportive elements of the body, including the nails, hair, and epidermis.

Klippel-Feil syndrome: Defects of the cervical vertebrae, resulting in a shorter-than-normal neck with limited motion and asymmetry in rotation and lateral flexion.

Klumpke's palsy: Damage (generally due to birth trauma) resulting in paralysis of the forearm. See also **Brachial palsy.**

Kyphosis: A spinal abnormality in which the curvature of the thoracic spine is excessively convex. Commonly called *hunchback.*

Lacrimal caruncle: The red area at the inner canthus of the eye.

Lanugo: A fine, soft, downy hair covering the fetus *in utero* and sometimes the neonate. It first appears at about 20 weeks gestation, covering most of the body including the face. Most of it disappears by 40 weeks gestation.

Large for gestational age (LGA): An infant whose weight falls above the ninetieth percentile for gestational age when plotted on a standard growth chart.

Lesion: Any discontinuity of tissue or change in the structure or function of an organ or part due to disease or trauma.

Light sleep state: See **Active sleep.**

Lipoma: A benign tumor composed of fat cells.

Lordosis: A spinal abnormality in which the curvature of the lumbar and cervical spine is excessively concave. Commonly called *swayback.*

Low birth weight: An infant who weighs less than 2,500 gm at birth.

Macrocephaly: Excessive head size (an occipital-frontal circumference above the ninetieth percentile for gestational age, with otherwise normal weight and length percentiles). Macrocephaly can be familial or it may be due to hydrocephalus or associated with dwarfism or osteogenesis imperfecta.

Macrodactyly: An enlarged finger or toe. It is seen in otherwise normal infants, or it may indicate neurofibromatosis.

Macroglossia: An abnormally large tongue.

Macrostomia: An abnormally large oral opening.

Macule: A discolored, flat, nonpalpable spot or patch less than 1 cm in diameter.

Malacia: Abnormal softening of tissues.

Malformation: A congenital defect arising from abnormal tissue. The cause of the tissue abnormality may be intrinsic (genetic) or extrinsic (environmental).

Manubrium: Uppermost portion of the sternum.

Mediastinum: A space within the chest cavity containing the heart, esophagus, trachea, mainstem bronchi, thymus, and major blood vessels.

Melanosis, transient neonatal pustular: Small pigmented macules (often surrounded by very fine white scales) caused by the rupture of superficial vesiculopustular lesions 12–48 hours after birth. The condition—seen in up to 5 percent of African-American and about 0.2 percent of Caucasian infants—is benign and generally resolves by three months of age.

Meningocele: A lesion associated with spina bifida in which more than one vertebra is involved. The meninges protrude through the bony defect and are covered by a thin atrophic skin. The spinal roots and nerves are normal.

Metatarsus adductus: A common congenital foot anomaly caused by intrauterine positioning. It may be positional (flexible) or structural (fixed). In the structural type (with bony abnormalities), there is limited abduction of the forefoot, and the heel is in a valgus position. In the positional type, the forefoot abducts easily, and the heel is in a varus or neutral position.

Microcephaly: Abnormal smallness of the head (an occipital-frontal circumference below the tenth percentile for gestational age), generally due to poor brain growth.

Micrognathia: An abnormally small lower jaw, seen in Robin sequence and other syndromes.

Micropenis: Abnormally small penis. Micropenis suggests congenital hypopituitarism when seen with certain other anomalies or conditions. Also called *penile hypoplasia.*

Microstomia: An abnormally small oral opening. It may be seen with some trisomies.

Midclavicular line: A reference line (used to describe the location of physical findings) passing vertically through the clavicle.

Midsternal line: A reference line (used to describe the location of physical findings) bisecting the suprasternal notch.

Milia: Multiple yellow or pearly white papules about 1 mm in size. These epidermal cysts, found on the brow, cheeks, and nose of up to 40 percent of newborns, are caused by accumulation of sebaceous gland secretions and spontaneously resolve during the first few weeks of life.

Miliaria: Changes in the skin caused by obstruction of the sweat ducts. **Miliaria** is generally associated with excessive warmth and/or humidity and is classified into four types, based on severity. **Miliaria crystallina** occurs when sweat escapes into the epidermal stratum corneum, causing formation of clear, thin vesicles 1–2 mm in diameter. **Miliaria rubra,** commonly called prickly heat, presents as small erythematous papules and occurs when continued obstruction of the sweat ducts causes release of sweat into adjacent tissues of the epidermis. **Miliaria pustulosa** occurs with continued occlusion of the sweat ducts, as leukocytes infiltrate the vesicles. Unresolved **miliaria pustulosa** can lead to **miliaria profunda,** secondary infection of the deeper dermal portions of the sweat glands.

Mongolian slant: Description of an eye in which the outer canthus is higher than the inner canthus.

Mongolian spot: A large gray or blue-green macule or patch caused by melanocyte infiltration of the dermis. This pigmented lesion, generally found on the buttocks, flanks, or shoulders, is seen in up to 90 percent of African-American, Oriental, and Hispanic and up to 10 percent of Caucasian infants.

Monosomy: A form of chromosomal aneuploidy in which one chromosome of a pair is missing.

Mottling: Blotchy skin showing areas of different color. It may indicate cardiogenic shock in the neonate.

Mucocele: A mucous retention cyst (distended cavity containing mucus) presenting as a translucent or bluish swelling under the tongue.

Murmur: A prolonged heart sound caused by turbulent blood flow. Documenting the timing, location, intensity, radiation, quality, and pitch are all important to the evaluation of the origin of a murmur, as is the age of the newborn. There are two types of murmurs: *innocent* and *pathologic.*

Murmur, continuous: A pathologic murmur, heard through both systole and diastole, present in about a third of premature infants with a PDA and also in full-term or premature infants with arteriovenous fistulas.

Murmur, continuous systolic (crescendo systolic): An innocent murmur heard in up to 15 percent of newborns, beginning within the first 8 hours of life. It is best heard in the upper left sternal border.

Murmur, early soft midsystolic ejection: An innocent murmur often heard in premature infants, beginning within the first week or two of life and disappearing by the eighth week. Medium-to-high-pitched, it is best heard in the upper left sternal border, with wide radiation.

Murmur, loud systolic ejection: A pathologic murmur that presents within hours of birth, generally due to aortic or pulmonary stenosis or coarctation of the aorta.

Murmur, systolic ejection: An innocent murmur heard in more than half of all newborns, beginning within the first day of life and lasting up to a week. It can be described as "vibratory" and is best heard along the mid- and upper left sternal border.

Murmurs, innocent: Innocent murmurs have no pathologic cause within the heart or great vessels. They are generally systolic, symptomless, and common in normal newborns during the first 48 hours of life when they are associated with decreasing pulmonary vascular resistance and with closure of the PDA. They include **systolic ejection murmurs, continuous systolic (crescendo systolic) murmurs,** and **early soft midsystolic ejection murmurs.**

Murmurs, pathologic: Pathologic murmurs are due to cardiovascular disease. When they present is dependent on their cause and on normal changes associated with transitional circulation. Many do not appear until pulmonary vascular resistance falls. Absence of a murmur does not rule out CHD; as many as a fifth of the infants who die from CHD by one month of age do not have murmurs. Pathologic murmurs include **loud systolic ejection murmurs** and **continuous murmurs.**

Muscle tone, phasic: The brief, forceful contraction of a muscle in response to a short-duration, high-amplitude stretch. In the newborn, phasic tone is evaluated by testing the resistance of the extremities to movement (scarf sign and arm and leg recoil) and by assessing the activity of the deep tendon reflexes (biceps and patellar reflexes).

Muscle tone, postural: The long-duration, low-amplitude stretch of a muscle in response to gravity. In the newborn, the traction response (pull-to-sit maneuver) is used to evaluate postural tone. Depressed postural tone is called *hypotonia.*

Myelomeningocele: A lesion associated with spina bifida in which bilateral broadening of the vertebrae or absence of the vertebral arches is seen. The lesion is most often seen in the lumbar spine and is characterized by protrusion of meninges and spinal roots and nerves, along with fusion of remnants of the spinal cord and an exposed neural tube. The higher the defect on the spine, the greater the degree of paralysis. Hydrocephalus is frequently seen with a myelomeningocele, especially in the Arnold-Chiari malformation.

Necrosis, subcutaneous fat: A hard, nonpitting, sharply circumscribed subcutaneous nodule that appears during the first weeks of life, grows larger over several days, and then resolves spontaneously over several weeks. Color will vary. Possible causes include trauma, cold, or asphyxia. Intervention may be necessary if the condition is associated with hypercalcemia.

Neonatal Behavioral Assessment Scale (NBAS): An examination tool developed by T. B. Brazelton to assess behavior in the term infant.

Neonatal torsion of the testis: A condition in which a testis and its tunica vaginalis rotate in the scrotal sac, inguinal canal, or abdomen. Torsion of a descended testis presents with reddish to bluish coloring of the scrotal skin and a nontender or mildly tender mass. Torsion is difficult to identify if the testis has not descended.

Nevus, pigmented: A dark brown or black macule commonly seen on the lower back or buttocks. Although pigmented nevi are generally benign, malignant changes occur in up to 10 percent of these lesions.

Nevus, port wine: A flat, nonblanching pink or reddish purple lesion with sharply delineated edges directly beneath the epidermis. The port wine nevus generally appears on the face, consists of dilated capillaries, and varies in size from small to covering almost half the body. Although usually unilateral, on occasion it crosses the midline. It neither grows in size nor resolves spontaneously. Port wine nevi located over the branches of the trigeminal nerve may be associated with Sturge-Weber syndrome.

Nevus, sebaceous: A small yellow or yellowish-orange papule or plaque consisting of immature hair follicles and sebaceous glands. It is commonly found on the scalp or face.

Nevus simplex: An irregularly bordered pink macule that blanches with pressure and becomes more prominent with crying. Found most often on the nape of the neck, the upper eyelids, the bridge of the nose, or the upper lip, the nevus simplex is composed of dilated capillaries and is seen in up to 50 percent of newborns. Its common name is *stork bite.*

Nipple line: A reference line (used to describe the location of physical findings) passing horizontally through the nipples.

Nipples, supernumerary: Accessory nipples—raised or pigmented areas 5-6 cm below the normal nipples. In Caucasian infants, they may be associated with congenital anomalies.

Nodule: An elevated palpable lesion, solid and circumscribed (a papule) greater than 1 cm in diameter.

Normal variants: Minor differences in the appearance of the features between races, but that are normal for the race. Also called *minor variants.*

Nystagmus: A rapid, searching movement of the eyeballs seen in some newborns until three to four months of age. Occasional nystagmus is normal in the otherwise normal neonate; persistent is abnormal and may indicate loss of vision.

Observation: A physical assessment technique involving careful visual attention to, and notation of the status of external body parts and systems, for the purpose of forming a judgment. Also called *inspection.*

Occipital-frontal circumference (OFC): Measurement of the neonate's head taken over the occipital, parietal, and frontal prominences, avoiding the ears. This growth parameter is used, with the infant's gestational age, to determine whether the infant's head is small, appropriate, or large for gestational age In the term infant, the normal OFC is 31–38 cm.

Oligohydramnios: The presence of less than 500 ml of amniotic fluid at term or 50 percent of normal volume at any time during pregnancy. The intrauterine compression caused by the lack of fluid may produce unusual flattening of the facial features in the newborn.

Omphalocele: Protrusion of abdominal contents through a defect at the umbilicus. A thin, translucent membrane covers the protrusion, and may rupture at delivery. Omphalocele is seen more often in male infants, especially premature males, and is usually associated with trisomies 13, 18, and 21; Beckwith-Wiedemann syndrome; or congenital heart disease.

Omphalomesenteric duct: Persistence in the newborn of this embryological duct between the ileum and the umbilicus, with seepage of ileal liquid from the opening.

Ophthalmoscope: A hand-held device, containing lenses and a mirror, that produces a beam of light for inspection of the interior of the eye. In physical examination of the newborn, it is used to assess pupillary constriction and the red reflex. It can also be used to inspect the anterior vascular capsule of the lens to determine gestational age.

Opisthotonus: Marked extensor hypertonia, with arching of the back. It may be seen with bacterial meningitis, severe hypoxic-ischemic brain damage, and massive intraventricular hemorrhage.

Orchiopexy: Surgical fixation of an undescended testis in the scrotum. Generally done between 9 and 18 months of age.

Organization: An infant's ability to integrate physiologic (heart rate, respiratory rate, oxygen consumption, digestion) and behavioral (state, motor activity) systems in response to the environment. Preterm infants show decreased organizational abilities.

Organomegaly: Enlargement of one or more internal organs.

Ortolani maneuver: A procedure for evaluating hip stability in the newborn. After flexing the infant's knee and hip, grasp the thigh and first abduct with a lifting motion and then adduct the leg. If a clunk is felt as the femoral head passes over the acetabulum, the infant may have congenital hip dysplasia.

Otoscope: A device used to inspect the ears. Due to the presence of vernix in the neonate's ear canal, the device is normally not used in newborn examinations.

Outer canthal distance: The measurement between the outer canthi of the two eyes.

Pallor: Paleness of the skin in the newborn may indicate compromised cardiac status. The paleness may be due to vasoconstriction and to shunting of blood away from the skin to vital organs or anemia.

Palpation: A physical assessment technique involving application of pressure to the skin with the fingertips or part of the palm to assess the condition of underlying body parts.

Palpebral fissure: The eye opening.

Papule: An elevated palpable lesion, solid and circumscribed, less than 1 cm in diameter.

Patch: A discolored, flat, nonpalpable spot (a macule) greater than 1 cm in diameter.

Patent ductus arteriosis (PDA): A cardiac abnormality marked by failure of the ductus arteriosis to close after birth. In a left to right shunt blood flows from the aorta to the pulmonary artery, resulting in recirculation of arterial blood through the lungs.

Patent urachus: Persistence of an embryological communication between the urinary bladder and the umbilicus, with passage of urine through the umbilicus.

Percussion, direct: A physical assessment technique involving striking the body surface sharply and listening to the sound produced, to determine the condition of an underlying body part. In *indirect (mediate)* percussion, the examiner places the middle finger of the left hand on the area to be assessed and then strikes the finger with the middle finger of the other hand. Although not generally employed in examination of the abdomen, percussion can distinguish areas of tympanic (resonant or bell-like) sound from areas of dull sound. Tympanic sounds are present over the organs that contain air; increased tympany suggests abnormal amounts of air. Dull sounds are percussed over the liver, spleen, and bladder. Extended areas of dullness suggest organ enlargement; dullness in unusual areas may indicate masses. Shifting dullness is heard with ascites. It is of limited value in examination of the neonate's chest due to its small size, but can be useful in distinguishing between air, fluid, and solid tissue in some situations. Changes in resonance indicate changes in the consistency of the underlying tissue.

Perfusion, peripheral: Cardiac perfusion to the skin.

Perinatal history: Record of occurrences in the life of the mother, the fetus, and the newborn.

Perinatal period: Definitions of the length of the perinatal period vary; it extends from about week 20 or 28 of gestation until one week to one month after birth.

Perineum: Area between the scrotum and anus in the male and the vulva and anus in the female. It should be smooth in newborns. Dimpling suggests genetic anomalies or fistulas.

Periodic breathing: A series of respirations followed by a pause of up to 20 seconds.

Periosteum: Fibrous membrane covering the bones.

PERL: A notation standing for "pupils equal and reactive to light."

Petechia (plural: petechiae): A pinpoint-sized hemorrhagic spot on the skin.

Phenotype: Genetically and environmentally determined physical, biochemical, and physiological characteristics of an individual or group.

Phimosis: An irretractable foreskin. It may not be diagnosed until the infant reaches three months of age.

Pigeon chest: An abnormality of the bony structure of the chest in which the sternum protrudes. It is seen in infants with Marfan syndrome and rickets.

Pinna: The part of the ear that projects from the head. Formation, amount of cartilage present, and recoil when folded and released are considered indicators of gestational age.

Pit, ear: A slight depression anterior to the tragus. It may lead to a congenital preauricular sinus or fistula. Ear pits may be familial or associated with other anomalies.

Plagiocephaly: Asymmetrical skull shape caused by craniosynostosis (premature fusion) of the sutures on one side of the skull.

Plantar flexion: Flexing the foot toward the planter surface.

Plantar surface: The sole of the foot. Creases appear on the plantar surface of the foot between 28 and 30 weeks gestation and cover the surface at or near term. Therefore, plantar surface creasing is one indicator of gestational age.

Plaque: A fusion or coalescence of several papules (solid, circumscribed, elevated palpable lesions less than 1 cm in diameter).

Plethora: Ruddy appearance of the skin in a newborn. Plethora may indicate a high level of red cells to blood volume.

Pleural cavities: Two potential spaces (left and right) within the chest cavity enclosed by a serous membrane called the **pleura.** A portion of the pleura called the **parietal pleura** lines the walls of the thoracic cavity; the portion called the **visceral pleura** envelops the lungs.

Pneumothorax: Accumulation of air or gas in the pleural space.

Polycythemia: A condition in which the infant's central hematocrit is greater than 65. A polycythemic infant is pink at rest but plethoric to purplish when crying. The ruddy coloring can sometimes be mistaken for cyanosis (because the unsaturated hemoglobin in the blood of the infant may mask the saturated hemoglobin, making the infant appear purplish).

Polydactyly: A congenital anomaly marked by one or more extra digits on the hands or feet. There appears to be a familial tendency to polydactyly, and it is more common in African-American infants than in those of other races. The extra digit may be only a skin tag or a floppy appendage or it may appear normal.

Popliteal angle: The angle between the lower leg and the thigh posterior to the knee. The popliteal angle decreases with advancing gestational age.

Positional deformity: A flexible deformity of an extremity with no bony abnormality involved. It is caused by intrauterine positioning and generally corrects without treatment.

Postterm: An infant born at 42 or more weeks gestation.

Precordium: The area of the anterior chest over the heart. In the full-term newborn after the first few hours of life, the precordium should be quiet; a bounding precordium is characteristic of left-to-right shunt lesions (PDA or ventricular septal defect). In premature infants, the precordium is more active due to decreased subcutaneous tissue.

Preterm: An infant born at less than 38 weeks gestation.

Priapism: Constant erection of the penis, an abnormal finding that may indicate a spinal cord lesion.

Pronation: The turning of the body or a body part face down; as the hand so that the palm is facing down.

Prone: Positioned face down.

Proptosis: Abnormal protrusion or bulging of the eyeball. Also called *exophthalmos.*

Prune belly syndrome: A rare congenital deficiency of the abdominal muscles marked by a protruding, thin-walled abdomen covered with wrinkled skin. It occurs more frequently in males and is associated with renal and urinary tract abnormalities.

Pseudohermaphroditism: A condition in which the gonads are of one sex but one or more morphologic criteria are of the opposite sex. In **female pseudohermaphroditism,** the infant is genetically and gonadally female, with partial masculinization. In **male pseudohermaphroditism,** the infant is genetically and gonadally male, with the presence of some female characteristics.

Pseudostrabismus: The appearance of strabismus (crossed eyes) due to a flat nasal bridge or the presence of epicanthal folds.

Ptosis: Paralytic drooping of the eyelid in which the upper lid droops when the eyes are fully open.

Pulse deficit: A difference between the heart rate counted by a peripheral pulse and that counted by auscultation. A pulse deficit is frequently seen with ectopic rhythms.

Pulse pressure: The difference between the systolic and the diastolic blood pressure. For term infants, the average difference is 25–30 mmHg; for premature infants, it is 15–25 mmHg. Wide pulse pressures can indicate large aortic runoff, as in PDA. Narrow pulse pressures are seen with peripheral vasoconstriction, heart failure, and low cardiac output.

Pupillary reflex: Contraction of the pupil when the eye is exposed to bright light.

Pustule: An elevation of the skin filled with cloudy or purulent fluid.

Quiet alert state: A wakeful state of infant consciousness characterized by interaction with the environment. The infant focuses on stimuli and presents an alert appearance, especially in the eyes. Motor activity is minimal. In this state, preterm infants may show hyperalertness (inability to terminate fixation on a stimulus).

Rachitic rosary: In a newborn with rickets, a series of small lumps can be felt along the edge of the sternum during palpation. The lumps are enlarged costal cartilages.

Radiation: The transmission of a body sound to another location.

Rales: See **Crackles.**

Ranula: A cystic tumor, presenting as a translucent or bluish swelling beneath the tongue, caused by obstruction of a salivary duct or a mucous gland.

Recoil, arm or leg: Test used to evaluate phasic muscle tone. The infant's arm or leg is gently extended. In premature infants of 28 or fewer weeks gestation, minimal resistance is normal. Resistance increases with gestational age.

Red retinal reflex: Reflection of a clear red color from the retina when a bright light is direct-

ed at the newborn's lens. The reflex is a pale color in dark-skinned infants.

Reflex, anocutaneous: An autonomic nervous system reflex. *Stimulus:* Cutaneous stimulation of the perianal skin. *Normal response:* Contraction of the external sphincter. Also called *anal wink.*

Reflex, Babinski: A developmental reflex. *Stimulus:* Stroke the sole of the infant's foot. *Positive response:* Extension of the great toe and spreading of the other toes.

Reflex, biceps: A motor reflex that is most active during the first two days after birth and when the newborn is alert. *Stimulus:* Place thumb over insertion of infant's biceps tendon, flex newborn's arm, and tap thumb with reflex hammer. *Normal response:* Infant flexes biceps muscle.

Reflex, corneal: A peripheral sensory reflex. *Stimulus:* Blow air on the infant's eye or touch the cornea gently with a piece of cotton. *Normal response:* The infant blinks.

Reflex, Moro: A developmental reflex that is normally completely present at birth only in term neonates. This reflex may be elicited by sudden movement of surface infant is on, loud noise, or causing the head to drop approximately 30°. *Stimulus:* Hold infant supine, supporting head a few centimeters above bed, withdraw supporting hand and allow the infant to "fall back" to it. *Normal response:* As infant's head falls, infant extends and abducts arms and opens hands; then adducts and partially flexes arms, and makes fists. Infants greater than 32 weeks gestation may cry out. Premature infants do not complete the reflex by adducting and flexing the extremities, nor do they cry. Complete lack of the reflex is abnormal; asymmetric response may indicate a localized neurologic defect (such as a brachial plexus injury).

Reflex, palmar grasp: A developmental reflex that is normally present at birth in both term and preterm infants. *Stimulus:* Stroke infant's palm with a finger. *Normal response:* Infant grasps finger and tightens grasp on attempt to withdraw finger.

Reflex, patellar (knee jerk): A motor reflex that is most active during the first two days after birth and when the newborn is alert. *Stimulus:* Tap infant's patellar tendon just below kneecap, with newborn's knee flexed and supported. *Normal response:* Infant extends knee and contracts quadriceps.

Reflex, rooting: A developmental reflex that is normally present at birth in both term and preterm infants. *Stimulus:* Stroke infant's cheek and corner of mouth. *Normal response:* Infant turns head toward stimulus and opens mouth.

Reflex, startle: Resembles Moro reflex but is more limited. See **Reflex, Moro.**

Reflex, stepping: A developmental reflex that becomes more active 72 hours after birth. *Stimulus:* Hold infant upright with soles of feet touching a flat surface. *Normal response:* Alternate stepping movements.

Reflex, sucking: A developmental reflex that is normally present at birth in both term and preterm infants. (It is weaker in preterm neonates.) *Stimulus:* Touch infant's lips. *Normal response:* Infant opens mouth and makes sucking movements.

Reflex, tonic neck: A developmental reflex that is normally present at birth only in term neonates. *Stimulus:* With infant supine, turn infant's head to one side. *Normal response:* Extension of upper extremity on side to which head is turned and flexion of upper extremity on opposite side. Lack of response or a marked response with minimal head turning is abnormal. Also called *fencing position.*

Reflex, truncal incurvation (Galant): A developmental reflex. *Stimulus:* Suspend infant ventrally, supporting anterior chest wall in palm of hand. Apply firm pressure parallel to spine in thoracic area with thumb or cotton swab. *Positive response:* Infant flexes pelvis toward side of stimulus.

Reflexes, developmental: Reflexes that do not require functional brain above the diencephalon. Those present in most newborns include the sucking, rooting, palmar grasp, tonic neck, Moro, stepping, truncal incurvation, and Babinski reflexes. Also called *primary* or *primitive* reflexes.

Respiratory distress syndrome (RDS): A condition of the newborn most often occurring in premature infants, but may be seen at term, marked by breathing difficulties and cyanosis and having as it's origin a deficiency of surfactant and structural immaturity.

Retinoblastoma: A retinal tumor. Lack of a red reflex in a newborn could indicate its presence.

Retraction: A drawing in of the chest during respiration. Immediately after birth, substernal or intercostal retractions are common; if they persist, they may indicate respiratory problems. Suprasternal retraction, especially with gasping or stridor, may indicate obstruction of the upper airway.

Rhonchi: Adventitious breath sounds lower in pitch and more musical than crackles. Although seldom heard in the neonate, they may be auscultated if secretions or aspirated foreign matter is present in the large airways.

Rotation, neck: Turning of the face to the side.

Rub: Adventitious breath sound resembling the rubbing of a finger over a cupped hand held near the ear. Rubs are often heard in newborns during mechanical ventilation; they are also associated with inflammation of the pleura.

Ruga (plural: rugae): A ridge, wrinkle, or fold. Rugae first appear on the front of the scrotal sac at about 36 weeks gestation, covering the sac by 40 weeks. In the term male infant, the scrotum is fully rugated; the preterm male has few or no rugae.

Scale: Exfoliation of dead or dying bits of skin. Scale can also result from excess keratin production.

Scaphocephaly: Long, narrow head shape caused by craniosynostosis (premature fusion) of the sagittal suture, limiting lateral growth of the skull.

Scapula: One of the pair of triangular bones at the back of the shoulder articulating with a clavicle. Commonly called the *shoulder blade.*

Scarf sign: A test for newborn gestational age involving gently pulling the arm of a supine infant across the chest and around the neck as far as possible posteriorly. The older the infant, the greater the resistance to this maneuver.

Sclera: The white portion of the eyeball.

Sclera, blue: Unusual blue coloring of the white portion of the eyeball. It is seen with a variation of osteogenesis imperfecta and certain other abnormalities.

Scoliosis: A congenital deformity of the spine in which vertebrae fail to form and/or segment. It is embryonic in origin. If undetected, it can affect neurologic function as well as appearance. Congenital scoliosis may be associated with genitourinary tract anomalies, Klippel-Feil syndrome, and Sprengel deformity.

Seizure: An abnormal series of movements (neurologic in origin) characterized by alternate muscular contraction and relaxation of unequal amplitude. The movements are less rapid than those seen in jitteriness. They do not occur in response to stimuli and cannot be stopped by flexing and holding the affected limb; may be accompanied by abnormal eye movements. See also **Jitteriness.**

Sensory threshold: An infant's level of tolerance for stimuli. Infants who exceed their sensory thresholds (are overstimulated) exhibit signs and symptoms of stress. Low sensory thresholds are generally seen in preterm infants and in infants with neurological impairment.

Sequence: A single defect as the cause for other anomalies (the "snowball" effect).

Simian crease: A single transverse palmar crease. It may be found in normal newborns, but when seen with short fingers, an incurved little finger, and a low-set thumb, it is suggestive of Down syndrome.

Sinus, dermal: A posterior neural tube defect occurring along the midline of the back, frequently in the lumbar region. It may present as a dimple surrounded by tufts of hair or lipomas or may terminate in subcutaneous tissue, a cyst, or a fibrous band. It may also extend into the spinal cord and be associated with spina bifida.

Sinus, preauricular: An abnormal channel located in front of the pinna (auricle) of the ear. If it communicates with the internal ear or the brain, chronic infection is likely.

Skin tag: A small skin outgrowth. Those occurring anterior to the tragus are thought to be embryological remnants of the first branchial arch. Skin tags may be familial or associated with other anomalies.

Small for gestational age (SGA): An infant whose weight falls below the tenth percentile for gestational age when plotted on a standard growth chart.

Spermatocele: A retention cyst, palpable as a mass on the epididymis.

Spina bifida: The mildest form of posterior neural tube defect, with the malformation arising from lack of or incomplete closure of the posterior portion of the vertebrae. The meninges and spinal cord are normal. The defect is covered with skin (which may be dimpled), and it is most common in the lower lumbar and lumbosacral area. See also **Sinus, dermal.**

Split: Term describing a heart sound in which two components can be heard. The "splitting" is caused by the asynchronous closure of the two valves that create the sound. The rapid newborn heart rate makes splitting difficult to auscultate. In newborns splitting is usually not heard in S1. S2 is generally single at birth but is split in two-thirds of infants by 16 hours of age and in four-fifths by 48 hours of age. Wide splitting of S2 is abnormal, however.

Sprengel deformity: A congenital anomaly of the shoulder girdle, marked by some hypoplasia and malrotation of the scapula, which gives it an elevated appearance. Shoulder abduction and flexion are limited. This deformity is more often unilateral, but can be bilateral. It is often associated with congenital spinal anomalies, Klippel-Feil syndrome, and renal anomalies.

State (of consciousness): One of six levels of consciousness seen in infants. There are two sleep states *(deep* and *light),* one transitional state *(drowsiness),* and three awake states *(quiet alert, active alert,* and *crying).* Behavioral assessment evaluates the newborn's ability to control his state, move smoothly from one state to another, and maintain alertness when in an awake state. Term infants may use changes in state to control environmental input.

Stenosis, anal: Constriction or obstruction of the anorectal canal. Signs include passage of small, thin stools, progressive abdominal distention, and finally vomiting.

Stenosis, pyloric: Obstruction of the pyloric orifice of the stomach, usually presenting about 3 weeks of age, rarely before the fourth or fifth day of life. If present, it is palpable immediately after feeding or vomiting as an ovoid mass between the umbilicus and the right lower costal margin. Signs of pyloric stenosis (upper quadrant distention and visible peristalsis) in the absence of a palpable

mass may indicate duodenal or jejunal obstruction in the neonate.

Sternocleidomastoid muscle: The muscle that flexes the vertebral column and rotates the head.

Stethoscope: An acoustical device used to auscultate (listen to) sounds within the body. In the neonate, these include heart, lung, venous, arterial, and intestinal sounds. A neonatal stethoscope generally has a double head composed of a flat diaphragm (for auscultating high-frequency sounds) and a bell (for auscultating low-frequency sounds). It does not magnify sound but simply eliminates environmental noise.

Strabismus: The appearance of crossed eyes in the newborn due to muscular incoordination.

Streeter dysplasia: See **Congenital constricting bands.**

Stridor: A high-pitched hoarse adventitious breath sound heard during inspiration or expiration at the larynx or upper airways. In the newborn, stridor indicates partial obstruction of the airway. It may also be heard in infants with edema of the upper airway after extubation.

Structural deformity: A fixed (or rigid) deformity involving bony abnormalities. It generally requires surgical intervention.

Subcutaneous tissue: Layer of fatty tissue underlying the dermis, which insulates the body, protects the internal organs, and stores calories.

Sucking blister: Intact or ruptured vesicle or bulla sometimes seen on the lips, fingers, or hands of the newborn. The cause is vigorous sucking, *in utero* or after birth.

Sunset sign: Eyelid retraction and a downward gaze in which the sclera is visible above the iris. The sign is often seen in infants with hydrocephalus.

Supination: Turning of the body or a body part face up; as of the hand so that the palm is facing up.

Supine: Positioned face up.

Suprasternal notch: An indentation on the upper border of the sternum.

Suture: A fibrous joint between bones of the skull. The **metopic suture** extends midline down the forehead between the two frontal bones and intersects with the **coronal suture,** which separates the frontal and parietal bones. The **sagittal suture** extends midline between the two parietal bones to the back of the head, where it intersects with the **lambdoidal suture,** which separates the parietal and occipital bones. The **squamosal suture** extends above the ear and separates the temporal from the parietal bone.

Sutures, overriding: Head molding may cause the edge of the bone on one side of a suture to feel as if it is on top of (overriding) the edge of the opposite bone. Overriding is commonly seen in the lambdoidal suture, with the parietal bone on top of the occipital. Overriding sutures must be differentiated from craniosynostosis (premature fusion of a suture).

Symmetrically growth retarded: An infant who has not grown at the expected rate—that is, who ranks at less than the tenth percentile for gestational age on standard growth charts—for *all three* growth parameters: weight, length, and occipital-frontal head circumference.

Symphysis, pubic: Midline cartilaginous joint connecting the pubic bones.

Syndactyly: Congenital webbing of the fingers and toes, frequently familial in origin. The more severe the webbing, the greater the likelihood of underlying bony abnormalities.

Syndrome: A recognizable pattern of anomalies, often of more than one system, that is historically based and leads to a diagnosis.

Systole: The period of contraction of the heart, particularly of the ventricles.

Tachycardia, sinus: A heart rate greater than 180–200 beats per minute in the newborn. Simple tachycardia, originating in the sinus node of the heart, normally occurs in response to a stimulus that increases demand on the heart. When the stimulus is removed, the rate gradually returns to normal.

Tachycardia, supraventricular (SVT): A heart rate greater than 200–300 beats per minute in the newborn. Without immediate intervention, it can lead to cardiovascular collapse.

Tachypnea: Excessively rapid and shallow respirations. In the neonate, persistent respirations of greater than 60 per minute may indicate TTN, RDS, meconium aspiration, pneumonia, hyperthermia, or pain.

Tap: A sharp, well-localized point of maximum cardiac impulse, usually associated with pressure overload or hypertrophy.

Temperament: The way in which an infant interacts with the environment. S. Chess and A. Thomas identify three categories of temperament: easy, difficult, and slow-to-warm.

Teratogenic agent: An extrinsic factor—either environmental or maternal—that causes abnormalities in fetal development. Examples include infection, metabolic disorders, and exposure to drugs or alcohol, heavy metals, many chemicals, and radiation.

Term: An infant born between the beginning of week 38 and the end of week 41 of gestation.

Testicular torsion: See **Neonatal torsion of the testis**.

Thorax: The chest. The thoracic cavity is bounded by the sternum, 12 thoracic vertebrae, 12 pair of ribs, and the diaphragm.

Thrill: A low-frequency, palpable murmur that resembles holding one's hand on a purring cat. Thrills are uncommon in the newborn. If present, their location can aid in identification of cardiac problems.

Thrush: An oral fungal infection characterized by adherent white patches on the tongue and mucous membranes and caused by *Candida albicans.*

Thyroglossal duct cyst: A cyst on the embryological duct between the thyroid and the back of the tongue.

Torticollis: An anomaly affecting the sternocleidomastoid muscle, more often on the right side. It is not usually seen until about two weeks of age, when it can be palpated as a firm, immobile mass 1–2 cm in diameter in the midportion of the muscle. Undetected, it produces facial asymmetry and limited neck rotation.

Traction response (pull-to-sit maneuver): Tests the ability of the infant's muscles to resist the pull of gravity. When the normal term infant's hands are grasped and he is slowly pulled from a supine to a sitting position, the infant contracts the shoulder and arm muscles, and then flexes the neck, with the head lagging behind the body only minimally. The infant also flexes the elbows, knees, and ankles. When the infant reaches the sitting position, the head remains erect briefly before falling forward. Neck flexion is not seen in infants of less than 33 weeks gestation.

Transient tachypnea of the newborn (TTN): A condition of the newborn marked by excessively rapid respirations. The underlying pathology is usually retained fetal lung fluid; tachypnea subsides as fluid is absorbed or expelled.

Transillumination: A physical assessment technique involving shining light through body tissues. The area being examined is placed between the light and the observer. If a pneumothorax is suspected in the neonate, transillumination can allow comparison of the left, right, upper, and lower aspects of the chest and illuminate air pockets with a lantern-like glow. If the infant's head is an unusual size or shape or if the neurologic examination is abnormal, transillumination can help identify the reason. It is useful for identification of abnormal findings in the scrotum. Masses filled with clear fluid appear translucent with illumination; solid or blood-filled masses do not transilluminate.

Trisomy: A form of chromosomal aneuploidy characterized by the presence of 47 chromosomes. It is generally caused by nondisjunction (failure of the egg or sperm to divide the genetic material equally). The most common autosomal trisomies are of chromosome 21 (Down syndrome), chromosome 18, and chromosome 13.

Urethral meatus: Opening of the urethra on the body surface, located directly below the clitoris in female infants and at the center of the end of the penile shaft in males. Anterior displacement of the meatus at or on an enlarged clitoris suggests pseudohermaphroditism in a female infant. Hypospadias and epispadias are placement abnormalities seen in male infants.

Uvula, bifid: A split uvula. It may be associated with other congenital anomalies.

Valgus: Bent outward or twisted away from the midline of the body.

Varicocele: Abnormal dilation of the spermatic cord veins in the scrotum. The mass feels like a bag of worms, is seen more often on the left side, and suggests obstruction above the scrotal sac.

Varus: Turned inward.

Vernix caseosa: A greasy white or yellow material, composed of sebaceous gland secretions and exfoliated skin cells, that covers the newborn infant's skin. Vernix develops during the third trimester of intrauterine growth, gradually decreasing in amount as the fetus approaches 40 weeks gestation. Because vernix may be present in the newborn's auditory canal, otoscopic examination is not done immediately after birth.

Very low birth weight: An infant who weighs less than 1,500 gm at birth.

Vesicle: An elevation of the skin filled with serous fluid and less than 1 cm in diameter.

Vesicular breath sounds: Normally found over the entire chest, except over the manubrium and the trachea. During expiration, vesicular sounds are soft, short, and low-pitched; during inspiration, they are louder, longer, and higher pitched.

Werdnig-Hoffmann disease: A disorder of the lower motor neurons, causing flaccid weakness of the extremities as well as tongue fasciculation.

Wheal: A reddened, solid elevation of the skin caused by a collection of fluid in the dermis.

Wheezes: Adventitious breath sounds, usually louder on expiration than on inspiration, that are higher in pitch than rhonchi. They are usually heard only in newborns with BPD.

Whorl, hair: Spiral hair growth pattern commonly seen in the posterior parietal region of the newborn's scalp. Absence of or abnormal location of a whorl can indicate abnormal brain growth.

Witch's milk: Milky secretions engorging the breasts of some infants at birth, due to the influence of maternal estrogen. The secretions generally disappear in one to two weeks, and the enlargement subsides over several months.

Xiphoid process: Sword-shaped cartilaginous projection at the end of the sternum.

Glossary compiled and verified using the following sources:

- *Dorland's Medical Dictionary*, 26th ed. 1981. Philadelphia, Pennsylvania: WB Saunders.
- *Stedman's Medical Dictionary*, 25th ed. 1990. Baltimore, Maryland: Williams & Wilkins.
- *Mosby's Medical, Nursing and Allied Health Dictionary*, 3rd ed. 1990. St. Louis, Missouri: Mosby-Year Book.
- Kenner C, Brueggemeyer A, and Gunderson LP, eds. 1993. *Comprehensive Neonatal Nursing: A Physiologic Perspective.* Philadelphia, Pennsylvania: WB Saunders.
- Polin RA, and Fox WW, eds. 1992. *Fetal and Neonatal Physiology,* vols. 1 and 2. Philadelphia, Pennsylvania: WB Saunders.
- Taeusch HW, Ballard RA, and Avery ME, eds. 1991. *Schaffer and Avery's Diseases of the Newborn,* 6th ed. Philadelphia, Pennsylvania: WB Saunders.
- Seeley RR, Stephens TD, and Tate P, eds. 1992. *Anatomy and Physiology,* 2nd ed. St. Louis, Missouri: Mosby-Year Book.
- Blackburn ST, and Loper DL, eds. 1992. *Maternal, Fetal, and Neonatal Physiology: A Clinical Perspective.* Philadelphia, Pennsylvania: WB Saunders.
- *Miller-Keane Encyclopedia and Dictionary of Medicine, Nursing, and Allied Health,* 5th ed. 1992. Philadelphia, Pennsylvania: WB Saunders.

Index

caput succedaneum, 57
cephalhematoma, 57, 57f
to clavicles, 122
to eyes, 60
facial signs of, 58
forcep marks, 46, 46f
genital, 106
to humerus, 122
intraventricular hemorrhage and, 157
to legs, 127
liver or spleen rupture and, 99
musculoskeletal problems and, 118
to neck, 128–129
neurologic assessment and, 138, 139
to nose, 63f
respiratory rate and, 69
to scalp, 57, 57f
spinal cord injury with, 151–152
subarachnoid hemorrhage and, 155
subdural hemorrhage and, 155, 156
See also Hypoxic-ischemic encephalopathy
Bladder. *See* Urinary bladder
Blink reflex, 147t
Blisters, sucking, 46, 47f, 215
Blood gases, cord, 190t, 192
Blood group, antepartum testing, 14t
Blood group incompatibilities, hepatomegaly
and, 99
Blood pressure, 88–90, 88f, 89f
coarctation of the aorta and, 100
extremity, indications for assessing, 2
monitoring methods, 88–90
normal values, 89f, 90
pulse pressure, 212
Blood pressure cuff size, 88, 88f
Blood testing
antepartum testing intervals, 14t
intrapartal, 190t, 192
"Blueberry muffin" spots, 50
Body position. *See* Posture
Bones
absence of, 130, 131f, 173t
cranial, 54, 55f, 195
elasticity of, 117
hypertrophy of, in Klippel-Trenaunay-
Weber syndrome, 49
Botulism, infantile, 144
Bounding pulses, 82
Bowel sounds, 98
defined, 195–196
in lung auscultation, 74
BP. *See* Blood pressure
BPD. *See* Bronchopulmonary dysplasia
Brachial palsy, 130, 130f
defined, 196
neurologic assessment and, 139, 144
perinatal history and, 118
signs of, 122
Brachial pulse, 80f, 81
Brachycephaly, 56, 56f, 196
Bradycardia
defined, 196
fetal, monitoring for, 191
with intraventricular hemorrhage, 157
periodic breathing and, 70
sinus, 83–84
subdural hemorrhage and, 156

Bradypnea, defined, 69, 196
Brain anatomy, intracranial hemorrhage and,
155f, 156f
Brain atrophy, maternal drug use and, 151t
Branchial cleft cyst, 65, 176t
Branchial sinus, 65, 196
Brazelton, T. B.
behavioral assessment scale by, 160
cost of attention, 164
Breasts
accessory nipples, 173t, 208
enlarged, 70–71
gestational age criteria, 23t, 26f, 30, 32f–33f
palpation of, 74
Breathing problems
nose malformations and, 62
periodic breathing, 70, 210
See also Respiration assessment; Respiratory
distress
Breath sounds, 71–74, 72f, 73t, 74t
mechanical ventilation and, 75, 76
Breech delivery
congenital hip dysplasia and, 130
craniotabes and, 57
genital bruising with, 106, 106f, 107
head shape and, 54, 183t
musculoskeletal disorders and, 118
positional deformities from, 120, 121f
ruptured spleen and, 99
spinal cord injury with, 151–152
Bronchial breath sounds, 72, 73t, 196
Bronchopulmonary dysplasia (BPD)
breath sounds with, 73, 74t
defined, 196
Bronchovesicular breath sounds, 72, 73t, 196
Brow presentation, facial trauma from, 58
Bruising
as birth trauma sign, 138, 47, 57, 58
forcep marks, 46, 46f, 58
hyperpigmented macules vs, 44–45
See also specific parts of body
Bruits
in abdominal vessels, 98
defined, 196
in skull, 55, 141–142
Brushfield spots, 62, 196
Bulla, defined, 41, 196
Buttocks
hyperpigmented macules on, 44, 44f
pigmented nevus on, 45
tuberous sclerosis lesions on, 46

C

Café au lait spots, 40, 45, 45f, 138, 176t
defined, 196–197
Caffeine, maternal use of, 85
Calcaneovalgus, 183t
Calcium channel blockers, maternal use of, 12t
Candida albicans, 49
Candida diaper dermatitis, 49, 197
Candidiasis (thrush), 49, 64, 217
Canthus, defined, 197
inner canthal distance, 204
outer canthal distance, 209
Capillary filling time, 80, 197

Capurro, H. et al, gestational age criteria by,
22
Caput, defined, 197
Caput succedaneum, 57, 197
Carbamazepine, maternal use of, 180t
Cardiac abnormalities
genitourinary anomalies and, 104
maternal anticonvulsants and, 9
Cardiac arrhythmia, 84–85
Cardiac failure
respiratory quality with, 69
skull ausculation and, 55
Cardiac lesions, respiratory quality with, 69
Cardiac obstruction, weak or absent pulses
with, 82
Cardiac output
apical impulse and, 82
supraventricular tachycardia and, 84
Cardiac rhythm and regularity, 84–85
Cardiac volume overload, heaves with, 83
Cardiogenic shock, mottling of skin with, 80
Cardiomyopathy
S4 heart sound with, 86
syndromes associated with, 79t
Cardiopulmonary disorders, maternal, 16t
Cardiovascular assessment, 77–90
auscultation, 77, 83–88, 83f
blood pressure, 2, 88–90, 88f, 89f, 100, 212
breathing patterns, 80
history taking, 77–78
liver palpation as part of, 88
murmurs and. *See* Murmurs
observation, 2t, 77, 78–80, 82–83
peripheral pulses, 80f, 81–82, 81f
point of maximal impulse (PMI), 3, 82–83,
83f
prune belly syndrome and, 109
skin and mucous membranes, 79–80
timing of, 77
Cardiovascular drugs, maternal use of, 12t
Carpenter syndrome, congenital heart defects
with, 79t
Cataracts, congenital, 61–62, 62f, 173t, 174f
Catheter irritation, premature ventricular beats
and, 85
Catheter method of BP measurement, 90
Caucasian infants
congenital hip dysplasia and, 130–131
hyperpigmented macules in, 44
"normal" findings and, 175
polydactyly and, 135
transient neonatal pustular melanosis in, 45
Caudal regression syndrome, voiding
dysfunctions and, 112
Caudocephalad, defined, 197
Cavernous hemangioma, 48–49, 48f, 192, 203
Central cyanosis
defined, 79, 199
implications of, 5, 80
Central nervous system problems
abdominal movement and, 93
apnea and, 70
bladder distention and, 100
bradypnea with, 69
hypotonia and, 143
maternal drug use and, 151, 151t
port wine facial hemangiomas and, 138–139

Cephalhematoma, 57, 57f, 138, 141, 197
Cephalosporins, maternal use of, 12t
Cerebellar abnormalities, 151t
Cerebral infarction, maternal cocaine use and, 151t
Cerebral injury
  facial weakness and, 149t
  tone abnormalities and, 144
Cerebral irritation, ankle clonus and, 142
Cerebral palsy, perinatal history and, 118
Cerebrohepatorenal syndrome, congenital heart defects with, 79t
Cervical cytology, antepartum testing, 14t
Cesarean delivery
  head shape and, 54
  respiratory rate and, 69
CHARGE association, congenital heart defects with, 79t
CHD. *See* Congenital heart disease; Congenital hip dysplasia
Chest assessment, 67
  anomalies, 173t, 176t
  auscultation, 71–74, 72f, 73t, 74t
  inspection, 68–71, 70t, 71f, 82–83, 82f
  landmarks and structure, 67–68, 68f
  mechanical ventilation and, 75–76, 75t
  palpation, 74–75
  percussion, 74
  transillumination, 75
Chest circumference, 70, 119
Chief complaint, 14
Chin, anomalies of, 173t
Chlamydia, maternal, 16t
Chlordiazepoxide, maternal use of, 180t
Chlorpropamide, maternal use of, 180t
Choanal atresia, bilateral, 63, 173t, 195
Cholesterol-reducing drugs, maternal use of, 181t
Chordee, 110f, 111, 111f, 173t, 197
Chorioamnionitis, 16t
Chorionic villus sampling, 14t, 187
Chromosomal aneuploidy, 177–179, 197
Chromosomal disorders, 177f
  antepartum tests for, 187, 189–190
  cri du chat syndrome, 139, 198–199
  cutis aplasia and, 50
  cutis marmorata and, 42
  ear defects with, 59f, 60
  eye anomalies with, 61
  eye signs of, 61, 62
  hypoplasia and, 110–111
  microcephaly and, 141
  mouth abnormalities with, 63
  nail defects with, 51
  nose signs of, 63
  omphalocele and, 95
  symmetrical growth retardation and, 37
  See also Congenital anomalies; Genetic disorders; specific disorders
Circumcision, penile malformations and, 112
Circumference. *See* Chest circumference; Occipital-frontal head circumference
Circumoral cyanosis, 41–42, 62, 79, 199
Clavicles, 67, 68f
  cleidocranial dysostosis, 129–130, 129f
  defined, 197
  inspection of, 122

palpation of, 65, 74, 122
Cleaners, as teratogens, 182t
Cleft lip/palate, 63, 173t, 176t
  defined, 197
  with Trisomy 13, 179f
Cleidocranial dysostosis, 129–130, 129f, 197
Clinical expertise, development of, 1
Clinodactyly, 173t, 176t
Clitoris, 107f
  gender ambiguity and, 115
  gestational age criteria, 26f, 31, 108
  hypertrophy of, 204
Clomiphene, maternal use of, 180t
Clonazepam, maternal use of, 180t
Clonus
  ankle, 142
  defined, 142, 197
Clubfoot (Talipes equinovarus), 128, 132f, 133–134, 173t, 183t
  congenital hip dysplasia and, 131
  defined, 197
Coagulation abnormalities, intraventricular hemorrhage and, 157
Coarctation of the aorta
  femoral pulses and, 81–82, 100
  murmurs with, 88
  syndromes associated with, 79t, 80
Cocaine, maternal use of, 13t, 151t, 180t
Codeine, maternal use of, 12t
Coloboma, 60–61, 62, 173t, 176t, 197
Color of skin, 2t, 5, 23t, 26f, 30, 30f, 41–43
  in cardiovascular exam, 79, 80
  respiratory status and, 68
Coma, with tentorial laceration, 156
Conception/ovulation date, gestational age and, 22t
Congenital anomalies
  antepartum testing for, 187–191
  deformations, 175, 183, 183t, 185f, 199
  disruptions, 175, 184, 184f, 185f, 200
  of eyes, 61–62
  facial signs of, 58–59
  of feet, 129
  genitourinary anomalies and, 103–104
  hair signs of, 57–58
  of lower extremities, 130–134, 131f–134f
  malformations, 175, 176–183, 184, 206
    positional deformities vs, 120
  mouth signs of, 63
  musculoskeletal, 123, 124, 128–134. *See also* specific anomalies
  nail defects, 51
  of spine, 123, 124, 124f, 128f, 129
  supernumerary nipples with, 71
  umbilical vessels and, 96
  of upper extremities, 129–130, 129f–131f
  See also Chromosomal disorders; Dysmorphogenesis; specific anomalies; specific parts of body
Congenital constricting bands (Streeter dysplasia), 133f, 134, 184, 184f, 198
Congenital heart disease (CHD)
  blood pressure and, 90
  defined, 198
  genitourinary anomalies and, 103–104
  history taking and, 77–78, 78t, 79t
  murmurs and, 86, 87

observation for, 78–79
  omphalocele and, 95
  premature atrial beats with, 85
  premature ventricular beats with, 85
Congenital heart disease, maternal, 16t, 77, 78
Congenital hip dysplasia, 118, 125, 127, 130–131, 198
Congenital infections, of skin, 49–50
Congestive heart failure
  liver palpation and, 99
  respiratory distress and, 80
  skull ausculation and, 55
  supraventricular tachycardia and, 84
Conjunctiva, 60f
Consanguinity, 17f, 18
Consciousness. *See* State
Consistency, importance of, 1
Consolability, 160, 161, 163f, 164, 167, 198
Consolidation, defined, 198
Constricting bands, congenital (Streeter dysplasia), 133f, 134, 184, 184f, 198
Continuous murmurs, 87, 88, 207
Contraction deformities of limbs, urogenital defects and, 103, 104f
Contraction stress test, 188–190
Coping ability, assessing preterm infant for, 160
Cord blood gases, 190t, 192
Cordocentesis, 192
Corneal reflex, 148, 212
Cornelia de Lange syndrome
  congenital heart defects with, 79t
  cutis marmorata and, 42
  eyebrow signs of, 61
Coronal suture, 54, 55f, 56, 216
Corticosteroids, maternal use of, 13t, 182t, 190
Costal cartilage, palpation of, 75
Costal margin, 68f, 98f
Cost of attention, 164, 198
Coumadin. *See* Warfarin
Crackles, 72–73, 74t, 198
Cranial bones, 54, 55f, 195
Cranial nerve I (olfactory nerve), 147
Cranial nerve II (optic nerve), 147, 148t
Cranial nerve III (oculomotor nerve), 147t, 148, 148f, 156
Cranial nerve IV (trochlear nerve), 147t, 148, 148f
Cranial nerve V (trigeminal nerve), 147t, 148
Cranial nerve VI (abducens nerve), 147t, 148, 148f
Cranial nerve VII (facial nerve), 147t, 148–149, 149t
Cranial nerve VIII (auditory nerve), 147t, 149
Cranial nerve IX (glossopharyngeal nerve), 147t, 149
Cranial nerve X (vagus nerve), 147t, 149
Cranial nerve XI (accessory nerve), 147t, 149
Cranial nerve XII (hypoglossal nerve), 147t, 149
Cranial nerve assessment, 147–149, 147t
Craniosynostosis, 56–57, 56f, 141, 173t, 183t, 198
Craniotabes, 57, 183t, 198
Cranium bifidum, 152
Creases, miliaria in, 43

Cremasteric reflex, defined, 198
Crepitus, palpating sternum for, 75
Crescendo systolic murmur, 87, 207
Cri du chat syndrome, 139, 198–199
Crossed extension reflex, 145f
Crouzon syndrome, craniosynostosis and, 56
Crust, defined, 41, 199
Crying
 assessing, 1, 63
 as avoidance behavior, 161, 165, 165t
 bulging fontanel and, 54
 cranial nerve dysfunction and, 149
 cyanosis and, 80
 defined, 199
 during exam, 5
 facial movements during, 59, 139, 149
 overstimulation and, 163f, 164, 165, 165t
 quality of, 139
 tremors with, 120
Cryptorchidism, 112–113, 199
Cubitus valgas, 176t
Cutis aplasia, 50–51, 50f, 57, 57f, 173t, 194
Cutis marmorata, 42, 199
Cyanosis, 68, 79–80
 central, 79, 80
  defined, 199
  implications of, 5, 80
 circumoral, 41–42, 62, 63
  defined, 79, 199
 peripheral. *See* Acrocyanosis
 polycythemia and, 42, 79
Cyclophosphamide, maternal use of, 12t, 180t
Cyst, defined, 41
Cystic fibrosis, maternal, 16t
Cystic hygroma, 64f, 65, 173t, 204
Cytomegalovirus, maternal, 16t, 182t

D

Danazol, maternal use of, 180t
Dandy-Walker syndrome, 141, 151t
Darwinian tubercle, 59f, 60, 199
Deep sleep state, 161, 199
Deep-tendon reflexes, 142, 151
Defects, polygenic, 177, 177f, 199
Defects, single-gene, 176–177
 defined, 199
 symmetrical growth retardation and, 37
Deformations, 175, 183, 183t
 defined, 199
 in malformation sequence, 185f
 positional deformities, 120, 211
 structural, defined, 215
Dehydration
 skin turgor and, 98
 sunken fontanel with, 54
Delivery
 intrapartal monitoring, 190t, 191–192
 timing of exam after, 4
Delivery history, 15
 head shape and, 54
 reviewing, 4
 skin assessment and, 40
 See also Birth trauma; Perinatal history
Demographic information, high-risk
  pregnancy factors, 11t
Depigmentation lesions, 176t

defined, 199
 tuberous sclerosis and, 139
Dermal sinus
 defined, 214
 in spina bifida, 152–153
Dermatoglyphics, 176t
Dermis, 40, 199
DES (diethylstilbestrol), 13t, 180t
Developmental reflexes, defined, 213
Diabetes mellitus, maternal
 antepartum testing with, 14t, 188, 190
 asymmetrical growth retardation and, 37
 congenital heart disease and, 77
 implications of, 4, 16t, 182t
Diaper dermatitis, Candida, 49, 197
Diaphragm, 67, 69
 paralysis of, 139
Diaphragmatic hernia
 auscultation and, 74
 CHD and, 79
 defined, 199
 embryonic development and, 171
 percussion with, 74
 respiratory quality with, 69
Diastasis recti, 95–96, 176t, 199–200
Diastole, defined, 200
Diazepam, maternal use of, 180t
Diethylstilbestrol (DES), 13t, 180t
Differential diagnosis, visual, 5–6
"Difficult" babies, identifying, 168
DiGeorge syndrome, congenital heart defects
  with, 79t
Digoxin, maternal use of, 12t
Dimples, spinal, sinuses vs, 152–153, 176t
Direct percussion, 4, 210
Dislocations
 of hip, 125–126
 of knee (genu recurvatum), 131f, 132
Disorganization, signs of, 164
Disruptions, 175, 184, 184f, 185f
 defined, 184, 200
 in malformation sequence, 185f
Distractibility, in temperament assessment,
  167
Distress, observations of, 2t
Disulfiram, maternal use of, 180t
Diuretics, maternal use of, 12t, 182t
Dolichocephaly, 56
"Doll's eye" maneuver, 148, 148f, 149
 defined, 200
 intraventricular hemorrhage and, 157
 subdural hemorrhage and, 156
Doppler ultrasound
 for blood pressure measurement, 89
 for gestational age assessment, 22t
Doppler velocimetry, 188
Dorsalis pedis pulse, 81, 81f
Dorsiflexion, defined, 119, 200
Dorsiflexion angle of foot, gestational age and,
  138f
Double outlet right ventricle (DORV),
  syndromes associated with, 79t
Down syndrome. *See* Trisomy 21
Doxepin, maternal use of, 180t
Doxycycline, maternal use of, 181t
Drowsiness, 161, 162f, 200

Drugs. *See* Medications, maternal; Substance
  abuse
Drug withdrawal, 151
 deep-tendon reflexes and, 142
 jitteriness and, 140
Dubowitz, L. M. S., 21, 22, 137
Dubowitz, Dubowitz, and Goldberg scoring
  system, 21, 22, 23t–24t, 25
 timing recommendations for, 34, 36
Dubowitz, V., 21, 22, 137
Dubowitz and Dubowitz neurologic
  evaluation, 137
Dullness, in abdomen, 101
Duodenal obstruction, signs of, 93
Dwarfism, macrocephaly and, 54
Dysmorphogenesis, 171–186
 defined, 200
 initial examination of, 171
 major vs minor anomalies, 175
 normal/unusual/abnormal continuum, 172,
  175–176
Dystopia canthorum, 176t

E

Early soft midsystolic ejection murmur, 87,
  207
Ears, 7, 59–60, 59f
 gestational age criteria, 23t, 26f, 30, 33f, 210
 malformations of, 173t, 176t, 183t
  urogenital defects and, 103, 104f
 normal, 58f, 59, 60f
 observation of, 2t
 pit in, 210
"Easy" babies, identifying, 168
Ebstein's anomaly, splitting of heart sound S2
  with, 85
Ecchymosis, defined, 41, 200
Ectodermal dysplasia, nail defects with, 51
EDC. *See* Expected date of confinement
EDD. *See* Expected date of delivery
Edema, 80
 assessing for, 40, 41
 breath sounds with, 73, 74t
 defined, 200
 gestational age criteria, 23t
 transillumination of chest and, 75
Ejection clicks, 86, 200
Ejection murmurs, systolic, 87, 88, 207
Elbow, 122, 122t
 congenital absence of the radius, 130, 131f
 in neurologic assessment, 138f, 139
Ellis-van Creveld syndrome, congenital heart
  defects with, 79t
Embryonic development, malformations and,
  171, 172f
Embryonic period, defined, 200
Encephalocele, 58, 152, 173t, 174f
 defined, 200
 maternal cocaine use and, 151t
Encephalopathy, 151
 defined, 200–201
 perinatal asphyxia and. *See* Hypoxic-ischemic
  encephalopathy
 reflexes and, 142, 150t
Endocrine disorders
 gender ambiguity and, 115

Physical Assessment of the Newborn

TEST DIRECTIONS

1. Please fill out the answer form and include all requested information. We are unable to issue a certificate without complete information.
2. All questions and answers are developed from the information provided in the book. Select the **one best answer** and fill in the corresponding circle on the answer form.
3. Mail the answer form to: **NICU INK,®** 1410 Neotomas Ave., Suite 107, Santa Rosa, CA 95405-7533 with a check for $35.00 (processing fee) made payable to NICU INK® This fee is non-refundable.
4. Retain a copy of the test for your records.
5. You will be notified of your results within 6–8 weeks.
6. If you pass the test (70%) you will earn 30 contact hours (3 CEUs) for the course. Approved by the California Board of Registered Nursing, provider #CEP 6261; Florida Board of Nursing, provider #27I 1040, content code 2505; Iowa Board of Nursing, provider #189; and Alabama Board of Nursing, provider #ABNP0169.

COURSE OBJECTIVES

After reading and studying the content, and taking the test the participant will be able to:

1. describe the principles of physical assessment as they apply to the neonatal physical examination.
2. outline the neuromuscular criteria as determined by the "new" Ballard gestational age examination.
3. define specific terms utilized when describing the skin.
4. list and describe common variations in newborn skin.
5. describe the normal parameters of the head, eyes, ears, nose, mouth, and neck examination.
6. identify the characteristic birth trauma findings associated with head, eyes, ears, nose, mouth, and neck.
7. define the physical landmarks and structure of the chest.
8. describe respirations by rate, quality, pattern, and auscultatory findings.
9. list what to look for in the maternal and family history that might indicate an increased probability of congenital heart disease.
10. describe the auscultatory assessment of the cardiovascular system.
11. describe the normal findings in the neonatal abdominal examination.
12. discuss techniques utilized to assess both superficial and deep structures when examining the neonatal abdomen.
13. describe the normal findings associated with the male and female genitourinary system.
14. identify abnormal genitourinary system findings and the assessment techniques used to delineate them.
15. describe the normal findings of the full-term infant's musculoskeletal system.
16. list the most common abnormalities found in the musculoskeletal system.
17. list the major reflexes that are present in the neonate and at what stage they appear and disappear.
18. describe the common anomalies encountered in the neurological examination of the neonate and discuss the implications to the infant.
19. discuss factors that influence infant behavioral responses.
20. identify the behaviors that define temperament and how they are used to describe a particular infant.
21. list the terminology used to describe variations in neonatal anatomy.
22. identify the common findings with specific teratogens and syndromes.
23. list and discuss common antepartal tests and their indications.
24. describe fetal heart rate abnormalities that may be found during intrapartal monitoring and the effect these deviations may have on the newborn.

---

1. The most important technique in physical assessment of the newborn is:
   a. auscultation
   b. palpation
   c. observation

2. Bimanual palpation is an appropriate technique for palpating the:
   a. kidneys
   b. liver
   c. spleen

3. To facilitate palpation, abdominal muscle relaxation can be achieved by:
   a. elevating the infant's hips off the bed
   b. examining the infant in a prone position
   c. rolling the infant to a side-lying position

4. The x-ray is commonly used in place of which technique of physical examination?
   a. auscultation
   b. palpation
   c. percussion

5. A large amount of transmitted light is seen during transillumination of an enlarged scrotum. This finding supports the diagnosis of:
   a. hydrocele
   b. inguinal hernia
   c. testicular torsion

6. The examiner performing a physical assessment of the infant of a diabetic mother should pay particular attention to which system?
   a. cardiovascular
   b. gastrointestinal
   c. genitourinary

7. Which of the following is the recommended approach for organizing a physical examination?
   a. auscultation, palpation, observation
   b. observation, auscultation, palpation
   c. palpation, observation, auscultation

8. To reduce sound distortion, stethoscope tubing should be no longer than:
   a. 10 inches
   b. 12 inches
   c. 14 inches

9. The risk for congenital heart disease is increased in the neonate who was exposed *in utero* to:
   a. anticonvulsants
   b. cocaine
   c. cephalosporins

10. Findings of decreased tone and activity in the newborn infant are consistent with a maternal history of:
    a. magnesium sulfate intake
    b. smoking
    c. systemic lupus erythematosus

11. Following identifying data, a complete history should begin with the:
    a. chief complaint
    b. mother's medical history
    c. past obstetrical history

12. During fetal movement counts, what number of movements per hour is considered acceptable?
    a. 2
    b. 3
    c. 4

13. A decreased α-fetoprotein identifies an increased risk of:
    a. anencephaly
    b. intrauterine growth retardation
    c. trisomy 21

14. The following parameter is included in the biophysical profile:
    a. gestational age assessment
    b. fetal weight estimation
    c. movement

15. Triple-marker testing for trisomy 21 has a prediction-rate accuracy of:
    a. 40 percent
    b. 50 percent
    c. 60 percent

16. A decreased level of human placental lactogen is indicative of:
    a. a chromosomal anomaly
    b. intrauterine infection
    c. uteroplacental insufficiency

17. Hemoglobin A_{1C} is a test used to evaluate pregnancies complicated by:
    a. diabetes
    b. hypertension
    c. systemic lupus erythematosus

18. Decreased beat-to-beat variability seen on a fetal monitor strip is indicative of:
    a. chorioamnionitis
    b. cord compression
    c. fetal hypoxia

19. Administration of propranolol to a laboring woman can result in what fetal heart rate pattern?
    a. decreased variability
    b. bradycardia
    c. tachycardia

20. Umbilical cord compression during uterine contractions results in:
    a. early decelerations
    b. late decelerations
    c. variable decelerations

21. To be considered normal, a fetal scalp pH should be greater than:
    a. 7.20
    b. 7.25
    c. 7.30

22. When ingested by the mother during pregnancy, a drug known to cause hearing loss in the newborn is:
    a. cefazolin
    b. phenobarbital
    c. streptomycin

23. An infant born to a woman with a primary CMV infection in the first trimester of pregnancy is at increased risk for:
    a. encephalitis
    b. hydrocephalus
    c. microcephaly

24. The new Ballard assessment tool overestimates gestational age by:
    a. 2–4 days
    b. 4–6 days
    c. 1 week

25. Eye examinations for the purpose of gestational age assessment should be done at:
    a. 0–48 hours of age
    b. 3–5 days of age
    c. 1 week of age

26. To assess an infant's posture, the infant should be positioned:
    a. prone
    b. side-lying
    c. supine

27. A square window is assessed by measuring the angle between the:
    a. ear and shoulder
    b. lower leg and thigh
    c. wrist and forearm

28. The scarf sign is scored according to the relationship between the elbow and the:
    a. ear
    b. midline of the body
    c. shoulder

29. The development of lanugo peaks at:
    a. 26–28 weeks
    b. 28–30 weeks
    c. 30–32 weeks

30. At term, plantar creases are found on what area of the foot?
    a. anterior two-thirds
    b. entire plantar surface
    c. half

31. In extremely premature neonates, the Ballard gestational age examination is most accurate when done:
    a. in the first 12 hours after birth
    b. 12–24 hours after birth
    c. 24–48 hours after birth

32. According to Amiel-Tison, neurologic evaluations should be done:
    a. one hour before feeding
    b. immediately before feeding
    c. one hour after feeding

33. If a neurologic assessment is unreliable because of asphyxia, gestational age can be assigned by:
    a. delaying the assessment for 48 hours
    b. estimating the neurologic score
    c. multiplying the physical assessment criteria by 2

34. A low birth weight infant is defined as one with a birth weight less than:
    a. 1,500 grams
    b. 2,000 grams
    c. 2,500 grams

35. An infant with a normal head circumference and a birth weight graphed at less than the 10th percentile would be classified as:
    a. AGA
    b. asymmetrically growth retarded
    c. symmetrically growth retarded

36. A congenital viral infection most commonly results in which of the following conditions?
    a. asymmetric growth retardation
    b. large for gestational age infant
    c. symmetric growth retardation

37. According to the new Ballard scoring system, which of the following infants would be considered most mature?
    a. abundant lanugo, 1–2 mm breast bud, pinna flat
    b. anterior transverse plantar crease; soft, ready, ear recoil; few scrotal rugae
    c. sparse lanugo, scrotum empty, flat areola

38. The outermost layer of the skin is the stratum:
    a. corneum
    b. keratin
    c. melanin

39. Sweat glands are found in the:
    a. dermis
    b. epidermis
    c. subcutaneous layer

40. A function of the subcutaneous layer of the skin is to:
    a. produce melanin
    b. produce skin oils
    c. store calories

41. The dermis and epidermis are attached by:
    a. fat cells
    b. fibrils
    c. keratinized cells

42. **Vernix caseosa is composed of skin cells and:**
    a. keratin
    b. sebaceous gland secretions
    c. sweat gland secretions

43. **A family history of neurofibromatosis should lead the examiner to check the infant for:**
    a. café au lait spots
    b. hairy nevus
    c. multiple hemangiomas

44. **During physical examination a term newborn is found to have loose skin folds elicited by pinching the skin. This finding indicates:**
    a. decreased subcutaneous fat
    b. a normal growth pattern
    c. tissue edema

45. **A blister greater than 1 cm in diameter is termed a:**
    a. bulla
    b. pustule
    c. vesicle

46. **A macule is:**
    a. flat
    b. fluid-filled
    c. raised

47. **The difference between a nodule and a papule is that a papule is:**
    a. elevated
    b. palpable below the skin
    c. well circumscribed

48. **Purpura refer to spots which are:**
    a. filled with serous fluid
    b. hemorrhagic
    c. semisolid

49. **A wheal originates in the:**
    a. dermis
    b. epidermis
    c. subcutaneous fat layer

50. **Circumoral cyanosis present at 18 hours after birth usually is indicative of:**
    a. anemia
    b. critical cardiac disease
    c. normal transitional changes

51. **Cutis marmorata refers to which of the following skin changes?**
    a. harlequin color change
    b. jaundice
    c. mottling

52. **Harlequin color changes can be alleviated by:**
    a. pressing the skin with the examiner's finger tips
    b. turning the infant
    c. warming the infant

53. **The papules found in erythema toxicum contain:**
    a. eosinophils
    b. neutrophils
    c. sebaceous secretions

54. **Milia located in the mouth are referred to as:**
    a. buccal cysts
    b. Epstein's pearls
    c. sucking blisters

55. **Sebaceous gland hyperplasia occurs secondary to:**
    a. androgen stimulation
    b. infection
    c. obstruction of the glands

56. **A warm humid environment can result in the development of:**
    a. erythema toxicum
    b. miliaria
    c. sebaceous nevus

57. **Hyperpigmented macules are most frequently seen over the:**
    a. arms
    b. buttocks
    c. scalp

58. **The most likely diagnosis for a neonate presenting at birth with superficial pustular lesions is:**
    a. infection of the sebaceous glands
    b. miliaria pustulosa
    c. transient pustular melanosis

59. **The rate of malignant changes occurring with pigmented nevus is approximately:**
    a. 10 percent
    b. 15 percent
    c. 20 percent

60. **Tuberous sclerosis presents with:**
    a. café au lait patches
    b. pigmented nevi
    c. hypopigmented macules

61. **Hypopigmented lesions are best seen under:**
    a. natural light
    b. ultraviolet light
    c. white light

62. Infants with multiple fat necrosis lesions should be monitored for:
    a. hypercalcemia
    b. hypoglycemia
    c. jaundice

63. The most common vascular birthmark is:
    a. nevus simplex
    b. port wine nevus
    c. strawberry hemangioma

64. Port wine nevi most commonly occur on the:
    a. arms
    b. face
    c. neck

65. A nevus flammeus associated with Sturge-Weber syndrome follows the distribution pattern of which nerve?
    a. facial
    b. olfactory
    c. trigeminal

66. The natural history of a strawberry hemangioma is that it will:
    a. begin to regress after six months
    b. continue to grow for 2–3 years
    c. remain static in size

67. Unlike a strawberry hemangioma, a cavernous hemangioma:
    a. always requires treatment
    b. has poorly defined borders
    c. regresses spontaneously

68. Diaper dermatitis caused by *Candida albicans* presents with:
    a. a petechial rash
    b. red macular eruptions
    c. white or yellow pustules

69. The skin rash seen in neonatal herpes:
    a. always precedes systemic illness
    b. begins with tender erythema
    c. ulcerates rapidly

70. Scalded skin syndrome results from what type of infection?
    a. *Candida albicans*
    b. cytomegalovirus
    c. *Staphylococcus aureus*

71. Blueberry muffin spots result from:
    a. dermal erythropoiesis
    b. vesicle eruptions
    c. scar tissue

72. The area of the skull most affected by cutis aplasia is over the _____ bone.
    a. occipital
    b. parietal
    c. temporal

73. A syndrome associated with nail atrophy is:
    a. Beckwith-Wiedemann
    b. trisomy 21
    c. Turner

74. The normal head circumference for a term infant is:
    a. 24–30 cm
    b. 31–38 cm
    c. 39–46 cm

75. Causes for macrocephaly include:
    a. Apert syndrome
    b. Down syndrome
    c. osteogenesis imperfecta

76. Transillumination of a normal neonate's skull should demonstrate a ring of light less than:
    a. 1 cm
    b. 2 cm
    c. 3 cm

77. The frontal and parietal bones are separated by which suture?
    a. coronal
    b. metopic
    c. sagittal

78. An increased anterior fontanel size can be seen in infants with:
    a. congenital adrenal hyperplasia
    b. hypothyroidism
    c. myasthenia gravis

79. The presence of a third fontanel is associated with:
    a. Down syndrome
    b. cutis aplasia
    c. microcephaly

80. Normal suture separation extends up to:
    a. 1 cm
    b. 2 cm
    c. 3 cm

81. Asymmetric skull growth is termed:
    a. brachycephaly
    b. plagiocephaly
    c. scaphocephaly

82. The flattened head shape seen in premature infants is termed:
    a. craniotabes
    b. dolichocephaly
    c. scaphocephaly

83. Craniosynostosis is commonly found with which of the following?
    a. breech positioning
    b. hyperthyroidism
    c. maternal diabetes

84. A cephalhematoma differs from caput succedaneum in that it is:
    a. diffuse and poorly defined
    b. is always evident at birth
    c. present for weeks following delivery

85. Abnormally placed hair whorls may be an indication of:
    a. mental retardation
    b. metabolic disorders
    c. neural tube defects

86. The most common location for an encephalocele is the _____ area.
    a. occipital
    b. parietal
    c. temporal

87. Pits, skin tags, and other minor ear malformations are usually located anterior to the:
    a. concha
    b. helix
    c. tragus

88. Low-set ears are defined as those whose insertion site fall below a line drawn from the:
    a. bridge of the nose to pupil of the eye and toward the ear
    b. inner to the outer canthus of the eye and toward the ear
    c. outer canthus of the eye to midtemple

89. A defect in the closure of a portion of the eye is termed a:
    a. coloboma
    b. glabella
    c. ptosis

90. Hypertelorism is the term given to:
    a. decreased palpebral fissure length
    b. slanted epicanthal folds
    c. widely-spaced eyes

91. Cornelia de Lange syndrome should be suspected in infants with:
    a. continuous eyebrows
    b. eyes with an antimongolian slant
    c. sparse eye lashes

92. For optimal evaluation of a neonate's eyes, the ophthalmoscope should be held _____ inches from the pupil.
    a. 6
    b. 8
    c. 10

93. During a normal eye exam, red light is reflected from the:
    a. lens
    b. iris
    c. retina

94. Brushfield spots can found on the:
    a. cornea
    b. iris
    c. sclera

95. Nystagmus is abnormal when it persists beyond:
    a. 4 months
    b. 6 months
    c. 8 months

96. Congenital glaucoma may present with:
    a. exophthalmos
    b. nystagmus
    c. strabismus

97. An infant who is cyanotic at rest and pink when crying should be suspected of having:
    a. bilateral choanal atresia
    b. dislocated septum
    c. microstomia

98. The combination of a thin upper lip, smooth philtrum, and short palpebral fissure is seen in infants with:
    a. Down syndrome
    b. fetal alcohol syndrome
    c. Noonan syndrome

99. Macroglossia is a feature of which of the following syndromes?
    a. Beckwith-Wiedemann
    b. Crouzon
    c. Pierre Robin

100. A benign bluish swelling under the tongue is a(n):
    a. eruption cyst
    b. Epstein pearl
    c. ranula

101. A cystic hygroma develops because of:
    a. branchial cleft cysts
    b. proliferation of hematopoietic tissue
    c. sequestered lymph channels

102. The neonate has how many pairs of true ribs?
    a. 5
    b. 6
    c. 7

103. A normal respiratory rate for a term infant is:
    a. 20–40 breaths per minute
    b. 40–60 breaths per minute
    c. 60–80 breaths per minute

104. Stridor might be expected in an infant with:
    a. atelectasis
    b. transient tachypnea
    c. a vascular ring

105. Expiratory grunting occurs when the infant attempts to:
    a. decrease air trapping
    b. increase intrathoracic pressure
    c. overcome an upper airway obstruction

106. The average chest circumference in a term infant is:
    a. 25 cm
    b. 29 cm
    c. 33 cm

107. The size of the breast bud in a term infant is normally:
    a. 0.5 cm
    b. 1 cm
    c. 1.5 cm

108. The distance between the infant's areola should be what in relationship to the chest circumference?
    a. less than ¼
    b. ¼ to ½
    c. ½ to ¾

109. The secretion of witch's milk indicates the presence of:
    a. infection
    b. lymph fluid
    c. maternal estrogen

110. Wide-spaced nipples are a feature of which of the following syndromes?
    a. Down
    b. Noonan
    c. Turner

111. Supernumerary nipples are typically located on a line drawn:
    a. horizontally through the true nipple
    b. vertically through the anterior axillary line
    c. vertically through the true nipple

112. Excessive nasal secretions should alert the examiner to the possibility of congenital:
    a. chlamydia
    b. gonorrhea
    c. syphilis

113. The transmission of breath sounds is decreased in the presence of:
    a. respiratory distress syndrome
    b. lung hyperinflation
    c. pneumonia

114. During expiration, vesicular breath sounds are:
    a. heard best over the trachea
    b. longer than on inspiration
    c. short and soft

115. Bronchovesicular breath sounds are normally heard over the:
    a. lower lung fields
    b. manubrium
    c. trachea

116. A maneuver which is useful in distinguishing upper airway sounds from lung sounds is to:
    a. listen through the infant's back
    b. place the stethoscope over the infant's nose and mouth
    c. use the bell of the stethoscope

117. Fine crackles originate in the:
    a. alveoli
    b. bronchioles
    c. large airways

118. Medium crackles have been compared to the sound of:
    a. the fizz of a carbonated drink
    b. rubbing a finger over a cupped hand
    c. rubbing a lock of hair between two fingers

119. Wheezes may be heard in neonates with which lung condition?
    a. narrowing of airway
    b. opening of collapsed alveoli
    c. secretions in small airways

120. Crepitus may be a sign of:
    a. consolidation
    b. narrowing of the airways
    c. pulmonary air leak

121. Rachitic rosary may be found in infants with:
    a. fractured clavicle
    b. osteogenesis imperfecta
    c. rickets

122. During transillumination, a false positive result may be obtained in the presence of:
    a. dark skin
    b. lung consolidation
    c. subcutaneous air

123. The opening of atelectatic alveoli during mechanical ventilation is thought to result in what type of breath sounds?
    a. course crackles
    b. rubs
    c. harsh

124. During high frequency ventilation, musical breath sounds indicate:
    a. air in the pleural space
    b. normal ventilation
    c. the presence of secretions

125. Maternal conditions which are known to affect the neonate's cardiovascular system include:
    a. myasthenia gravis
    b. Grave's disease
    c. systemic lupus erythematosus

126. The risk for congenital heart disease (CHD) in offspring of mothers with CHD is:
    a. 5–10 percent
    b. 10–15 percent
    c. 15–20 percent

127. A drug known to cause congenital heart disease is:
    a. lithium
    b. phenobarbital
    c. tetracycline

128. Rubella contracted by the mother during early pregnancy causes which of the following congenital heart defects?
    a. endocardial cushion defect
    b. pulmonary branch stenosis
    c. truces arteriosis

129. Extracardiac anomalies are accompanied by CHD in what percentage of infants?
    a. 10
    b. 20
    c. 30

130. An infant is said to be polycythemic when his central hematocrit exceeds:
    a. 50 percent
    b. 60 percent
    c. 65 percent

131. Central cyanosis becomes visible at what level of unbound hemoglobin?
    a. 5 gm/100 ml
    b. 10 gm/100 ml
    c. 15 gm/100 ml

132. An abnormal capillary filling time is one that exceeds:
    a. 2 seconds
    b. 3 seconds
    c. 4 seconds

133. Infants with Turner syndrome should be investigated for the presence of:
    a. coarctation of the aorta
    b. dextrocardia
    c. ventricular septal defects

134. To assess for aortic coarctation or stenosis, the strength of the femoral pulses should be compared to the:
    a. dorsalis pedis pulse
    b. left radial pulse
    c. right brachial pulse

135. In addition to a PDA, bounding pulses are found with what other heart lesion?
    a. total anomalous pulmonary venous return
    b. transposition of the great vessels
    c. truncus arteriosus

136. A 2 day old term infant with an active precordium should be suspected of having:
    a. left ventricular hypertrophy
    b. pulmonary stenosis
    c. a ventricular septal defect

137. The apical impulse is normally found in which intercostal space?
    a. 3rd
    b. 4th
    c. 5th

138. A displaced PMI can result from:
    a. lung consolidation
    b. pneumothorax
    c. pulmonary interstitial emphysema

139. Taps and thrills are best felt with the:
    a. back of the hand
    b. fingertips
    c. ulnar surface of the hand

140. Right ventricular hypertrophy is likely to result in which of the following findings?
    a. a heave
    b. a tap
    c. a thrill

141. For the purposes of auscultation, the pulmonic area is identified as being at the:
    a. fourth intercostal space, left midclavicular line
    b. second intercostal space, left sternal angle
    c. second intercostal space, right sternal angle

142. When untreated, SVT results in:
    a. ballooning of the aorta
    b. congestive heart failure
    c. pulmonary hypertension

143. Premature atrial beats may occur as a result of:
    a. hypokalemia
    b. irritation from a central line
    c. sepsis

144. The first heart sound results from:
    a. closure of the mitral valve
    b. ejection of blood from left ventricle
    c. closure of the aortic valve

145. The second heart sound is best heard over the:
    a. aortic area
    b. mitral area
    c. tricuspid area

146. S3, if heard, occurs because of:
    a. narrowed pulmonary arteries
    b. rapid ventricular filling
    c. turbulent aortic flow

147. Wide splitting of S2 occurs with:
    a. Ebstein anomaly
    b. tricuspid atresia
    c. patent ductus arteriosus

148. S4 is heard with conditions such as:
    a. cardiomyopathy
    b. critical pulmonary stenosis
    c. mitral valve prolapse

149. Ejection clicks are normal:
    a. at 12 hours of age
    b. at 72 hours of age
    c. when heard after S2

150. A high-pitched murmur occurs with:
    a. ASD
    b. mitral stenosis
    c. VSD

151. The most common innocent murmur is a:
    a. continuous systolic murmur
    b. pulmonary branch stenosis murmur
    c. systolic ejection murmur

152. A Grade III systolic ejection murmur occurs with:
    a. aortic stenosis
    b. mitral regurgitation
    c. patent ductus arteriosus

153. Right-sided heart failure should be considered when the liver is palpated at what level below the costal margin?
    a. 1 cm
    b. 2 cm
    c. 3 cm

154. The most common cause of an elevated BP reading in the neonate is:
    a. renal disease
    b. recording BP during crying
    c. using a cuff that is too small

155. A diagnosis of coarctation of the aorta is supported by which of the following systolic blood pressure readings?

	upper limb	lower limb
a.	52	37
b.	40	42
c.	48	26

156. A pulse pressure of 28 in a preterm infant is:
    a. suggestive of a PDA
    b. indicative of congestive heart failure
    c. normal

157. Dichotomous movements of the abdomen and chest are suggestive of:
    a. intestinal obstruction
    b. peritoneal irritation
    c. pyloric stenosis

158. A newborn presenting with visible peristalsis should be investigated for:
    a. duodenal obstruction
    b. pneumoperitoneum
    c. pyloric stenosis

159. Which of the following congenital malformations occurs in association with Down syndrome?
    a. bladder exstrophy
    b. gastroschisis
    c. omphalocele

160. The usual location for a gastroschisis is:
    a. at the umbilicus
    b. to the left of midline
    c. to the right of midline

161. A common finding in bladder exstrophy is:
    a. duodenal atresia
    b. epispadias
    c. posterior urethral valves

162. A term Caucasian infant with an umbilical hernia should be checked for:
    a. congenital heart disease
    b. hypothyroidism
    c. urinary tract anomalies

163. The differential diagnosis for a painful mass palpated just below the sternum includes:
    a. enlarged spleen
    b. epigastric hernia
    c. pyloric stenosis

164. In a healthy term infant the umbilical cord normally falls off by day:
    a. 14
    b. 18
    c. 21

165. A single umbilical artery is a hallmark for anomalies of which system?
    a. cardiovascular
    b. gastrointestinal
    c. respiratory

166. An omphalomesenteric duct connects the umbilicus to the:
    a. liver
    b. ileum
    c. urinary bladder

167. Persistent serosanguinous discharge from the umbilicus is indicative of a:
    a. granuloma
    b. peritoneal fistula
    c. urachal cyst

168. Anal sphincter tone can be determined by:
    a. checking the rectum for the presence of stool
    b. eliciting an anal wink
    c. observing for stool oozing from the anus

169. There is an increased risk of intestinal obstruction in infants born to women with:
    a. diabetes
    b. Grave's disease
    c. pregnancy-induced hypertension

170. In a term infant, bowel sounds are normally heard by _____ minutes after delivery.
    a. 15
    b. 30
    c. 60

171. In an infant with a soft abdomen, hyperactive bowel sounds heard following a feeding usually represent:
    a. early obstruction
    b. gastroenteritis
    c. a normal pattern

172. An infant with a persistent bruit should be investigated for abnormalities of the:
    a. inferior vena cava
    b. liver
    c. pancreas

173. Flexing the infant's knees and hips causes the:
    a. abdominal muscles to relax
    b. kidneys to move anteriorly
    c. liver to drop below the costal margin

174. The spleen normally doesn't extend more than _____ cm below the left costal margin.
    a. 1
    b. 2
    c. 3

175. A cystic mass palpated in the abdomen usually arises from the:
    a. kidney
    b. liver
    c. spleen

176. The right kidney is difficult to palpate because it is:
    a. behind the head of the pancreas
    b. covered by the liver
    c. located more posterior than the left

177. The bladder is palpated just above the:
    a. inguinal canal
    b. ischial spine
    c. symphysis pubis

178. Percussion that does not demonstrate tympany below the left costal margin is suggestive of:
    a. duodenal atresia
    b. esophageal obstruction
    c. pneumoperitoneum

179. Physical findings suggestive of urogenital defects include:
    a. flattened facies
    b. polyhydramnios
    c. vaginal skin tags

180. Congenital anomalies frequently found in combination with GU anomalies include:
    a. coloboma
    b. duodenal atresia
    c. tracheoesophageal fistula

181. On physical exam, an infant is noted to have a palpable subumbilical mass. This infant should be further evaluated for a/an:
    a. distended bladder
    b. multicystic kidney
    c. undescended testis

182. Rugae begin to form on the scrotum at:
    a. 32 weeks
    b. 34 weeks
    c. 36 weeks

183. The testes begin to descend into the inguinal canal at:
    a. 26–28 weeks
    b. 28–30 weeks
    c. 30–32 weeks

184. Transplacentally acquired maternal hormones result in which of the following findings in a newborn male?
    a. edema of the genitalia
    b. penile discharge
    c. redness of the genitalia

185. The presence of a nonretractable foreskin is referred to as:
    a. cryptorchidism
    b. epispadias
    c. phimosis

186. The average penile length for a term neonate is:
    a. 2 cm
    b. 3.5 cm
    c. 5 cm

187. The presence of posterior urethral valves can result in:
    a. ascites
    b. bladder prolapse
    c. bowel obstruction

188. Hydroureter, hydronephrosis, and renal dysplasia frequently occur with:
    a. bladder exstrophy
    b. multicystic kidney disease
    c. prune belly syndrome

189. Which of the following physical findings is associated with urogenital defects?
    a. low set ears
    b. presence of extra digits
    c. single umbilical artery

190. The fetal bladder is connected to the umbilical cord via the:
    a. retroperitoneal fistula
    b. umbilical ureter
    c. urachus

191. In the male infant, incomplete development of the anterior urethra results in:
    a. bladder exstrophy
    b. epispadias
    c. hypospadias

192. A higher risk of endocrine or chromosomal anomalies occurs in infants with which type of hypospadias?
    a. balanic
    b. penile
    c. perineal

193. Curvature of the penis resulting from the growth of fibrous tissue is referred to as:
    a. chordee
    b. epispadias
    c. urachal patency

194. Circumcision is contraindicated in infants with (a):
    a. hypospadias
    b. patent urachus
    c. phimosis

195. An infant with a weak urine stream should be investigated for the presence of:
    a. chordee
    b. posterior urethral valves
    c. undescended testes

196. Neurogenic bladder is a complication of:
    a. hydronephrosis
    b. myelomeningocele
    c. prune belly syndrome

197. Testes undescended at birth usually descend by:
    a. one month of age
    b. two months of age
    c. three months of age

198. Cryptorchidism carries an increased risk of:
    a. hydrocele
    b. malignancy
    c. testicular torsion

199. A common complication of an inguinal hernia is:
    a. bowel obstruction
    b. cryptorchidism
    c. pyelonephritis

200. An infant presenting with a swollen, discolored, and tender scrotum should be investigated for:
    a. hydrocele
    b. priapism
    c. testicular torsion

201. Hydrocolpos is a condition which can result from a/an:
    a. imperforate hymen
    b. prolapsed ovary
    c. urogenital sinus

202. A Problem with sexual differentiation should be suspected in a female infant presenting with:
    a. clitoral hypertrophy
    b. hydrometrocolpos
    c. inguinal hernia

203. Additional accuracy in performing newborn measurements can be obtained by:
   a. overlapping paper tape edges
   b. folding a paper tape in half lengthwise
   c. using a tape with a slight stretch

204. A term newborn infant should be expected to regain birth weight by:
   a. 7 days of age
   b. 14 days of age
   c. 21 days of age

205. The average term infant's head circumference is:
   a. 12–13 inches (30.5–33 cm)
   b. 13–14 inches (33–35.5 cm)
   c. 14–15 inches (35.5–38 cm)

206. When comparing a term infant's chest and head circumferences, the chest circumference is normally:
   a. 4 cm less than the head
   b. 2 cm less than the head
   c. 2 cm more than the head

207. The hand with the palm facing up is said to be:
   a. adducted
   b. pronated
   c. supinated

208. When in plantar flexion, the forefoot is:
   a. higher than the ankle
   b. in line with the ankle
   c. lower than the ankle

209. Out-turned feet would be said to be in which position?
   a. inverted
   b. valgus
   c. varus

210. A newborn who presents with legs of unequal length should be assessed for the presence of:
   a. achondroplasia
   b. congenital tuberculosis
   c. intra-abdominal neoplasms

211. In term infants, the upper body segment should not be more than _____ times the length of the lower body segment.
   a. 1.5
   b. 1.7
   c. 1.9

212. In a term infant, the presence of tremors while at rest is abnormal after:
   a. 4 days of age
   b. 5 days of age
   c. 6 days of age

213. Normally, the newborn's neck should rotate:
   a. 60 degrees
   b. 80 degrees
   c. 100 degrees

214. After the clavicle, the bone most commonly fractured at delivery is the:
   a. femur
   b. humerus
   c. radius

215. When examining the hands of a newborn with neurofibromatosis, one may expect to find:
   a. macrodactyly
   b. polydactyly
   c. simian creases

216. Term newborn infants normally have a flexion contracture of the hips that measures:
   a. 25–30 degrees
   b. 30–35 degrees
   c. 35–40 degrees

217. A reliable maneuver for ruling out congenital hip dysplasia is:
   a. Allis's
   b. Ortolani
   c. Palliser

218. During testing, a dislocatable hip will produce which of the following sensation/"sound"?
   a. click
   b. clunk
   c. snap

219. Pain elicited on passive movement of the legs is a sign of:
   a. avulsion of the femoral epiphysis
   b. congenital hip dysplasia
   c. tibial torsion

220. An orthopedic consultation should be obtained for a newborn with:
   a. anterior bowing of the tibia
   b. flat feet
   c. inturned feet

221. Clubfoot can be differentiated from a positional foot deformity by moving the foot into:
   a. dorsiflexion
   b. plantar flexion
   c. rotation

222. A decreased number of cervical vertebrae are present in which syndrome?
   a. Noonan's
   b. Klippel-Feil
   c. Sprengel

223. A mass in the sternocleidomastoid muscle is present with congenital:
     a. kyphosis
     b. scaphocephaly
     c. torticollis

224. Scoliosis develops on the basis of a:
     a. chromosomal defect
     b. failure of vertebral formation
     c. vertebral fusion

225. A hypoplastic malrotated scapula results in:
     a. cleidocranial dysostosis
     b. lordosis
     c. Sprengel deformity

226. Brachial plexus injuries most commonly result in paralysis of the:
     a. lower arm
     b. upper arm
     c. whole arm

227. Anomalies usually accompanying congenital absence of the radius include:
     a. hypoplastic or absent thumb
     b. overlapping digits
     c. shortening of the humerus

228. Congenital hip dysplasia is more common with:
     a. breech positioning
     b. multiple gestation
     c. male gender

229. Congenital absence of a long bone most commonly affects the:
     a. fibula
     b. tibia
     c. ulna

230. The most common congenital foot anomaly is:
     a. genu recurvatum
     b. metatarsus adductus
     c. talipes equinovarus

231. The highest incidence of clubfoot occurs in infants of what race?
     a. Asian
     b. Caucasian
     c. Polynesian

232. The most widely accepted theory to explain Streeter dysplasia is:
     a. amniotic bands
     b. familial tendency
     c. oligohydramnios

233. Early correction of syndactyly may be necessary to:
     a. assist with parental bonding
     b. prevent deterioration in function
     c. reestablish blood supply

234. An infant with a number of café au lait spots should be investigated for the presence of:
     a. Down syndrome
     b. neurofibromatosis
     c. tuberous sclerosis

235. Sturge-Weber syndrome should be suspected in a neonate with a:
     a. depigmented area of skin
     b. facial hemangioma
     c. hairy nevus

236. A deletion of the short arm of the fifth chromosome results in which of the following findings?
     a. catlike cry
     b. facial asymmetry
     c. macrocephaly

237. Erb's palsy results from damage to spinal roots at:
     a. C-2 to C-4
     b. C-5 to C-6
     c. C-8 to T-1

238. The presence of Bell's palsy results in
     a. absence of movement in one hand
     b. facial weakness
     c. respiratory distress

239. As the neonate matures, tone increases in which direction? From the:
     a. center of the body to the periphery
     b. head to the legs
     c. legs to the head

240. In the preterm neonate, frog-leg posture should disappear by :
     a. 34 weeks
     b. 36 weeks
     c. 38 weeks

241. Lying with extended extremities should be considered abnormal in infants greater than:
     a. 32 weeks
     b. 34 weeks
     c. 36 weeks

242. In a term infant, jitteriness may occur in the presence of:
     a. hypocalcemia
     b. hypochloremia
     c. hyponatremia

243. The neurologic examination of a neonate shows a normal anterior fontanel with widened sutures. This finding suggests:
    a. craniosynostosis
    b. hydranencephaly
    c. intrauterine growth retardation

244. Posterior ballooning of the skull is seen in infants with:
    a. Dandy-Walker syndrome
    b. hydranencephaly
    c. hydrocephalus

245. A brief, forceful contraction in response to a short stretch is termed:
    a. abnormal tone
    b. phasic tone
    c. postural tone

246. Tendon reflexes that can be tested in the neonate include the _____ reflex.
    a. biceps
    b. tonic neck
    c. triceps

247. Exaggerated deep tendon reflexes may be present in neonates with:
    a. drug withdrawal syndrome
    b. intrauterine infection
    c. metabolic disorders

248. Postural tone is best assessed by which of the following maneuvers?
    a. heel-to-ear
    b. eliciting a grasp
    c. pull-to-sit

249. Lower limb strength is evaluated by checking the:
    a. Babinski reflex
    b. extensor tone
    c. stepping reflex

250. An infant demonstrating weakness of the limbs that is more pronounced in the upper limbs should be evaluated for injury to which cerebral area?
    a. frontal
    b. occipital
    c. parasagittal

251. Fasciculations may be observed in infants with:
    a. congenital myasthenia gravis
    b. muscular dystrophy
    c. Werdnig-Hoffmann disease

252. An infant presenting with opisthotonus should be suspected of having:
    a. bacterial meningitis
    b. infantile botulism
    c. a motor neuron disorder

253. In a neonate with normal response to a doll's eye maneuver, turning the head to the left will cause the infant's eyes to:
    a. remain in midline
    b. turn to the left
    c. turn to right

254. An infant presenting with stridor may have sustained damage to which cranial nerve?
    a. IX
    b. X
    c. XI

255. The harlequin sign appears as a result of:
    a. autonomic vasomotor instability
    b. eliciting the Herring-Breuer reflex
    c. overstimulation of sympathetic nervous system

256. In the term infant, focal ischemic damage to the middle cerebral artery results in:
    a. hemiparesis
    b. speech impairments
    c. weak lower limbs

257. Fixed positioning and limited movement of a limb is termed:
    a. arthrogryposis
    b. fasciculation
    c. opisthotonus

258. A dermal sinus is most commonly seen in which region of the spine?
    a. lumbar
    b. sacral
    c. thoracic

259. A myelomeningocele is differentiated from a meningocele by the presence of _____ in the sac.
    a. cerebral spinal fluid
    b. meninges
    c. spinal roots

260. The most benign form of intracranial hemorrhage in a term infant is a:
    a. intraventricular bleed
    b. subarachnoid bleed
    c. subdural bleed

261. A tentorial laceration results in bleeding in the:
    a. ventricles
    b. subarachnoid space
    c. subdural space

262. The most common cause of hydrocephalus following an intraventricular hemorrhage is:
    a. blockage of the aqueduct of Sylvius
    b. inflammation of the arachnoid villi
    c. overproduction of CSF

263. When an IVH occurs in a term neonate, the most likely site is the:
    a. Choroid plexus
    b. germinal matrix
    c. subependymal tissue

264. A complete NBAS assessment takes:
    a. 15 minutes
    b. 30 minutes
    c. 60 minutes

265. Which of the following is a cause for concern in the term neonate?
    a. abrupt changes in state
    b. inability to self-console
    c. crying during light sleep

266. According to Brazelton, the "cost of attention":
    a. determines if the infant will become hyperalert
    b. is the time it takes an infant to recover from stimulation
    c. varies according to the infant's maturity

267. Signs of stress in a neonate include:
    a. apnea
    b. bringing hands to midline
    c. falling asleep

268. The organized infant is one who:
    a. abruptly changes state in response to stimulation
    b. habituates to stimuli
    c. releases stress by crying

269. A strategy to support a disorganized infant is to:
    a. contain the infant's extremities during caregiving
    b. introduce a combined program of auditory and visual stimulation
    c. space caretaking activities over short regular intervals

270. The level of tolerance for a stimulus is termed:
    a. cost of attention
    b. organizational pattern
    c. sensory threshold

271. Approach behaviors include:
    a. dilated pupils
    b. extended arms
    c. rapid breathing

272. Successful habituation in a term infant usually occurs after how many repetitions?
    a. 5–9
    b. 10–14
    c. 15–19

273. Problems with habituation may interfere with:
    a. achieving an alert state
    b. feeding
    c. providing time out signals

274. A term infant should be able to horizontally follow an object:
    a. 30 degrees
    b. 60 degrees
    c. 90 degrees

275. Preterm infants should be able to fixate on simple patterns by:
    a. 28 weeks
    b. 30 weeks
    c. 32 weeks

276. In determining temperament, regular sleep-wake patterns would show evidence of:
    a. adaptability
    b. distractibility
    c. rhythmicity

277. The rate of dysmorphogenesis for newborn infants is estimated to be _____ per 100 live births.
    a. 1–2
    b. 3–4
    c. 4–5

278. Most serious anomalies develop during which trimester?
    a. 1
    b. 2
    c. 3

279. Diaphragmatic hernia usually occurs during which period following conception?
    a. 0–6 weeks
    b. 6–12 weeks
    c. 12–18 weeks

280. Features which differ among ethnic groups are termed:
    a. family traits
    b. minor anomalies
    c. normal variants

281. Infants with three minor anomalies have a _____ percent probability of having a major anomaly.
    a. 3
    b. 11
    c. 90

282. An example of a malformation occurring because of polygenic transmission is:
    a. osteogenesis imperfecta
    b. spina bifida
    c. Turner syndrome

283. An infant with 45 chromosomes is said to have:
    a. monosomy
    b. polyploidy
    c. trisomy

284. The most frequent cause of trisomy is:
   a. breakage
   b. nondisjunction
   c. translocation

285. An example of a sequence effect in congenital malformations is:
   a. Down syndrome
   b. neural tube defects
   c. Potter syndrome

286. An example of an association in congenital malformations is:
   a. diaphragmatic hernia
   b. prune belly syndrome
   c. VATER

287. A teratogen known to cause facial anomalies and limb defects is:
   a. heroin
   b. phenytoin
   c. tetracycline

288. The teratogenic effects of warfarin sodium include:
   a. eye abnormalities
   b. exstrophy of the bladder
   c. neural tube defects

289. Clinical features of trisomy 18 include:
   a. lymphedema
   b. polydactyly
   c. rocker bottom feet

290. Chromosome analysis of a female infant presenting with webbed neck, blue sclera, low posterior hair line, and lymphedema would be expected to show:
   a. 44X
   b. 46 XXY
   c. 47 XX

ANSWER FORM: Physical Assessment of the Newborn

Please completely fill in the circle of the **one best answer** using a dark pen.

Questions are numbered vertically.

1. a. ○ b. ○ c. ○ 16. a. ○ b. ○ c. ○ 31. a. ○ b. ○ c. ○ 46. a. ○ b. ○ c. ○ 61. a. ○ b. ○ c. ○ 76. a. ○ b. ○ c. ○ 91. a. ○ b. ○ c. ○ 106. a. ○ b. ○ c. ○ 121. a. ○ b. ○ c. ○ 136. a. ○ b. ○ c. ○ 151. a. ○ b. ○ c. ○

2. a. ○ b. ○ c. ○ 17. a. ○ b. ○ c. ○ 32. a. ○ b. ○ c. ○ 47. a. ○ b. ○ c. ○ 62. a. ○ b. ○ c. ○ 77. a. ○ b. ○ c. ○ 92. a. ○ b. ○ c. ○ 107. a. ○ b. ○ c. ○ 122. a. ○ b. ○ c. ○ 137. a. ○ b. ○ c. ○ 152. a. ○ b. ○ c. ○

3. a. ○ b. ○ c. ○ 18. a. ○ b. ○ c. ○ 33. a. ○ b. ○ c. ○ 48. a. ○ b. ○ c. ○ 63. a. ○ b. ○ c. ○ 78. a. ○ b. ○ c. ○ 93. a. ○ b. ○ c. ○ 108. a. ○ b. ○ c. ○ 123. a. ○ b. ○ c. ○ 138. a. ○ b. ○ c. ○ 153. a. ○ b. ○ c. ○

4. a. ○ b. ○ c. ○ 19. a. ○ b. ○ c. ○ 34. a. ○ b. ○ c. ○ 49. a. ○ b. ○ c. ○ 64. a. ○ b. ○ c. ○ 79. a. ○ b. ○ c. ○ 94. a. ○ b. ○ c. ○ 109. a. ○ b. ○ c. ○ 124. a. ○ b. ○ c. ○ 139. a. ○ b. ○ c. ○ 154. a. ○ b. ○ c. ○

5. a. ○ b. ○ c. ○ 20. a. ○ b. ○ c. ○ 35. a. ○ b. ○ c. ○ 50. a. ○ b. ○ c. ○ 65. a. ○ b. ○ c. ○ 80. a. ○ b. ○ c. ○ 95. a. ○ b. ○ c. ○ 110. a. ○ b. ○ c. ○ 125. a. ○ b. ○ c. ○ 140. a. ○ b. ○ c. ○ 155. a. ○ b. ○ c. ○

6. a. ○ b. ○ c. ○ 21. a. ○ b. ○ c. ○ 36. a. ○ b. ○ c. ○ 51. a. ○ b. ○ c. ○ 66. a. ○ b. ○ c. ○ 81. a. ○ b. ○ c. ○ 96. a. ○ b. ○ c. ○ 111. a. ○ b. ○ c. ○ 126. a. ○ b. ○ c. ○ 141. a. ○ b. ○ c. ○ 156. a. ○ b. ○ c. ○

7. a. ○ b. ○ c. ○ 22. a. ○ b. ○ c. ○ 37. a. ○ b. ○ c. ○ 52. a. ○ b. ○ c. ○ 67. a. ○ b. ○ c. ○ 82. a. ○ b. ○ c. ○ 97. a. ○ b. ○ c. ○ 112. a. ○ b. ○ c. ○ 127. a. ○ b. ○ c. ○ 142. a. ○ b. ○ c. ○ 157. a. ○ b. ○ c. ○

8. a. ○ b. ○ c. ○ 23. a. ○ b. ○ c. ○ 38. a. ○ b. ○ c. ○ 53. a. ○ b. ○ c. ○ 68. a. ○ b. ○ c. ○ 83. a. ○ b. ○ c. ○ 98. a. ○ b. ○ c. ○ 113. a. ○ b. ○ c. ○ 128. a. ○ b. ○ c. ○ 143. a. ○ b. ○ c. ○ 158. a. ○ b. ○ c. ○

9. a. ○ b. ○ c. ○ 24. a. ○ b. ○ c. ○ 39. a. ○ b. ○ c. ○ 54. a. ○ b. ○ c. ○ 69. a. ○ b. ○ c. ○ 84. a. ○ b. ○ c. ○ 99. a. ○ b. ○ c. ○ 114. a. ○ b. ○ c. ○ 129. a. ○ b. ○ c. ○ 144. a. ○ b. ○ c. ○ 159. a. ○ b. ○ c. ○

10. a. ○ b. ○ c. ○ 25. a. ○ b. ○ c. ○ 40. a. ○ b. ○ c. ○ 55. a. ○ b. ○ c. ○ 70. a. ○ b. ○ c. ○ 85. a. ○ b. ○ c. ○ 100. a. ○ b. ○ c. ○ 115. a. ○ b. ○ c. ○ 130. a. ○ b. ○ c. ○ 145. a. ○ b. ○ c. ○ 160. a. ○ b. ○ c. ○

11. a. ○ b. ○ c. ○ 26. a. ○ b. ○ c. ○ 41. a. ○ b. ○ c. ○ 56. a. ○ b. ○ c. ○ 71. a. ○ b. ○ c. ○ 86. a. ○ b. ○ c. ○ 101. a. ○ b. ○ c. ○ 116. a. ○ b. ○ c. ○ 131. a. ○ b. ○ c. ○ 146. a. ○ b. ○ c. ○ 161. a. ○ b. ○ c. ○

12. a. ○ b. ○ c. ○ 27. a. ○ b. ○ c. ○ 42. a. ○ b. ○ c. ○ 57. a. ○ b. ○ c. ○ 72. a. ○ b. ○ c. ○ 87. a. ○ b. ○ c. ○ 102. a. ○ b. ○ c. ○ 117. a. ○ b. ○ c. ○ 132. a. ○ b. ○ c. ○ 147. a. ○ b. ○ c. ○ 162. a. ○ b. ○ c. ○

13. a. ○ b. ○ c. ○ 28. a. ○ b. ○ c. ○ 43. a. ○ b. ○ c. ○ 58. a. ○ b. ○ c. ○ 73. a. ○ b. ○ c. ○ 88. a. ○ b. ○ c. ○ 103. a. ○ b. ○ c. ○ 118. a. ○ b. ○ c. ○ 133. a. ○ b. ○ c. ○ 148. a. ○ b. ○ c. ○ 163. a. ○ b. ○ c. ○

14. a. ○ b. ○ c. ○ 29. a. ○ b. ○ c. ○ 44. a. ○ b. ○ c. ○ 59. a. ○ b. ○ c. ○ 74. a. ○ b. ○ c. ○ 89. a. ○ b. ○ c. ○ 104. a. ○ b. ○ c. ○ 119. a. ○ b. ○ c. ○ 134. a. ○ b. ○ c. ○ 149. a. ○ b. ○ c. ○ 164. a. ○ b. ○ c. ○

15. a. ○ b. ○ c. ○ 30. a. ○ b. ○ c. ○ 45. a. ○ b. ○ c. ○ 60. a. ○ b. ○ c. ○ 75. a. ○ b. ○ c. ○ 90. a. ○ b. ○ c. ○ 105. a. ○ b. ○ c. ○ 120. a. ○ b. ○ c. ○ 135. a. ○ b. ○ c. ○ 150. a. ○ b. ○ c. ○ 165. a. ○ b. ○ c. ○

166. a. ○ 178. a. ○ 190. a. ○ 202. a. ○ 214. a. ○ 226. a. ○ 238. a. ○ 250. a. ○ 262. a. ○ 274. a. ○ 286. a. ○
 b. ○   b. ○   b. ○   b. ○   b. ○   b. ○   b. ○   b. ○   b. ○   b. ○   b. ○
 c. ○   c. ○   c. ○   c. ○   c. ○   c. ○   c. ○   c. ○   c. ○   c. ○   c. ○

167. a. ○ 179. a. ○ 191. a. ○ 203. a. ○ 215. a. ○ 227. a. ○ 239. a. ○ 251. a. ○ 263. a. ○ 275. a. ○ 287. a. ○
 b. ○   b. ○   b. ○   b. ○   b. ○   b. ○   b. ○   b. ○   b. ○   b. ○   b. ○
 c. ○   c. ○   c. ○   c. ○   c. ○   c. ○   c. ○   c. ○   c. ○   c. ○   c. ○

168. a. ○ 180. a. ○ 192. a. ○ 204. a. ○ 216. a. ○ 228. a. ○ 240. a. ○ 252. a. ○ 264. a. ○ 276. a. ○ 288. a. ○
 b. ○   b. ○   b. ○   b. ○   b. ○   b. ○   b. ○   b. ○   b. ○   b. ○   b. ○
 c. ○   c. ○   c. ○   c. ○   c. ○   c. ○   c. ○   c. ○   c. ○   c. ○   c. ○

169. a. ○ 181. a. ○ 193. a. ○ 205. a. ○ 217. a. ○ 229. a. ○ 241. a. ○ 253. a. ○ 265. a. ○ 277. a. ○ 289. a. ○
 b. ○   b. ○   b. ○   b. ○   b. ○   b. ○   b. ○   b. ○   b. ○   b. ○   b. ○
 c. ○   c. ○   c. ○   c. ○   c. ○   c. ○   c. ○   c. ○   c. ○   c. ○   c. ○

170. a. ○ 182. a. ○ 194. a. ○ 206. a. ○ 218. a. ○ 230. a. ○ 242. a. ○ 254. a. ○ 266. a. ○ 278. a. ○ 290. a. ○
 b. ○   b. ○   b. ○   b. ○   b. ○   b. ○   b. ○   b. ○   b. ○   b. ○   b. ○
 c. ○   c. ○   c. ○   c. ○   c. ○   c. ○   c. ○   c. ○   c. ○   c. ○   c. ○

171. a. ○ 183. a. ○ 195. a. ○ 207. a. ○ 219. a. ○ 231. a. ○ 243. a. ○ 255. a. ○ 267. a. ○ 279. a. ○
 b. ○   b. ○   b. ○   b. ○   b. ○   b. ○   b. ○   b. ○   b. ○   b. ○
 c. ○   c. ○   c. ○   c. ○   c. ○   c. ○   c. ○   c. ○   c. ○   c. ○

172. a. ○ 184. a. ○ 196. a. ○ 208. a. ○ 220. a. ○ 232. a. ○ 244. a. ○ 256. a. ○ 268. a. ○ 280. a. ○
 b. ○   b. ○   b. ○   b. ○   b. ○   b. ○   b. ○   b. ○   b. ○   b. ○
 c. ○   c. ○   c. ○   c. ○   c. ○   c. ○   c. ○   c. ○   c. ○   c. ○

173. a. ○ 185. a. ○ 197. a. ○ 209. a. ○ 221. a. ○ 233. a. ○ 245. a. ○ 257. a. ○ 269. a. ○ 281. a. ○
 b. ○   b. ○   b. ○   b. ○   b. ○   b. ○   b. ○   b. ○   b. ○   b. ○
 c. ○   c. ○   c. ○   c. ○   c. ○   c. ○   c. ○   c. ○   c. ○   c. ○

174. a. ○ 186. a. ○ 198. a. ○ 210. a. ○ 222. a. ○ 234. a. ○ 246. a. ○ 258. a. ○ 270. a. ○ 282. a. ○
 b. ○   b. ○   b. ○   b. ○   b. ○   b. ○   b. ○   b. ○   b. ○   b. ○
 c. ○   c. ○   c. ○   c. ○   c. ○   c. ○   c. ○   c. ○   c. ○   c. ○

175. a. ○ 187. a. ○ 199. a. ○ 211. a. ○ 223. a. ○ 235. a. ○ 247. a. ○ 259. a. ○ 271. a. ○ 283. a. ○
 b. ○   b. ○   b. ○   b. ○   b. ○   b. ○   b. ○   b. ○   b. ○   b. ○
 c. ○   c. ○   c. ○   c. ○   c. ○   c. ○   c. ○   c. ○   c. ○   c. ○

176. a. ○ 188. a. ○ 200. a. ○ 212. a. ○ 224. a. ○ 236. a. ○ 248. a. ○ 260. a. ○ 272. a. ○ 284. a. ○
 b. ○   b. ○   b. ○   b. ○   b. ○   b. ○   b. ○   b. ○   b. ○   b. ○
 c. ○   c. ○   c. ○   c. ○   c. ○   c. ○   c. ○   c. ○   c. ○   c. ○

177. a. ○ 189. a. ○ 201. a. ○ 213. a. ○ 225. a. ○ 237. a. ○ 249. a. ○ 261. a. ○ 273. a. ○ 285. a. ○
 b. ○   b. ○   b. ○   b. ○   b. ○   b. ○   b. ○   b. ○   b. ○   b. ○
 c. ○   c. ○   c. ○   c. ○   c. ○   c. ○   c. ○   c. ○   c. ○   c. ○

Physical Assessment of the Newborn

Name _____
        Please Print

Address _____

City _____ State _____ Zip _____

Nursing License # _____ State(s) of License _____

Social Security #_____ Phone # _____
      (Alabama participants only)   (optional)

Mail a $35.00 processing fee payable to NICU INK.®

NICU INK,® 1410 Neotomas Ave., Suite 107, Santa Rosa, CA 95405-7533.

Foreign Participants: International Money Order drawn on U.S. Bank only. Thank you.